"This book offers a way of life which, if followed consistently, can provide renewed energy, increased vitality, and the greater satisfaction that comes from living a full and useful life. It teaches how life can be made richer and more fruitful in every way. . . ."

"How wonderful to discover the rare values that only a healthy and active life can provide. The purpose of this book is to guide the reader toward the attainment of these objectives."

—Max Warmbrand, N.D., D.O.

"It is my firm belief that Dr. Warmbrand, in this encyclopedia, has given a clear concept of a method of treating the sick, a method that contains within itself the heart and soul of all healing."

—Joseph L. Kaplowe, M.D.

# FREE CATALOG
# OF HEALTH BOOKS

A wide selection of fine books on Vitamins and Minerals; Nutrition; Natural Healing Methods; Organic Foods; Vegetarian, Macrobiotic, Reducing, and other Special Diets; Exercise & Fitness; Yoga, and many other health-oriented subjects is on sale at the store where you bought this book.

A giant 32-page "Health Books Catalog" listing over 2,000 of these books is available to you absolutely free. Just send name and address to:

**HEALTH BOOKS CATALOG
AURORA BOOK COMPANIONS
Box 5852—Dept. "E"
Denver, Colorado 80217**

*Distributed By*
**The NUTRI-BOOKS Corp.**
**Denver, Colorado**

ENCYCLOPEDIA OF

# HEALTH

## AND

# NUTRITION

(Original title: *The Encyclopedia of Natural Health*)

A complete one volume guide to
Natural Health Knowledge
combining the soundest principles of
folk medicine and modern health science

## MAX WARMBRAND, N.D., D.O.

PYRAMID BOOKS  NEW YORK

**THE ENCYCLOPEDIA OF HEALTH AND NUTRITION**
**(Original title: *The Encyclopedia of Natural Health*)**

A PYRAMID BOOK
Published by arrangement with The Julian Press, Inc.

Pyramid edition published July, 1974
  Second printing September, 1974

ISBN: 0-515-03413-4

Printed in the United States of America

Pyramid Books are published by Pyramid Communications, Inc. Its trademarks, consisting of the word "Pyramid" and the portrayal of a pyramid, are registered in the United States Patent Office.

PYRAMID COMMUNICATIONS, INC.
919 Third Avenue
New York, New York 10022, U.S.A.

# CONTENTS

Author's Preface  viii

Section One: A HEALTHY DIGESTION: THE KEY TO A HAPPY LIFE

Introduction  15

1  When Your Stomach Starts Talking,
   It's Time to Listen!  19
2  Get Acquainted With Your Digestive Organs  31
3  When the Stomach Becomes Inflamed  36
4  The Whys and Wherefores of Ulcers  53
5  Constipation: A Most Common Disorder  69
6  Ulcerative Colitis: A Life-Threatening Disease  82
7  Your Liver and Your Digestion  100
8  Your Gallbladder and Your Digestion  112
9  Your Nerves and Your Digestion  124
10  Heart Attacks and Indigestion  128
11  Oxygen: The Breath of Life  133
12  Symptom-Relieving Drugs Lead to
    More Diseases  137
13  The Curse of Chemical Pollutants
    and Additives  140
14  A Résumé of Facts Worth Knowing  146
15  Conclusion  151

Section Two: DISEASES OF THE RESPIRATORY SYSTEM

1  The Common Cold  155
2  Influenza  159
3  Pneumonia  162
4  Bronchitis  172
5  Bronchial Asthma  176
6  Allergy and the Respiratory Diseases  185

Section Three: DIABETES: A METABOLIC DISORDER

1  What We Know About Diabetes  193
2  Diabetes in Children  207
3  A Program for the Care of Diabetes  209

Section Four: ARTHRITIS AND OTHER RHEUMATIC DISEASES

Introduction  217
A Plea to Members of the Medical Profession  220
1  Facts About Arthritis  222

2   Fallacious Concepts   232
3   Fundamental Changes Necessary   234
4   The Effects of Drugs   245
5   Cortisone: The Failure of Another Dream   254
6   Gout and What We Know About It   259
7   The Transition Period   263
8   Nutrition in the Treatment of Arthritis   269
9   Building a Clean Body   280
10  The Basic Program of Treatment   284
11  Only Nature Cures   296
12  Stories That Tell the Story   298
13  The Theory of Infection   308
14  Our Theory Confirmed   314
15  Conclusion   318

Section Five: THE PREVENTION AND CONTROL OF HEART DISEASE

Preface   323
Introduction   325
1   Our Greatest Health Hazard   328
2   The Fascinating Story of the Circulatory System   333
3   The Three Major Types of Heart Disease   342
4   Metabolism: A Factor in Heart Disease   351
5   The Role of Nutrition   369
6   Chemical Additives in Our Food   387
7   The Smoking Question   394
8   Effects of Alcohol   402
9   Dangers of Obesity   405
10  Nervous Tension   413
11  Rheumatic Fever   417
12  How About the Drugs Used in Heart Disease?   428
13  Stories That Tell the Story   437
14  Why These Measures Are Helpful   447
15  Physical Exercise and Heart Disease   450
16  A Sample Program   455
17  A Decalogue of Health for the Heart Sufferer   461
18  Prevention Possible   463
19  Eating for Health   467
20  A Final Summary: The Do's and Don't's
      of Correct Eating   469

Index of Names   473
Index of Subjects   481

## PUBLISHERS' NOTE

*This volume is called an encyclopedia not because it is an alphabetic compendium, but because it is, as the great medical authority Galen used the term, "A complete round or course of learning." Dr. Warmbrand deals not only with the facts, but how the facts relate to the people who must use and are affected by the facts. What happens in the medical laboratory under relatively sterile and static conditions is not necessarily true of what happens in the living human physiology. The field of study in this encyclopedia is the living human being as he exists and functions in all phases of his orbit: physiologic, biologic, and social. The laboratory is recognized and utilized not as the means for total proof but as another method of observing and diagnosing the health and illnesses of man.*

# AUTHOR'S PREFACE

Natural Health is a science with a history as old as thinking man himself. It is the study of man's most successful fundamental survival habits and practices. It is the science that incorporates the best and most practical of these into a way of life whereby the continuing needs of mankind to survive in a constantly changing Universe can best be served. In essence, it is a science which seeks the best possible health under real, possible conditions.

Natural Health is not opposed to any of the established healing systems; rather it complements them. It points out the fallacies of present-day indiscriminate healing practices and adheres to the fundamental principles that underlie all sound healing systems. It supports the position of those physicians who are endeavoring to discard commonly held fallacies for those procedures which are necessary if the continuing deterioration in health is to be checked and a healthier pattern of living is to be established.

Natural Health bases its philosophy and approach to the problems of health on the two fundamental principles enunciated by the famous Greek physician Hippocrates, known in history as the Father of Medicine. It recognizes the historic role that the physician has occupied in the life of man and emphasizes the direction he must take if he is to maintain his enviable position in society.

The first principle, recognized as the basic principle of all healing professions, is expressed by the well-known phrase "vis medicatrix naturae," Nature Cures. This principle establishes the fact that healing is the prerogative of the organism and is brought about by the inherent curative powers of the body.

The second principle, "la nocere," promulgates the idea that the measures that are employed in the treatment of disease *must do no harm*. The first principle is the science of natural health. The second principle enunciates the discipline tha must govern the operation of all healing professions.

The conscientious physician who is aware of these basic principles does not practice his profession routinely; he is constantly in search of greater knowledge and will always strive to make his procedures conform to these two fundamental principles. Sound physiologic and hygienic measures of rehabilitation and a wholesome nutritional program are essential parts of this type of practice.

Outstanding medical authorities repeat this time and time again. The following statement by Dr. Lyman Wilbur, Dean Emeritus, Stanford University, appearing in a feature article in the *Journal of the American Medical Association* emphasizes this point: "Medicine based on pills and potions is becoming obsolete. . . . Biologic thinking is replacing empiricism . . . those treatments involving the use of heat, cold, water, electricity, movement and massage, having striking biologic responses, including effects on psychic reactions, are more potent than many of the drugs gathered through many centuries by trial and error."

The thought that medicine must adjust its practice to conform to natural law has been repeatedly stressed. Dr. Walter Estell Lee pointed this out some years ago in his *Surgery of the Extremities:* "The trouble with our profession is that it persists in too much meddlesome therapy—using the term in its broadest sense—to the detriment of Nature. We are losing sight of the patient himself and many of us are substituting machine-made diagnosis for clinical acumen, ready to use advertised remedies for intelligent cooperation with Nature, fads for facts," he stated.

Dr. Thomas Francis, Jr., School of Public Health, University of Michigan, recently made it clear that medicine as practiced to-day is far from providing the answers to our health problems, and emphasized the need for a complete re-evaluation.

"We are scarcely on the threshold of understanding the problems of either health or disease," declared Dr. Francis, and then pointed out that "our current ability to detect and identify disorders depends largely on their severity; *what we consider incipient is an already far-advanced biological imbalance.*" He then explained that we need *a program of true prevention* based upon: (1) Protection from chemical and physical exposure; (2) Prevention by correction of dietary deficiency or excess; and (3) Prevention of infectious disease by specific measures and sanitay social procedures.

Profound changes are now taking place in medical thinking, and the trends toward natural health have never been more evident. Dr. Leonard W. Larsen, recently elected President of the American Medical Association dwelled considerably in his inaugural address on what he chose to call the true professional spirit, and while doing this called attention to the fact that Hippocrates *"taught facts and scientific methods based on natural study and rational inquiry."* He reminded us further that *"he (Hippocrates) fostered the concept of the patient as a whole person, rather than just a conglomeration of many separate parts."*

"The really good doctor guided by the professional spirit will always remember that medicine exists for just one purpose—to serve humanity—and he will strive for excellence in meeting that purpose," Dr. Larsen continued, and then expressed the thought that "the true physician always continues the search and the striving."

In offering an explanation of what is meant by the true professional spirit, Dr. Larsen pointed out that it "emphasizes conformity to the principles of scientific truth and ethical conduct," but then stressed the fact that "it also recognizes the rights and the potentialities of the rebel or maverick who may have a new idea, a differen method, a fresh viewpoint."

The foregoing are not isolated statements. They are among thousands of similar statements made every year by outstanding medical authorities. They prove the need for a complete re-evaluation of many of our present-day health practices and the need for a return to fundamental Hippocratic principles.

All sound healing procedures fill a need in present-day society. To provide the best for the ailing and benefit all mankind, however, they should complement one another. While there are many disagreements that separate the various healing professions, it should not be too much to expect that those who are truly motivated by the ideal of service will select the best, and that out of this will arise new vistas and greater knowledge.

The purpose of this book is to make available to the reader information and knowledge that is essential, if the increase in chronic and degenerative diseases is to be reversed and a superior standard of health and well-being is to be established. The ideas stressed relate to man's habits of living, and outstanding medical as well as nonmedical authorities subscribe to the principles upon which is based the advice embodied in this volume.

The need to obtain skilled professional help and advice in case of serious ailment is constantly repeated. The information embodied in this volume, is faithfully adhered to, can improve health to the degree to which man has always aspired. This book offers a way of life which, if followed consistently, will provide renewed energy, increased vitality, and the greater satisfaction that comes from living a full and useful life. It teaches how life can be made richer and more fruitful in every way. Nevertheless, it points out that in case of illness the counsel and management of the experienced doctor is essential.

The skilled doctor is trained to render the services that are needed in case of ill health, and the great majority of doctors devote their life to the study of how they may best serve their patients in case of need. The reader must always remember that training and experience often make the difference between success and failure in attaining results.

The skilled doctor possesses the knowledge and experience to meet the challenge of the moment. However, to fulfill his true mission, he must also possess the qualities that enable him to serve in his true calling, that of a teacher and guide. To obtain the greatest amount of good, the individual in need of professional help should seek these qualifications in his doctor.

In these days when the specter of fatal disease fills us with great anxiety and, like the sword of Damocles, hangs as a continuing threat, it is essential that we acquire the knowledge that will help us counteract the rise in chronic and degenerative diseases and promote a healthier and more beneficial standard of living. The dedicated physician encourages the acquisition of this knowledge and, when his patient recovers, urges that sound living practices be followed so that a high standard of health be continued.

Health has many facets. It involves not only the need for good physical care but also a sound and constructive mental attitude.

Medical research has taken the spotlight in recent years with a continuous flow of information regarding disease. This, and the continuous increase in chronic and degenerative diseases, has done much to make the public disease-conscious. To see the picture in its total reality, however, it is essential that, alongside with our awareness of disease, we also develop a health consciousness. "How we think is how we are" is more than a philosophical phrase. It is well known, biologically as well as philosophically, that in man the psyche is the inspiration of action. Therefore, if one's psychology is exclusively in the direction of fear, the physical expression will tend to be repressed. On the other hand, if the approach embraces the positive view, we are not only fully aware of the dangers that confront us, but also recognize the measures that have to be applied to overcome them.

We must make sure not to make the mistake of going to the extreme where we recognize the role of the mind, and neglect essential physical needs. While the mind plays a vital role in proper direction and evaluation, the physical self with all its needs must never be overlooked, if we are to maintain our well-being and be at our best through a long and fruitful life.

The physical expression of life and living can be joyful and uplifting; yet this is often forgotten. Physical joy and exhilaration are as much a part of our heritage as are our religion and philosophy. To enjoy the wonders of our physical being is as necessary as the good food we must eat to better survive, and the ideals which lead us onward.

The beauty and rhythm of our physical existence contribute much to a richer and more complete life. There is a spiritual quality of joy in the physical flight of birds. Observe the grace in the movements of the domestic cat when it periodically stretches almost every part of its body. The human organism too, can express grace and charm in the fulfillment of its many physical activities. The tingle in our toes, the current and flow of life which courses though our being, the feeling of exhilaration when we relax and breathe deeply, are all part of the wholeness and beauty of our physical existence.

What a glorious existence when each day can mean a new beginning, a new life! What riches and fulfillment when every step toward renewed health and increasing mental and spiritual accomplishments is taken not merely as an end in itself but as a means toward a further awareness and participation in the fuller act of living! How wonderful to discover the rare values that only a healthy and active life can provide. The purpose of this book is to guide the reader toward the attainment of these objectives.

*New York, August* 1961                    MAX WARMBRAND

# Section One:

# A HEALTHY DIGESTION:
# THE KEY TO A HAPPY LIFE

# INTRODUCTION

Many years ago, an ancient sage said, "To eat is human, to digest divine!" Within the scope of this pithy quotation, he seems to have pinpointed the creative role that digestion plays in the life-giving cycle of nutrition and health.

It is well recognized that many disorders begin in the digestive tract. Improper digestion in its chronic form leads to defective assimilation of food and causes faulty nutrition, which nearly always precedes the onset and development of those derangements that have been assigned the names of many specific gastrointestinal diseases.

The need for this section is, therefore, clearly evident, since a well-functioning digestive system as a prerequisite for health is recognized by all who have devoted time and thought to this subject.

The simple lucid style that runs through all the pages that follow is striking and impressive. The author has made an exhaustive study of the digestive system and its disorders, as is revealed by his numerous references, and has presented to the layman, as well as to the physician, a therapeutic contribution of tremendous import and value.

Dr. Warmbrand shows that the same pattern is present in all digestive disorders, and points to irritation, malnutrition or nutritional deficiencies, and tensions as major factors. These factors, singly or in combination, give rise to an inflammatory process, characterized by plethora or an increased blood supply at the site or sites of trauma, representing the natural tendency to counteract the irritation and repair the damage. Persistence of the inflammatory state produces the sclerotic areas or scars, which again reveal the attempt of nature to heal and repair. In those cases where the tissues have lost the power of repair, necrosis or breakdown of tissue, called ulcers, develops as an expression of this defective reparative process.

Dr. Warmbrand makes it clear that there is a relationship between all digestive disorders, for a breakdown in one organ of digestion affects all the others. He further explains the effect of impaired digestion on the entire organism, showing the interrelation between the defect in the digestive system and other ailments with which it is apparently not associated.

To counteract the digestive disorders, Dr. Warmbrand advocates no miracle remedies. His is a program that promotes rehabilitation and repair by a well-planned program of nutrition and other simple but proved restorative measures.

Almost all morbid conditions are fundamentally related, the relationship having its origin in a common cause, which is due mainly to a disturbance or derangement of the entire metabolism through improper nutrition as well as other adverse or debilitating influences.

The failure to comprehend or to accept the unity and oneness of the living organism has been one of the stumbling blocks in medical progress. From a forgotten source comes the concept that a knowledge of the whole cannot be obtained by summations from inductions based upon studies of its parts, because the behavior of the whole is not a linear sum of the functions of the parts. Conversely, a knowledge of the nature of the parts cannot be derived by making deductions from generalizations about the whole. Man is more than an aggregate of the sum of a brain, lung, heart, liver, kidney, and cells. He is a dynamic synthesis whose totality is far greater than the sum of its parts. This grand totality, life, can never be comprehended by analysis of its fragments, isolated and alone, for how can the test tube and microscope reveal the nature of man and life any more than the knowledge of the properties of a drop of water can reveal to us an understanding of the river or the sea?

An Indian philosopher captured this thought in "he who sees but ONE in all the changing manifestations in the Universe, to him belongs eternal truth, and to him alone," summing up this thought in a most striking manner.

The artificial division of diseases has led to the treatment of parts of the living organism, and treatment of separate diseases has led to the concept of specifics and to the use of the myriad of drugs manufactured to-day. In comparison with the progress made in surgery in all its phases, particularly in cardiovascular, plastic, orthopedic, and brain surgery, medicine is at a relative standstill, especially in reference to the diseases of degeneration. This static position will persist until the orthodox medical world awakens and recognizes the role of defective nutrition, as well as the effects that chemical fertilizers, poisonous food additives, and poison sprays have upon your health.

The author specifically points out that, in addition to nutrition, other hygienic factors, such as exercise adapted to each case, bathing, adequate rest, and tranquillity are components needed to set in motion the natural healing force inherent in all living organisms.

To provide real benefit, science must be guided by nature. It must reach out for the hand of Mother Nature, and be led. Life is a phenomenon, and it is not the analytical but the phenomenological panorama of all living organisms that must be observed if one is really to understand life. What a paradox that physical laws are so faithfully and strictly adhered to, while the laws of biology and physiology are so obviously ignored, particularly in the fields of agriculture and nutrition!

Sir Stanton Hicks dealt with the indifference displayed on the subject of nutrition by stating that "food is not only an article of commerce and industry; it is the stream of life itself" and then commented, "Why we should sanctify human life . . . while remaining . . . indifferent to the sources of that life is surely a modern paradox."

The surgeon who declared humbly that "I sew the wound, but God heals it" recognized fully the curative force inherent in nature. The least that we, as physicians, can do is to avoid that which will obstruct this natural tendency to cure and to heal.

The removal of a tumor and the excision of an ulcer take from the body the end results of a pathological process, yet give nothing to the organism to prevent the recurrence of these morbid states.

Laxatives, antacids, tranquilizers, and soporifics are not the total answer to the quest for health. We physicians must reorient ourselves and then make a total re-evaluation of our entire therapeutic armamentarium. Let scientific man descend humbly from his self-erected pedestal. Let him see that the transgression upon immutable laws has brought about much suffering, and let him realize that only by a return to nature can he ever hope to be healthy again.

Perhaps, when the laboratory can produce the petal of a rose or the blade of grass, science will deserve the right to assume the superior attitude prevailing today. Scientific research must be subservient to Natural Law, and must not assume to be its master.

It is my firm belief that Dr. Warmbrand, in this encyclopedia, has given a clear concept of a method of treating the sick, a method that contains within itself the heart and soul of all healing. We must always hold before us the concept of totality—a concept that reveals to us that, within each fruit and all products of the good earth, there has been created a total universe wherein all elements in their proper orbit stand in perfect relationship, for this is the wisdom of nature.

The use of fragments isolated from their natural source may be beneficial and necessary at times, but the widespread use of synthetics, particularly coal tar products, to replace the natural element, has its origin in erroneous thinking, and constitutes a violation of law.

We physicians must recognize this error and take our rightful place as leaders in the struggle against disease. We must never overlook the fact that preventive medicine embraces more than the use of sera, vaccines, and wonder drugs. We must always keep in mind the somber warning of statistics, which clearly indicates the rising rate of the incidence of malignant states, and in addition points out that within a few generations almost every life will be doomed to terminate in this dreadful malady, if some other degenerative process has not superseded this cruelest killer of them all.

We must plan an active program of enlightenment, which will become a campaign against the great army of carcinogens that gain entry into their victims not only by ingestion, but also by inhalation, and which, by cumulative action, bring about the destruction of life.

In this section of his encyclopedia, as in all his writings, Dr. Warmbrand makes a powerful plea for healthful living, a plea based on the methods of nutrition and total rehabilitation. It is my sincere hope that its message will find its way to every physician who has taken the oath to give his best to all who come to him for help.

Joseph L. Kaplowe, M.D.

# 1

## WHEN YOUR STOMACH STARTS TALKING, IT'S TIME TO LISTEN!

### Facts About Indigestion

What would you think of a driver who drove his car at an excessive rate of speed, but tried to cover up his recklessness by blotting out the speedometer? You would surely think that he was irresponsible, wouldn't you?

It seems to us that when a sufferer from a stomach or other digestive disorder takes his antacid or other symptom relieving remedies, he acts just as foolishly and irresponsibly as the reckless automobile driver, since in taking these remedies he merely blots out the symptoms of the disorder but accomplishes nothing so far as eradicating the disease is concerned. As a matter of fact, by depending on these drugs, he actually lays the foundation for infinitely more serious disorders.

It should be obvious that the most sensible procedure in these cases would not be to turn to remedies that temporarily relieve the symptoms, and thereby provide a false sense of well-being, but to find out how the disorder developed and what changes must be made to bring about real correction.

Whenever our digestion goes wrong, we are warned of it by some very annoying symptoms. Heartburn, sour stomach, bad taste, halitosis, belching, nausea, vomiting, cramps, fullness or discomfort in the abdomen, a choking or constriction in the throat, debility and weakness—all are signals that something has gone wrong with our digestion, and that attention is necessary if we are to protect ourselves against further destructive changes.

These symptoms are commonly known as indigestion, and while some persons mistakenly assume that indigestion is a disease, it is well to emphasize that this term merely describes the various symptoms we have enumerated above, and should not be regarded as the actual disease.

These symptoms occur as a rule in conjunction with

various disorders of the digestive system, such as inflammation and ulcers of the stomach, constipation, spastic or ulcerative colitis, gallbladder and liver diseases. Also, they often show up in connection with diseases of the heart, the blood vessels, the circulation, the blood, the kidneys, the nervous system, as well as with emotional disorders.

That these symptoms can make life intolerable is well known. It should be obvious, however, that our major objective should be not to camouflage the symptoms of the disease, which is what will happen when "antacid" or "alkaline" remedies are used to obtain symptomatic relief, but to determine what the person suffers from, how the ailment has been brought on, and what must be done to eliminate it or bring it under thorough and effective control.

Our aim should be not merely to obtain temporary relief, but to bring about complete and permanent correction. This can be done only when the causes of the disease are determined and removed, and measures that will restore normal functioning are employed.

## How Digestive Disorders Devolop

If you agree that the wisest procedure is not to resort to measures that provide mere relief, but to discover and eliminate the causes of the disorder, then you will realize that our first step must be to find out how these disorders are brought on.

This is why a discussion of the various influences that lead to the onset of these disorders is necessary here. For clarity as well as convenience we may group these influences under the following headings:

### 1. Superficial or Surface Irritants

These include the various substances which, when taken into the digestive system, act as irritants or excitants to the mucosal lining or surface tissues of the digestive tract. Among these substances we include spices and condiments, highly stimulating or acid-causing foods, extremely hot or cold foods, and such irritating substances as coffee, tea, and alcohol, as well as chemicals and drugs of all kinds.

## 2. Deep-Tissue Irritants

Here we group the toxins or irritants that are taken up by the bloodstream and carried to the deeper tissues of the digestive organs. These toxins include many of the irritating substances that we have enumerated under the first heading, which the organs of the body have been unable to eliminate or render harmless, as well as some of the toxic by-products of body metabolism. We shall go into this subject more fully in another chapter.

## 3. Nervous and Emotional Tensions

That nervous and emotional tensions play a vital role in the onset of digestive disorders is well known. It is common knowledge that nervousness or tensions may kill off all desire for food. On the other hand, those who feel tense, anxious, and insecure often turn to food and drink as an emotional outlet, and often consume vast quantities of food and drink not needed for the body. They thus overburden the digestive system and lay the foundation for digestive diseases. It is also well known that tension can cause heartburn, as well as gas with pains and distress. Experience has proved that the worried and harassed businessman often ends with ulcers of the stomach or some other distressing or dangerous digestive disorder.

## 4. Wrong Food and Faulty Eating Habits

That a faulty diet can contribute to digestive disorders should be apparent. Many of us are aware that fried, greasy, and highly spiced foods are harmful to the digestion. Unfortunately, only relatively few persons realize that most of the foods and beverages consumed in the average household are highly deficient in essential food elements. The white flour and white sugar products, the refined cereals, and the great variety of pickled, processed, and chemically preserved foods that make up the greater part of the conventional diet may supply us with many calories, but they fail to provide the wholesome body-building elements needed to maintain the functional integrity of the body, as well as a healthy digestion. It should be apparent that these foods can set off a series of chain reactions that ultimately lead to malfunctioning and, in time, to a vast amount of deterioration.

## Disagreements Must Not Confuse Us

In enumerating the various factors that contribute to the onset of digestive disorders, we do not wish to imply that there is complete unanimity of opinion on all these points. To be more specific, we find, for instance, that some popular writers disregard the effects of surface or superficial irritants or, at most, concede that they play only a minor role. They proceed on the assumption that the organs of digestion are able to overcome the irritants or minimize their effect and, therefore, need not be regarded as a major influence.

While superficially this contention may seem reasonable, since the various substances we have enumerated among surface or superficial irritants are included almost routinely in the diets of most persons without any apparent harmful effects, a closer analysis will disclose how shallow such reasoning is, since it disregards the long-term of cumulative irritating and weakening influences. The fact that these substances can be used for long periods of time without causing any great discomfort merely demonstrates that the body possesses a powerfully built-in protective mechanism, but does this give us the right recklessly to dissipate or abuse it?

Then, there are those who overlook or disregard completely the harm caused by the irritating or toxic substances that circulate in the bloodstream. Dr. William Boyd, Professor of Pathology of the University of Toronto, must have had them in mind when, in his *Pathology of Internal Diseases,* he emphasizes that we must discard the idea that gastritis (stomach inflammation) is merely the result of surface irritation. He points out that this disease involves not only the surface tissues but also the deeper tissues, and writes that "inflammation of this deep portion will be produced by an irritant brought by the bloodstream rather than by one acting from the surface."

Then there are those who blame most digestive disorders solely or primarily on nervous tension, and disregard or minimize the role of faulty nutrition. Considering this point, we wish to emphasize that, while it is evident that anxiety and the tensions or stresses of modern daily living affect the digestive system and often precipitate or trigger the onset of digestive disorders, it is a great fallacy to overlook or disregard the other influences that undermine the health of the digestive organs and lead to their breakdown.

We are grateful to Dr. Sara M. Jordan for pointing out that while only 10 per cent of our population develop ulcers, a much larger percentage lives under conditions of stress and strain. She states further that while we find many ulcer sufferers "among people who shoulder the greatest responsibilities and burdens," we also find "ulcer victims among the shirkers, those people who think the world owes them a living."[1]

That refined and devitalized foods and faulty eating habits contribute to the development of digestive disorders should not require much speculation. Medical literature repeatedly refers to the fact that the contemporary American diet is high in "empty" calories, foods "rich in energy but low in essential nutrients," and that this often gives rise to deficiencies and metabolic disorders.

While dealing with this question, one cannot but be intrigued by a statement by one of our leading medical authorities that we are constantly being urged to consume more to provide a basis for our expanding economy, and that this in turn contributes to our expanding waistline! Whenever we permit ourselves to be induced to consume more food, especially that of the refined and processed type, we lay the foundation not only for an expanding waistline, but also for many deficiency diseases, and other diseases of the digestive system.

Dwelling on the question of an expanding waistline somewhat further, it is pertinent that a four-year study completed recently by the Society of Actuaries (life insurance statisticians) discloses that we have an entirely wrong

[1] *Today's Health*, June, 1959.

conception as to what constitutes normal weight, and that the ideal weight, the weight conductive to better health and a longer life, is actually 15 to 20 pounds below the so-called average normal weight.

While this fact has long been recognized in insurance circles and has been stressed for many years by the more progressive health authorities, we are nevertheless glad to see it reiterated, because many persons lose weight when they first change to a more wholesome diet, and then worry needlessly that they are depriving themselves of needed nourishment.

It is well to remember that stamina, endurance, and youthfulness go hand in hand with ideal weight, not over-weight, and that any increase in weight away from the ideal only reduces the vitally essential attributes of vigorous health.

## We Have Become a Nation of Drug Users

Tranquilizers, mood elevators, cortisone, the antibiotics, and a vast number of other drugs are commonly used for all kinds of real and imaginary ills, and anyone who questions the value of any of them is often regarded as a therapeutic nihilist or a misguided faddist.

That many of these remedies lead to digestive disorders is now becoming increasingly evident. Dr. Gordon McHardy of the Brown-McHardy Clinic and the Department of Medicine, Louisiana State University School of Medicine, in a paper read before the General Scientific Meeting at the 107th Annual Convention of the American Medical Association on June 24, 1958, dealt with this point in no uncertain terms. Here is what he said:

"The most widely used and probably most effective therapeutic agents today have been responsible for dramatic gastrointestinal reactions that have introduced new entities (of ailments) into the medical literature. *Thiazine-induced cholostatic jaundice, antibiotic-resistant staphlococcic pseudo-membranous enterocolitis, and steroid-activated or steroid-produced peptic ulcers have each offered frustrations to the therapist whose agent boomeranged so as to produce another illness* (my emphasis)."

In other words, such common disorders as jaundice, colitis, and ulcers are often the by-products of some of the most popular remedies in use today.

"The gastrointestinal tract is exceptionally susceptible to untoward reaction to certain therapeutic agents," Dr. McHardy said, and then went on to stress that these "hazardous gastrointestinal reactions" may result not only from such drugs as digitalis, colchicine, and atropine, but also from those that are used in the treatment of digestive disorders: "Among the more hazardous have been included those agents whose effects persist after discontinuance of the therapy and excretion of the drug; these are associated with appreciable illness and potential death."

Among the drugs used in gastrointestinal disorders, which can impair or damage the gastrointestinal tract, Dr. McHardy lists chlorpromazine, iproniazid (Marsilid), the arsenicals, the Rauwolfia compounds (tranquilizers), ACTH, cortisone and other cortisone-type hormones, the anticholinergics (remedies that inhibit the flow of secretions and the action of the digestive organs), as well as the opiates.

## Toxicity of Chemicals Used in Food Processing

Many persons are finally awakening to the fact that the chemicals used in agriculture and in food manufacturing can be extremely harmful. These chemicals tend to accumulate in the system, and while their damaging effects may not be immediately apparent, they can nevertheless have a detrimental effect upon the tissues of the body and, in time, contribute to the onset of serious disease. These chemicals have to be neutralized or rendered harmless by the liver and, like drugs, overtax the liver and impair its functional efficiency. When the liver is unable to render these substances harmless, they may find their way into the bloodstream and can trigger many disorders, including some that may involve the entire digestive system.

Many of our foremost authorities are beginning to be aware of the fact that chemical additives can be extremely dangerous to health. Only recently, a group of outstanding scientists from all over the world, meeting in Rome, announced that many of these chemicals are carcinogenic (cancer-producing) and, therefore, a menace to health. They listed among them many of the thickeners, sweeteners, flavorings, bleaches, preservatives, dyes, and cited in particular certain mineral oils and the paraffins used on food containers and as preservatives for fruits and vegetables. They condemned the use of poisonous anti-sprouting chemicals on potatoes, the use of pesticides in agriculture, the use of stilbestrol to fatten poultry and cattle, and the use of antibiotics in the treatment of livestock.

## Antibiotics and Digestive Upsets

Antibiotics can cause a great deal of harm. They often mask the symptoms of disease, but have no curative effect, and what is even worse, sometimes actually endanger the life of the patient. At times they cause severe anaphylactic reactions that can kill in minutes. Yet how many of us are aware that these drugs are often unknowingly taken into the system when milk from an antibiotically treated cow is used? How sure can we be that a stomach upset, blamed on an "allergy," has in reality not been caused by milk from a cow that has been treated with antibiotics?

We know that when raw milk is kept at a certain temperature it usually curdles and turns to sour milk. However, we have noticed that raw certified milk (the only raw milk available in large cities) kept at that temperature sometimes fails to curdle, and instead becomes spoiled and unfit for use. We have often wondered whether this was not because the milk came from a cow that had been treated with antibiotics. The living acidophilus bacteria in raw milk causes milk to ferment and make it curdle. The antibiotics used to suppress the action of bacteria are, however, not selective; they destroy not only harmful bacteria but also those that are beneficial.

## Insidious Effects Not Always Recognized

Those who possess a hardy constitution and are not, therefore, readily affected by these chemicals, should remember that some persons are more sensitive to certain drugs or chemicals than others, and that the life of some can actually be endangered when mere traces of these substances get into their systems. It is known that, even in the smallest doses, penicillin can be dangerous to some persons; the same is true about many other chemicals and drugs.

Moreover, even when we are not extremely sensitive, how can we be sure that the drugs are not being accumulated in the system and that their detrimental effects won't show up later? It is well known that a chemical or drug may be taken for years without any apparent harm, and then suddenly causes severe reactions and even death.

Dr. George P. Larrick, United States Commissioner of Food and Drugs, prepared a paper for the 12th Annual Meeting of the Dairy Products Improvement Institute, in which he stated that "residues of insecticides and penicillin used to treat ailing cows had been found in some milk supplies and constitute a potential health hazard."

Dr. Rankin who, in the absence of Dr. Larrick, read the paper before the Institute, mentioned that a panel of medical experts had reported to the Food and Drug Administration that penicillin in milk could be a real hazard to persons who are exquisitely sensitive to the drug.

Dr. Rankin pointed out further that "there also had been some disturbing reports recently that the wax materials used to coat cardboard milk containers . . . may not be entirely suitable for the purpose."[2] Since these waxes are also used on cucumbers, turnips, and various other vegetables and fruits, it should be apparent that this information is not of purely academic interest.

## The Circulating Toxins

When we talk of the toxins that circulate in the bloodstream and in the other body fluids, we broach a subject important not only in diseases of the digestive system, but in practically all other ailments of the body.

Many factors contribute to the accumulation of these toxins in the system. Poor nutrition, faulty or improper living habits, irritating or harmful drugs or chemicals, lack of fresh air, insufficient rest and sleep, in short all influences that impair bodily functioning contribute to it. It should be obvious that when a digestive disorder is the outgrowth of many abuses, it would be useless to expect

[2] *The New York Times,* February 20, 1959.

the modification of one or even several of the bad habits to bring about a complete correction. It should be clear that only when all the pernicious influences that have contributed to the onset of the disease have been removed can the disorder be completely eradicated or brought under effective control.

## Consequences Often Tragic

Sufferers from digestive disorders are invariably an unhappy lot. They cannot enjoy their meals and, as often as not, dread sitting down to the table for fear of the pains or discomforts that will follow. Yet, like the proverbial ostrich, many of them continue to follow their erroneous pattern of living, expecting to find relief in some remedy that they hope will obviate the need for a change in their habits of living.

That such an approach provides nothing but failure should be only too evident. Millions of people have discovered to their sorrow that while some of the commonly used remedies provide some measure of relief, the relief is not lasting and in the long run is usually followed by a recurrence of the symptoms and ultimately by more damage. The longer palliatives are used, the more severe the complications that usually follow.

So far as the effect of the commonly used antacid or alkaline remedies are concerned, it is well to point out that while their first effect is to neutralize the excessive amount of acid in the stomach, their secondary effect is in the nature of a rebound, actually causing an increased secretion of acid. The response of the body tissues to these remedies can be compared to the swing of a pendulum. Whenever you swing a pendulum in one direction, it invariably swings back in full force in the opposite direction. Harry Beckman, discussing the effects of the use of bicarbonate of soda, cites one study which showed that in one half of the patients examined this remedy "caused a rebound in gastric acidity to a point higher than would have been attained had the alkali not been administered." Discussing antacids generally, Beckman quotes Steigman and Fantus to the effect that the reduction of acidity through the use of these remedies "is neither great nor long lasting and may be followed by a rebound increase."[3]

Another point worth keeping in mind is that these remedies often cause a derangement of the acid-base balance that may lead to alkalosis, a condition vastly more dangerous than hyperacidity.

## The Penalty Can Be Great

From all that we have mentioned before, it should be apparent that, to overcome digestive disorders, the harmful influences that contribute to the onset of these disorders must be recognized and then controlled or eliminated. One may hope that our failure to do this may not always result in tragedy as did the case of one man who was finally diagnosed at the age of forty as having cancer. Unfortunately, by then the disease was inoperable. This man had suffered from heartburn since childhood, and had been advised to take the conventional bicarbonate of soda after meals to gain relief from it. Neither he nor his doctor realized what was the matter and so the patient continued with his usual pattern of living, allowing the insidious disease to develop. Whenever he suffered from heartburn, he simply resorted to his favorite remedy and quickly obtained symptomatic relief. He joked about the fact that he was always "prepared" with a supply of these powders in his pockets. The ultimate results in his case, however, were hardly funny.

We know that not all who take the usual acid or other symptom-relieving drugs are masking cancer. However, there is little to be happy about when one continues with unwholesome habits of living and then relies on these palliative measures for relief, since the trouble may be a major digestive disorder, such as peptic ulcer, colitis, or gallbladder trouble. Many of these diseases could be prevented if, instead of relying on these palliative measures, the necessary changes to check the inroads of the disease were made.

[3] Harry Beckman, *Treatment in General Practice.*

## Symptoms Often a Blessing

As such, the earlier digestive upsets can be a blessing, but
only if we recognize their implied warning and take the
steps necessary to prevent the spread of the destructive
process. Those who are unwilling to heed these warnings
and are satisfied instead with temporary relief will have
only themselves to blame for the dire results that follow.
They may end in the same way as the man who overtaxes
his horse in his effort to win the race but in the end loses
the horse.

## 2

# GET ACQUAINTED WITH YOUR DIGESTIVE ORGANS

The digestion of food starts in the mouth, is then continued in the stomach, and is finally completed in the small intestine.

It should not be difficult to understand why food must be eaten slowly and why it must be thoroughly chewed before it is swallowed. Chewing breaks the food into small particles and mixes it with the saliva. This inaugurates the first stages of digestion, the conversion of starch into simpler forms of sugar. This change is brought about by an enzyme in the saliva called ptyalin.

It is worth mentioning that the saliva, which starts the digestion of starches, is mildly alkaline.

## The Stomach

After the food has been chewed and swallowed, it enters the stomach, where the digestion of protein begins.

The stomach, when empty, is a small muscular organ that can hold about 2½ pints of food. Its muscles are pliale, however, and it can be stretched to accommodate vastly greater amounts. The millions of glands imbedded in the walls of the stomach secrete chemical substances that start the digestion of protein, and split some of the fats into fatty acids and glycerine.

Among those substances given off by the stomach glands that play an important role in stomach digestion is hydrochloric acid, which, in combination with the enzyme pepsin, starts the conversion of the various protein foods into the simpler amino acids, the building stones of the body tissues. Another enzyme, rennin, plays a special role in the digestion of the milk protein.

While the ptyalin-containing saliva that starts the digestion of starch is alkaline, the gastric juice that starts the digestion of protein is normally acid. Since starches require an alkaline medium for their digestion and the stomach juices are acid in nature, starch digestion ceases in the stomach.

## The Small Intestine

From the stomach the partly digested food is carried into the small intestine, where the last stages of digestion are completed.

The small intestine is about 1½ inches in diameter and about 25 feet long. Its walls, like those of the stomach, contain millions of glands that secrete enzymes needed for the digestion of various food elements. These intestinal enzymes, with the aid of the bile, which is secreted by the liver, and various enzymes secreted by the pancreas and carried to the small intestine by the pancreatic duct, complete the breakup of the various food elements and prepare them for absorption into the lymphatic system and the portal vein.

When the food reaches the small intestine, the fat is first emulsified by the bile and then acted upon by an enzyme known as lipase, while the enzyme trypsin completes the digestion of protein, and one known as amylopsin completes the digestion of the starches. While the secretions of the stomach are of an acid nature, the secretions of the small intestine are again alkaline.

It is well that these differences be kept in mind since they explain why some of the more thoughtful students of nutrition emphasize that concentrated starches and concentrated proteins should not be eaten together, but at separate meals. More conventional nutritionists reject this program, basing their rejection on the fact that both starches and protein are present in many foods, and that the digestive organs are usually able to handle these foods without any difficulty. What is often overlooked is the fact that foods containing both protein and starches in natural combination also possess the enzymes and other supportive elements needed for their digestion.

However, irrespective of whether this principle is accepted or rejected, it should be apparent that when several concentrated foods are eaten in the same meal, the digestive system tends to become overburdened. This practice should, therefore, be discouraged. This is of special importance when we are dealing with an active digestive disorder, or when the digestive system needs protection, strengthening, and rebuilding.

Students of anatomy divide the small intestine, for descriptive purposes, into three sections. The upper section, the part which connects with the distal or lower end of the stomach, is the duodenum; the middle section the jejunum; and the lower section, which connects with the large intestine, the ileum.

It is important that these divisions be kept in mind since an inflammation or ulcers in the distal or lower section of the stomach often extend into the upper section of the small intestine, the duodenum. The lower section of the small intestine, the ileum, had public attention at the time when President Eisenhower was operated upon for what is known as regional enteritis, or ileitis.

## The Absorption of Food

After the work of the small intestine has been completed, the digested portion of the food is picked up by countless millions of tiny velvety projections that cover the walls of the small intestine, and is carried to the liver. These tiny projections, known as the villi, contain blood as well as lymph vessels. The blood vessels of the villi absorb the products of the fully digested proteins and sugars and carry them to the liver. There the proteins are further modified to make them assimilable by the cells of the body, while the sugars are stored by the liver in the form of glycogen for future use. The lymph vessels of the villi absorb the digested fat and convert it into fatty tissues to be used as padding in different parts of the body, to protect the body against injuries and insulate it against cold, and to serve as an auxiliary source of energy.

## The Large Intestine

The food we eat contains both digestible and indigestible material. Furthermore, even digestible portions of the food are often not completely digested. The portions of the food that are indigestible or have not been completely digested are emptied into the large intestine and from there are ultimately expelled from the body.

The large intestine is 5 or 6 feet long and connects with the small intestine at the lower right side of the abdomen. From there, it extends upward until it reaches the lower ribs, then crosses over to the left side, and from there turns downward again. The portion on the right side extending upward is known as the ascending colon, the portion crossing over from the right to the left side as the transverse colon, while the portion on the left side that extends downward is known as the descending colon.

The part where the small and large intestines meet is shaped somewhat like a pouch, and is known as the saecum, while the end portion of the large intestine through which the undigested mass is finally expelled is known as the rectum.

The undigested mass normally reaches the large intestine in a semiliquid state. This mass contains not only the indigestible portions of the food, such as fibers, cellulose, etc., but also the digestible portions that have not been completely digested.

There are a number of reasons why digestible portions of the food reach the large intestine undigested or only partly digested. In some cases this happens because the food has not been chewed well enough. In other cases it is because too much food had been eaten, and the digestive system could not handle all of it. At certain times, the digestive organs are overtired and cannot do a complete job. In some cases an imbalance or an insufficient supply of the digestive secretions may interfere with the digestion. The intake of foods incompatibly combined and, therefore, overtaxing to the digestive system, may also be a contributory factor.

## When Residue Reaches the Large Intestine

As soon as the undigested mass reaches the upper part of the large intestine, a great deal of churning and mixing sets in. While this goes on, the fibers and other tough substances become softened and broken up. At the same time, some of the fluid is being extracted, converting the semiliquid material into a semisolid mass.

Billions of bacteria living in the large intestine invade the fibers and the cellulose of the vegetable foods and help to disintegrate them, while the undigested or incompletely digested portion of the protein undergoes certain putrefactive changes, setting free a number of toxic by-products. These toxic by-products are often damaging to the body unless they are promptly neutralized and rendered harmless by the liver, or are counteracted by the action of other bacteria in the colon.

When these changes are completed, the mass is then propelled onward by gentle wavelike contractions known as peristalsis, and is ultimately carried to the end portion of the intestine, the rectum, through which it is then expelled.

The stool, when eliminated, should be well formed, of a semisolid consistency, and brownish in color. The types of food eaten influence the coloring of the stool. A preponderance of heavy proteins may cause an increase in the dark brown color; where starches, especially grain starches, predominate, the stool is often light brown, while red foods such as beets often turn the stool a dark red color.

When watery, the stool has been eliminated too soon; this is diarrhea. When it is too solid, elimination has been delayed, inducing constipation.

The appearance of the stool often tells an interesting story. From its content, consistency, and shape we can tell whether the bowels are functioning normally, how well the food has been digested, whether too much food has been eaten, and whether the minerals as well as the other essential nutritional elements have been fully absorbed. We can also tell whether there is bleeding in the intestinal tract; the presence of pus is an indication of tissue breakdown somewhere in the digestive tract. The amount of fat present in the feces is a key to how well the pancreas and liver are functioning.

Thus, the stool may disclose a great deal about our habits and ways of living, as well as whether our digestive organs are functioning efficiently.

## 3

# WHEN THE STOMACH BECOMES INFLAMED

## Gastritis

Diseases of the stomach usually begin with inflammation. When the tissues of the stomach become inflamed and congested they are unable to digest food properly, and various symptoms of indigestion begin to appear.

We have already pointed out that irritating substances taken into the stomach, which that organ cannot handle, as well as toxins and irritants that circulate in the body and are carried by the bloodstream to the deeper tissues of the stomach, are often responsible for this disease. We further pointed out that nutritional deficiencies and nervous and emotional tensions also contribute to its development.

That faulty nutrition and careless eating habits play a part in its onset should be apparent. The diet of most persons is composed of large amounts of refined and processed foods, such as white flour, processed cereals, and white sugar products, and often includes excessive amounts of devitalized, concentrated foods, fried foods, coffee, tea, chocolate, liquor, artificially flavored soft drinks, and sharp spices and condiments. Furthermore, people as a rule eat too much, and too fast. They gulp their food down without chewing it, eat when not hungry, and pay very little attention to eating foods in physiologically compatible combinations.

All these enervating influences, individually and in combination, impair bodily functioning, lower the resistance of the individual, and ultimately undermine the health of the digestive organs.

In the early stages inflammation of the stomach or gastritis is usually a simple ailment and generally arises as a defense reaction on the part of the stomach tissues to irritants. It should be evident that at such time the disorder could easily be overcome, provided proper care were applied.

However, where the pernicious influences continue for any length of time or where the ailment is neglected or improperly treated, a great deal of damage can be done. Parts of the lining and the folds of the stomach may ultimately become thickened and hardened. Polyps develop. The functioning of the secretory glands becomes progressively impaired, causing first an increase and later a decrease in the flow of the gastric juices.

With further damage, some parts of the lining and deeper tissues of the stomach may begin to shrink or atrophy, while the secretion of the glands may diminish still further, or dry up completely.

Long-lasting cases of inflammation often give rise to serious malformations or lead to the development of ulcers and scars, while some cases may even break down to the point where they end with cancer.

Since cases vary, it should be apparent that, whenever possible, sufferers from digestive disorders should be under the care of a competent doctor. However, to obtain results it is essential that the doctor who is in charge of the case be not only able to determine the nature of the ailment, but that he also possess a complete understanding of how the recuperative forces of the body can be assisted to bring about recovery.

### An Over-All General Program

Since we are dealing with an inflamed stomach, it should be evident that the first requirement would be to give the stomach a chance to rest and quieten down. This is why we suggest that where the vitality of the patient permits, all foods should be excluded for from one to several days. Nothing but hot water flavored with a few drops of fresh juice, or some of the soothing bland herbal infusions or teas should be permitted at this time. These may be taken as often as desired.

## An Alternate Program

As an alternate program for those who are either unable or unwilling to abstain completely from food, we suggest a liquid diet for several days. In the milder or earlier cases of inflammation, freshly extracted ripe grapefruit juice, whole or diluted, or, when the grapefruit juice is not well tolerated, hot freshly made vegetable juice broth may be used. The juice or broth may be taken about every two hours or whenever the sufferer is hungry. Use only ripe sweet grapefruits, and make sure to squeeze the juice over a glass reamer. It should be squeezed immediately before it is taken, and should be taken without sugar or any other sweetening. It should never be chilled.

To prepare the vegetable broth, cut up various vegetables, such as carrots, celery, string beans, turnips, parsnips, and parsley. Add water to cover the vegetables completely. Then bring to a boil, and let them simmer until they are done. Only the clear broth should be taken for the first day or two, but later the vegetables may be mashed, strained through a colander, and then eaten.

Apple and grape juice are also highly satisfactory in these cases, and other fruit juices are often well tolerated. When in season, the freshly squeezed juice of the pomegranate, whole or diluted, is an ideal drink, and the same may be said of papaya juice where obtainable.

All fluids must be sipped slowly or should be taken with a spoon, a spoonful at a time.

## Milk Diet as an Alternative

In some cases, the inflammation may be of such a severe nature that even the bland juice or the vegetable broth proves irritating. In these cases, a milk diet is usually advisable at first. We start by using 8 ounces of ½ milk and ½ water about every two hours for the first day or two; and then switch to whole milk for a number of days thereafter. Only raw, skimmed milk should be used. Goat's milk, when available, is always preferable to cow's milk.

The milk too must be sipped slowly, or taken one spoonful at a time.

Acute cases are sometimes accompanied by nausea or vomiting. In these cases, all food, even the intake of liquids, must be stopped until the nausea or vomiting is completely eliminated. Small sips of pure, cool water are sometimes tolerated, but should be used only when needed to quench thirst or relieve dryness. Sucking a lemon or lime may provide relief from nausea.

## Other Helpful Measures

In addition to the modified fast, liquid or milk diet, other hygienic measures are usually necessary to promote elimination, induce relaxation, and promote rehabilitation and repair:

1. Warm, cleansing enemas should be taken once daily, whenever indicated or convenient. Only plain lukewarm water should be used for enemas. (Directions for the best way of taking an enema will be found at the end of this chapter.)

2. Tolerably hot baths in which one to two glasses of epsom salts have been added to the water are recommended. They should be taken once daily. These baths are best taken before retiring, but if they tend to disturb sleep, they may be taken upon arising. They should, however, always be followed by a period of rest. The patient must not stay in the bath for more than ten to fifteen minutes, or even less time if restlessness, nausea, or weakness appear.

3. An abundance of rest and sleep plus the avoidance of all tensions, anxieties, or emotional upsets, are imperative.

4. The patient's feet must be kept warm at all times.

These measures provide the digestive organs with a chance to rest, induce relaxation, encourage elimination, and promote rehabilitation and recuperation.

The fast or limited juice or milk is usually followed until the major symptoms have been brought under control; then a more generous diet can be instituted.

For milder cases of gastritis the following sample menu is suggested:

BREAKFAST   1.  Finely grated raw or heated apple or pear, or peeled, mashed raw peaches, or mangoes, blueberries, or ripe grapes (without seeds or skin);   2.

Very ripe, raw, baked, or broiled bananas. Baked soft well-ripened plantains (a Spanish variety of banana) may be used instead of bananas. The plaintains should never be eaten raw;    3. One glass of raw skimmed milk (sipped slowly or taken with a spoon).

OR

1.   Baked apple or applesauce, or stewed fresh peaches, or any other stewed fruit in season (unsweetened), or fresh blueberries;    2.   Buckwheat groats, or natural-brown or wild rice;    3.   1 glass of raw skimmed milk (as above).

NOON    1.   Any of the seasonal raw fresh fruits mentioned above, with about 4 ounces of a soft, bland cheese such as cottage cheese, pot cheese, farmer cheese, or ricotta, the Italian cottage cheese.

OR

1.   Small amounts of finely grated raw cucumber and carrot. (Pick fresh vegetables, and make sure that they are not waxed; otherwise, peel or scrape off skin);    2. Small portion of your favorite protein food (prepared simply and without spices or condiments);    3.   1 or 2 steamed vegetables, preferably from among carrots, parsnips, squash, turnips, eggplant, and okra. Other vegetables may be used later;    4.   If still hungry: A baked apple, applesauce, stewed fresh peaches, or any other fruit that is in season may be used for dessert.

DINNER    1.   Small amounts of finely grated raw cucumber and carrot;    2.   Potatoes, baked, boiled, or steamed in jacket (white or sweet potatoes or yams);    3.   1 or 2 steamed vegetables (of those mentioned above);    4.   And, if still hungry, baked apple or stewed fruit as above.

Omit seasonings of any kind. Do not add butter or salt to the vegetables, and do not use sugar or any other sweetening with your fruits or berries.

In the more severe cases, even small quanities of raw vegetables and raw fruits may be irritating, and may cause a recurrence of the distressing symptoms. In these cases, we have no alternative but to start with a diet composed primarily of soft, bland foods and exclude all raw foods and all food containing roughage, as well as other irritating foods.

## Misconceptions About Protein

The field of nutrition is burdened with numerous misconceptions and much misinformation on the subject of protein. Some persons are afraid that they will not get enough protein unless they include meat in their diet, while others have come to believe that they must use large quantities of protein if they are to be well fed.

Neither of these assumptions is correct. If you will just stop to think for a moment, you will realize that the cow which supplies us with milk, the most complete type of protein, obtains her protein from the grass she eats. We do not have to eat grass like the cow, but the green leafy vegetables such as turnip greens, escarole, chicory, dandelion, as well as string beans, green peas, and the root vegetables such as potatoes, carrots, beets, parsnips, and the fresh luscious fruits such as apples and grapes, supply some of the most valuable proteins.

It is true that the protein is present in these foods in a lesser concentration than it is in meat, fish, eggs, or cheese. Nonetheless even in smaller quantities these proteins are most desirable physiologically, and are easily utilized by the body.

We should always choose those proteins that are most easily digestible, and that provide a minimum of toxic by-products. The nutritionally enlightened person knows that the bland, soft cheese such as pot cheese, farmer's cheese, or ricotta, as well as lentils, green beans, and chick peas (garbanzos), provide ample and adequate protein to replace bodily loss. Those who wish to include meat in their diet can use chicken, lamb chops, lean meat, or lean fish. However, they must make sure that these foods are prepared without spices or condiments, and that they are either baked, boiled, or broiled, but not fried.

Furthermore, it is well to know that large quantities of much of these foods can lead to a great deal of harm. We must stress the fact that while an adequate supply of these foods is essential, they must not be used in excessive amounts.

## A Word of Warning

A word of warning is in place at this time: We pointed out above that no two cases of stomach trouble are alike, and therefore sufferers from inflammation or ulcers of the stomach should, whenever possible, obtain competent professional help. However, to obtain most effective results, it is essential that the physician in charge of the case possess a full grasp of the physiologically required principles stressed in this book, and has the necessary experience to apply them.

## Other Care Essential

In addition to planning the right diet, the other measures previously outlined must be continued, although in modified form, in accordance with the requirement of the particular case.

The warm cleansing enemas should be reduced, first to one every second day, and then to one every third day. They should then be continued twice a week until the bowels begin to move of their own accord at least twice daily. As soon as this is accomplished, the enemas should be discontinued or used only when needed to overcome flatulence (a gassy condition) or relieve a sense of discomfort.

The hot epsom salt baths may be continued. In most cases these baths will induce relaxation and promote sound sleep.

An abundance of rest and sleep is necessary. Sufferers from this disorder are often extremely nervous and greatly debilitated, and need much rest and sleep to recuperate. They must retire early and at the same time each day, and they must get as many hours of sleep as possible. A daily nap or rest period for at least one hour after the noon meal is very helpful.

Tension or emotional stress must be avoided. Fear, worry, anger, strain, resentment, and all forms of nervous tension play havoc with our health and must be eliminated if favorable results are to be attained.

## Where Raw Milk Is Obtainable

Those who live near a farm or close to persons who own a cow or goat should have no difficulty in obtaining raw milk, while those who live in the large cities can order raw certified (cow's) milk from the larger milk companies. The cream should be poured off before the milk is used.

Incidentally, in most cities raw milk is obtainable only by prescription. It is ironical that the inferior or processed types of milk can be purchased freely, while raw milk cannot be obtained except by prescription. However, one should have no difficulty in getting his doctor to cooperate on this matter.

## Is Cow's Milk the Ideal Food?

One of the prevalent nutritional misconceptions is that cow's milk is an ideal food for human beings. Yet, a few moments' thought should make us realize that this is not the case. Mother's milk is the ideal food for human babies and should be used in infant feeding. However, as soon as the child grows up and develops the ability to chew, the need for milk diminishes and becomes less important. Cow's milk has been adopted as a substitute for mother's milk in infant feeding when a mother is either unable or unwilling to nurse her baby. Though most children can handle it without difficulty, it is in no way nutritionally equal to or as easily digestible as mother's milk.

In the more advanced cases of stomach inflammation or in ulcers of the stomach, cow's or, whenever available, goat's milk may often be used to great advantage, since it is a bland and easily digestible protein food and absorbs the acid that the inflamed or irritated stomach glands secrete in large quantities. One of the cultured milks, such as sour milk, acidophilus milk, or buttermilk may often be used in place of sweet milk.

Soybean milk can often be used as a substitute for cow's milk or goat's milk. Soybean milk is obtainable ready prepared in all health and specialty food stores. In preparation for use, it should be diluted to half strength with water and then brought just to the boiling point, but should not be boiled. One-half teaspoon of honey may be added for sweetening.

Almond milk is another fine substitute for cow's milk. Almond milk can be prepared by dissolving one ounce of finely powdered blanched almonds in three ounces of boiling water. Mix well and then strain through a white cheesecloth.

## Raw Fruits and Raw Vegetables

While in the very acute or advanced cases of inflammation or ulcers of the stomach we have no alternative but to rely primarily, or even exclusively, upon bland steamed and baked vegetables, these foods *must* not be regarded as the best foods for regular use. These foods are used because they contain a minimum of roughage and, next to milk, are foods that a badly impaired stomach can handle without undue pain or discomfort. However, as soon as the acute stage subsides and the pains and discomforts have been overcome, our aim should be to start using raw fruit and vegetable juices and then follow with finely grated raw fruits and raw vegetables, since these are the foods that provide maximum nutrition for the weak and depleted tissues.

However, the mere absence of pain is no assurance that the damaged tissues have healed sufficiently to permit the use of fibrous foods. We can determine this only after using small quantities of these foods and observing their effect.

We start by adding one to two tablespoons of finely grated or scraped raw apple to the morning meal, and one to two tablespoons of finely grated cucumber to the noon and evening meals. When these foods cause no pain or discomfort, other fruits and vegetables may be gradually added. Ripe, raw peaches and grapes (without skin or pits) are then substituted for the grated apple, while grated carrots and finely chopped lettuce or escarole are next in line from among the many seasonal vegetables.

In due time a greater choice will be permitted. Once the inflammation has been overcome or the ulcers have healed, most foods will be easily digested and will cause no discomforts.

### These Meals Can Be Most Enjoyable

Persons who follow haphazard eating habits and who have never eaten many fruits or vegetables sometimes wonder at how enjoyable meals composed of these foods can be, and are usually pleasantly surprised with them. They find that with a little ingenuity and skill many tasty dishes can be prepared without spicy seasonings. The combination of various vegetables and the addition of bland herb flavorings such as thyme, sage, rosemary, marjoram, parsley, fennel, dill, and caraway seeds can do much to make these foods most enjoyable. (In Section VI recipes and suggestions for the preparation of meals with these herbs are given.)

### A Well-Balanced Program of Living

Once the inflammation has completely subsided, the aim should be to guard against a recurrence of the condition. It is a mistake to think that we can return to conventional foods and other unwholesome living habits, and get away with it. We must always remember that the same abuses that have brought on the disease in the first place can ultimately bring about its recurrence.

### The Hygienic Way of Living

The only protection we have against a recurrence of the disease is a wholesome, rational program of living. Such a program must be based upon the use of simple, unadulterated, and unrefined foods, the development of sensible eating habits, such as eating slowly, chewing the food well, eating only when hungry, controlling the intake of the food we eat, and making sure not to overeat. We also must be careful not to eat too many different kinds of food at one meal since this leads to overeating. Furthermore, an abundance of rest, sleep, and relaxation, moderate exercises, and other planned body-building activities, are important. This program also stresses the importance of eliminating all harmful and health-debilitating influences, such as the use of alcohol and tobacco, late hours, overexcitement, etc. Only a way of living based upon these principles can improve the health and strength of the individual and assure lasting results.

The health-appreciative person, he who recognizes the value of this way of life, realizes that to maintain a healthy digestive system and otherwise obtain maximum health benefits the inclusion of an abundance of raw fruits and vegetables in the diet is not only desirable but actually essential. He also becomes aware that all foods must be properly prepared since frying and overcooking destroy many of the valuable vitamins, minerals, and digestive enzymes, and diminish the nutritional value of carbohydrates, proteins, and all other food elements.

Once the digestion has been restored to normal, the quantity and the kind of food eaten are adjusted to meet the needs and desires of the individual. However, it is imperative that only simple, natural foods be used, and that all refined and processed foods such as white flour and white sugar products and the much publicized refined cereals; all sweets, such as cakes, pastries, malteds, ice cream, etc.; all stimulants such as coffee, tea, chocolate, alcohol, and the commercial soft drinks; all sharp and irritating spices, such as salt, pepper, mustard, eggs, as well as the fat meats and fish, and all fried foods, must be completely eliminated from the diet.

## Other Rules of Importance

Never compromise with the need for rest and sleep. Take walks regularly and exercise moderately once or twice a day. Get into the habit of relaxing at intervals during the day to counteract nervous tension. Develop calmness and composure. Be patient and tolerant, and don't let other people's foibles or weaknesses upset you. *Remember that resentment, hate, envy, fear, and jealousy hurt you most of all*. It is up to you to choose to live a healthy life and be proud of the fact that you have the good sense to do it!

*A Case History:* DAVID G.

Nothing illustrates more vividly the benefits that can be derived from this type of care than a case history. Out of the many cases of those who have been helped this way, we present that of David G. as an example.

David's history goes back 30 years, to when he was twenty-eight years old. By that time David had already been under the care of a physician for two years for stomach upsets. However, his condition seemed to be growing constantly worse. David recollects:

I became more constipated, my breath was foul, and I lost my pep. My stomach was like a gas tank. I couldn't sleep. If I did close my eyes, I had bad dreams. I became nervous, irritable, and jumpy. I felt that everyone was against me. My eyes began to twitch. People began to ask what was wrong with me.

One morning, I couldn't move my bowels, and I noticed my piles were out. I became alarmed because a young neighbor of ours had died a few weeks earlier of cancer of the rectum. I knew he had piles and had an operation recently. I had something to worry me now and didn't know what to do next.

I went to my local doctor who examined me and said that, organically, nothing was wrong, but that my nerves were in a bad way. I was told to calm down and not to worry needlessly. He gave me a diet, prescribed some medicine similar to the one I had been given before by the other doctor and told me to come back in about two weeks.

After two weeks, I went back to see him but I was a wreck. I felt I was getting worse day by day. He suggested that I take some tests.

After these tests, I was told that I had a nervous stomach and a new diet was prescribed. It was to consist of toast, sweet cream, milk, cheese, sour cream, lean meats, no fats, no fruits or vegetables.

But David did not seem to get any better. Then somebody called his attention to the fact that certain doctors who rely primarily on dietary and hygienic measures obtain excellent results in these cases and, in desperation, he decided to consult one of them.

We'll let David continue:

On my first visit, I was told to stop eating for three

days but if I got thirsty to have all the water I wanted, then for the next ten days to have either orange or grapefruit juice every two hours. I was also told that I must learn to relax, to rest as much as possible and to take it easy. Food alone would not be the cure unless I followed everything else so that I would be well again.

When I got home, my wife asked me what happened. I informed her of all I was to do. She in turn asked me if she should order the "box" as there would be nothing left of me if I followed such a rigid diet. Besides, how could I afford to take it easy?

I told her that I had tried everything up till now without results, and I did not want to be a sick husband ... and that I did not want to continue suffering. I told her that I wanted to get well and she agreed to help me. This made it easier for me. Courage, will power, faith, and my wife's willingness to see me through were all I needed.

At first, I lost a lot of weight and yet I went to work every day. Always being underweight and losing more weight made people question me all the more. However, I had less pain in my stomach and felt better without food than when I followed my previous diets.

After describing the diet and the other instructions that he was told to follow, which were similar to the program we have outlined above, David continued:

The first months of this rigid diet, and the exercises, did wonders for me. My body became more flexible and I was less tired. I had more strength, in spite of the fact that I had lost weight. I began to feel better and stronger each week that went by.

After three months of following the new routine, I began to see the light. I was being complimented on how well I looked and the improved color of my face.

I began to feel younger. I started each morning with a half-mile walk and gradually increased this to a mile every morning and evening. It was a bit difficult in the beginning to do so. As I continued walking, my breathing improved. I felt stronger and did not get dizzy any more. I still continue with my daily walks.

During the next ten years, I got stronger and felt younger from year to year. My mind was more alert. I had always been backward in business and always had someone thinking for me and doing things. As I became stronger, my mind began to be sharp and I had more faith and will power to do things. I began to be noticed.

I was called on to be a leader in my business and the people in my community wanted me to be president of the Board of Trade. I accepted. I was amazed how ably I handled important matters.

Whenever David became lax or careless, some of his old symptoms would return to remind him that he must not take chances with his health. He would quickly retrench and would begin to feel well again. He followed this program for about 25 years and stayed well.

Then pressure of business and family problems made him careless again, and again his digestive difficulties returned. David tried to make contact with the doctor who had treated him before, but by that time the doctor had retired from active practice and moved to another city. In desperation, David returned again to conventional medical treatment with its antacid palliatives and routines of soft diets. But, as before, improvements failed to come. David writes:

I began to be tired, my feet felt as though they were caving in, and I had no more pep. I couldn't digest my food because of the gases which traveled to my chest, and I became constipated. My breathing was poor.

For several hours after a meal, I would be belching. I would fall asleep for about a half hour and then awake with pain in my chest. I could not sleep. I lost weight and had a tired and drawn look on my face.

David was in despair. Finally, he located the doctor who had helped him. He made contact with him and, although retired from active practice, the doctor agreed to take him under his care again. The same program that helped him the first time brought about full recovery within a few months.

In concluding his story, David writes:

I have learned that one cannot cheat by wrong combinations, lack of rest, worry, and overwork, and expect to keep healthy.

I am grateful that I have learned at last how to relax,

not to worry, and to have peace of mind; and how and what to eat.

I have also learned that it is never too late to feel young and really alive again.

David's case history presents several object lessons. It illustrates that, even in very difficult cases, recovery is possible when the right regimen is followed, and furthermore illustrates how foolhardy it is to return to devitalizing living habits and invite a recurrence of suffering. We cannot reiterate too strongly the fact that the same unhealthy or unwholesome habits of living that initiated the disease in the first place will cause it to recur.

## Gastric Catarrh

In cases of gastritis of long standing, or where irritation has been going on for a long period of time, a great deal of mucus may accumulate in the stomach. These cases are sometimes diagnosed as gastric catarrh or catarrh of the stomach.

Mucus, which is secreted by the mucous membrane or inner lining of the body, serves a useful purpose. It acts as a lubricant and protects the tissues against the effects of irritating substances or toxins.

When the mucous membrane or inner lining of the stomach becomes badly irritated, it secretes excessive amounts of mucus and this protects the tissues against the harmful effects of the irritation. Overeating and eating too much of rich, concentrated foods are often a major cause of this condition, while the use of spices and condiments or the intake of drugs or chemicals is often a powerful contributory factor.

In these cases, the raw vegetables and raw fruits that contain too much roughage can be very irritating and must, therefore, be limited or even completely eliminated at first. Steamed and baked vegetables and stewed fruit, with moderate quantities of the light protein foods and easily digestible carbohydrates, must make up the bulk of the diet in these cases.

Furthermore, it is imperative that the intake of food be greatly restricted to guard against overeating. Incidentally, at this point it is well to mention that the more thoroughly the food is chewed and the fewer the combinations at any one meal, the less likely is the danger of overeating.

Only after the condition has been brought under control should the raw fruits and vegetables be added to the diet. They should be finely grated and used in small amounts at first, but the quantity may be gradually increased as the condition continues to improve.

## Soft, Bland Diet Imperative in These Cases

Sufferers from gastritis must follow a program that conforms to the suggestions we have outlined here or the condition is bound to grow worse. We remember the case of a woman who suffered from this disorder for many years and actually interfered with her recovery by adhering to a diet of raw fruits and raw vegetables, even after she had been warned that these foods were not advisable in her case.

This patient was extremely emaciated and wasted; her skin was coarse and wrinkled, her abdomen and its organs were dropped and sagging, she suffered greatly from nausea, pain, and distension. She could not understand why she failed to get well, since she had been careful in living only on what she considered to be the most nourishing and health-giving foods.

She was finally persuaded to change to a soft, bland, nonfibrous diet and, before very long, began to show a great deal of improvement.

After a time, small amounts of finely grated, raw vegetables and bland, raw fruits were added to her diet. The quantity of these foods was increased as her condition improved. It took a great many months before she recovered fully; but at last she began to realize that while raw fruits and raw vegetables are valuable foods, they can also do harm when used at the wrong time.

In cases of catarrhal gastritis, even normal quantities of otherwise suitable foods may be too stimulating and irritating and that is the reason why only the easily digestible and the readily assimilable bland foods must be used during the acute stage of the disease.

### Best Way to Take an Enema

Fill the enema bag with plain lukewarm water. Get into the knee-chest position or, if this is uncomfortable, lie flat on your back with the knees drawn up. Grease the nozzle with pure olive oil, insert it in the rectum, then let the water flow in slowly, but never use more than one half a bag at a time, or less if this amount causes pain or discomfort. If possible, retain the water for a few minutes and massage abdomen gently. Then expel and repeat. Always limit flow to ½ or ⅓ of the content of the bag.

The enema should always be regarded as an emergency measure. The long-range objective should be to establish normal bowel movements without any artificial help. To bring about this improvement as rapidly as possible, we suggest that the patient make it a practice to try to evacuate the bowels normally after each meal. Make sure not to strain, merely sit patiently for eight to ten minutes while giving the bowels a chance to function naturally. It may take some time before results begin to show up but patience will in most instances be well rewarded.

One technique that proves most effective when attempting to move the bowels is to make sure to be completely relaxed and to concentrate on some pleasant or interesting thoughts. Reading a magazine or a book while waiting to move the bowels often helps to bring about complete relaxation, providing the subject matter is not of too exciting a nature.

# 4

# THE WHYS AND WHEREFORES OF ULCERS

When an inflammation of the stomach persists, it often leads to the development of ulcers.

Ulcers develop when the affected part of the stomach fails to receive its normal blood supply and is deprived of the oxygen it needs to keep functioning. Tissues receive their oxygen from the blood and when any part of the stomach fails to obtain the oxygen it needs, it dies off. An interesting fact is that although the tissues of the stomach are composed of the same kind of tissue as the proteins we eat, they are fully protected against the digestive action of the hydrochloric acid and the protein digesting enzyme, pepsin, as long as they are supplied with the oxygen they need. However, when any part of the stomach is deprived of its oxygen, it loses its ingrown protective powers and becomes digested, the same as any other protein food.

## Size of Ulcers Varies

Ulcers of the stomach are known either as gastric or duodenal ulcers, depending upon where they are located. Those in the upper stomach are known as gastric ulcers, while those which are found in the lower portion of the stomach, and which sometimes extend into the small intestine, are known as duodenal ulcers. Basically the types are alike. They are named differently merely because of their location.

Some ulcers are extremely small, even pinpoint in size, while others may be very large. Some ulcers affect only the surface tissues, while in other cases the deeper tissues of the stomach are affected.

Small ulcers in close proximity to one another often coalesce and form large ulcers. If they are not healed, they ultimately penetrate into the deeper tissues and then develop into a much more serious problem. Perforation may result, and the patient's life may be endangered.

It should be evident from what we have stated earlier that the size of an ulcer and how far it progresses is usually controlled by the vitality and health of the tissues, and this, in turn, is determined almost entirely by our mode of living.

## Ulcer Pains Often Excruciating

The pains from ulcers are often excruciating,. The stomach acids irritate the sore and ulcerated areas, and cause the tissues to contract or go into spasm. This produces a great deal of suffering.

Frequent bland feedings, especially the use of acid-binding protein foods, often relieve these pains. This is because proteins use up the acids and relieve the irritation. This is the reason milk is often recommended in these cases and also why it is suggested that it be taken at frequent intervals or whenever the pains recur.

However, as long as the inflammation persists and the irritation continues, new quantities of acid continue to be poured out by the glands of the stomach, and then the pains recur. They usually reappear about one to two hours after a meal.

## Hemorrhages

In ulcers of the stomach, hemorrhages are a most serious problem. Bleeding takes place when an ulcer eats into or corrodes a blood vessel; or when mucus that has plugged up pinpoint ulcers has become loosened up and been washed away, laying bare a bleeding area; or when there is oozing of blood from weak or damaged tissues.

Bleeding from a superficial ulcer or from a small blood vessel may cease quickly and is more frightening than dangerous.

However, oozing of blood may continue from weak or damaged tissues, or bleeding may persist from denuded pinpoint ulcers, without being noticed except through an examination of the stool for what is known as occult blood. (The term occult blood usually refers to traces of blood found in the stool, in contradistinction to bleeding visible to the eyes. In medical terminology, this latter type of bleeding is known as *melena*.) Where bleeding continues, surgery may become necessary. However, there can be no guarantee that the bleeding will not return; only when the damaged tissues are rebuilt can we be certain of permanent results.

## The Deformed Stomach Wall

We have pointed out that when a stomach is inflamed for a long period of time it often becomes deformed or misshapen. The walls of the stomach become thickened and hardened and, in the more advanced cases, the tissues may shrivel up and waste away.

In these cases, some parts of the stomach may become stretched and dilated, while other parts may shrink and waste away. These changes cause varying degrees of obstruction which may lead to an unduly long retention of food in the stomach. In long-standing ulcer cases, these changes are often very pronounced.

Occasionally, the deformity presents a peculiar appearance similar to an hourglass, and this condition is known as an *hourglass stomach*. Scars or fibrous bands contract the center of the stomach, while the upper and lower ends of the stomach become distended, giving the stomach the appearance of an hourglass.

## Early Ulcers Can Heal Easily

While ulcers of the stomach present a more severe problem than the previously described inflammatory conditions, the early or simple stages of ulcer can nevertheless heal with little difficulty if proper care is provided.

In the more advanced cases, however, much more time and patience may be required before results are obtained. Irrespective, however, of whether the disease is in the early or more advanced stages it is important to realize that only when we provide the necessary tissue building foods, remove the underlying irritating influences, and restore the circulation to the affected part of the stomach can complete and lasting results be expected.

## Dietary Differences That Require Watching

While ulcers of the stomach are usually preceded by inflammation, and while the care in gastric inflammation and ulcers is in many ways similar, we wish to mention certain differences in the diet that must be strictly observed.

We have pointed out that in the earlier or milder cases of inflammation raw fruits and vegetables are permissable, provided they are finely grated and used in small quantities. This, however, is not true in ulcer cases. In these cases, only soft, bland, nonfibrous foods must be used, and raw fruits and raw vegetables may be added only after a certain amount of healing has taken place, and the stomach is able to handle them without any difficulty.

## How to Start

We begin the care of ulcers of the stomach essentially the same way as in inflammation. We recommend that whenever possible all solid food be completely eliminated for from one to several days and that only hot water or the soothing bland herb teas such as alfalfa, sage or camomile, flavored with a teaspoon of honey, be taken whenever the patient is hungry or thirsty. These liquids dilute and wash away the excess acid in the stomach and often provide relief.

However, in the more advanced cases of ulcer or where severe damage already exists, even plain hot water or the mild herb teas may cause pain. In these cases, the use of small quantities of milk is then indicated. We usually begin by using 8 ounces of ½ milk and ½ hot water about every two hours for the first two days, then ¾ milk and ¼ water for one or two days, and then whole skimmed milk.

However, in very severe cases the milk may at first have to be used only in very small quantities, sometimes not more than one or two ounces at a time—but that may be taken at more frequent intervals.

After the symptoms have subsided and hunger begins to assert itself, the quantity of milk may be increased and/or taken at more frequent intervals. Whenever possible, only raw skimmed milk should be used.

When on a milk diet, the bowels in some cases, may become irregular. Some patients will become constipated, while others will develop diarrhea. In constipation, the lukewarm water enema should be used for relief, while diarrhea can often be controlled when the quantity of milk is temporarily reduced or it is taken at less frequent intervals. Heating the milk, but not boiling it, also tends to control the diarrhea.

### A Soft, Bland, Nonfibrous Ulcer Diet

The milk may be continued anywhere from a few days to several weeks or until relief has been attained. Then, the patient is placed on a carefully regulated bland, soft, nonfibrous diet. The following is an example of such a diet:

BREAKFAST    1.  Baked or broiled ripe banana or plantain;    2.  8 ounces of raw skimmed milk, sipped slowly, or spoon-fed.

LUNCH    1.  1 or 2 steamed vegetables from among the following: potatoes, carrots, parsnips, turnips, squash, eggplant, okra;    2.  8 ounces of raw skimmed milk.

DINNER    1.  Potatoes (baked, boiled, or steamed) in jacket, and eaten without the skin;    2.  1 steamed vegetable of those mentioned above; 3.  8 ounces of raw skimmed milk.

Milk may also be taken between meals and before retiring. The milk should always be warmed, but not boiled. It should never be taken cold.

If the pains recur between meals, small quantities of whole skimmed or diluted milk (diluted ½ milk and ½ water) often provide relief. Freshly pressed grape juice diluted half and half with water is also often helpful.

All foods must be eaten slowly, should be taken in small quantities, and should be well chewed. It is better to eat more often than too much at any one meal.

In very severe cases, the steamed vegetables and the stewed fruits may at first have to be pureed to remove all fibers and coarse particles that might cause irritation of the inflamed area.

## Other Care Essential

While the diet in ulcer cases is of great importance, the other measures that we have outlined in the chapter on inflammation must also be carefully followed. Enemas should be taken at first every day, then every second day, finally every third day, and then should be continued every third or fourth day until the bowels begin to move at least twice daily.

Hot epsom salt baths should be taken, preferably before retiring. They have a relaxing effect on the body and usually induce sleep. However, as has been mentioned, hot baths may fail to relax the patient and as a result disturb sleep. Where this happens, the bath should be taken mornings, but should be followed with a period of rest. Make sure that you do not stay too long in the bath; and never force yourself to stay in it until you become restless, fatigued, or faint.

Plenty of rest and sleep are essential. Ulcer sufferers are highly nervous and irritable. Rest and sleep do much to strengthen the nervous system, and go a long way in rebuilding the health of the patient.

Deep breathing and simple leg exercises (described in the section on exercises) should be followed regularly, at least once a day, or whenever possible morning and night. These exercises should be done slowly and should never be continued beyond the point of fatigue.

Tobacco, alcohol, sweets, tea, coffee, chocolate, all soft drinks, as well as all condiments and spices and sharp stimulating foods must be excluded at all times. Not only do they interfere with the healing of the ulcers; they actually aggravate the condition.

## A Rational Diet

A soft, bland diet, free of roughage, is essential in ulcer cases. However, the foods that are to be used in these cases must have an alkaline base, must be easily digestible, and must provide all essential nutrient elements, such as the valuable vitamins, minerals, and digestive enzymes, as well as the easily digestible proteins and carbohydrates.

While it is true that at the onset the vitamin and mineral-rich raw fruits and vegetables may have to be omitted in most cases, it is still imperative that the diet provide at least a minimum of all the essential body and health-building elements, and it is for this reason that we urge that the easily digestible stewed fruits and steamed vegetables be included in the diet. These foods plus some of the dairy products and other easily digestible protein foods, as well as some of the whole grain foods, such as whole brown rice or whole finely ground buckwheat, will provide the nourishment that is needed in these cases in a manner that can be easily handled by sufferers from this disorder.

The more enlightened physicians are gradually beginning to realize that, because of their high cholesterol content, the dairy fat foods such as cream, butter, and fat cheeses are inadvisable in ulcer cases, and we hope that before long the harmful effects of the refined and processed foods will also become recognized and excluded from use.

The so-called Sippy diet, which is often prescribed by doctors in these cases, includes many high cholesterol and acid-producing foods, and, though it is soft and bland, is undesirable because of them.

Another point to bear in mind in connection with the Sippy diet is that it is usually used in combination with antacid remedies and occasionally causes a state of alkalosis. The *Journal of the American Medical Association,* April 1, 1961, in an editorial entitled "Milk-Alkali Syndrome," quotes from a "Syndrome Following Prolonged Intake of Milk and Alkali," by Burnett *et al.,* who pointed out that the milk and alkali treatment in ulcers can lead to a state of alkalosis with various other disorders such as high blood calcium, impairment in kidney function with retention of waste products in the blood, and damage to the cornea of the eye.

### Introducing Raw Fruits and Vegetables

While it is essential that in the great majority of these cases the soft, bland, nonfibrous foods be used at first, our ultimate aim should be to build up the health of the patient to the point where raw fruits and raw vegetables can be handled without any ill effects. However, these foods should be added only after the condition has improved sufficiently so that they can be digested without causing any suffering or distress.

To determine whether we have reached this stage, we start the same as in severe cases of inflammation, by using at first not more than one to two tablespoons of finely grated raw apple or ripe mashed peaches or mangoes with the breakfast meal, and one to two tablespoons of finely grated cucumber with the noon and evening meals. When obtainable, sweet Delicious or Golden Delicious apples are usually best.

If these foods are well tolerated, one to two tablespoons of finely grated carrots or finely chopped lettuce, preferably Romaine, is then substituted for the grated cucumber a few days later.

In time the quantity of these foods is gradually increased, or two of the three vegetables mentioned above are used together. Other tender, finely chopped or grated vegetables are added later, usually one at a time and in small quantities.

In most cases this program works out satisfactorily. Sometimes, however, when the stomach is still weak and sensitive, or when the ulcers are not entirely healed, a certain amount of distress may recur. This may also happen when the raw foods are introduced too soon or in too large quantities.

Where this happens, the raw fruit and vegetables must be discontinued, and the soft, bland, nonfibrous diet must again be resumed.

When the symptoms subside, the raw fruits and vegetables are again introduced but at a much more gradual pace and in smaller quantities to make sure that the pains or discomforts do not recur.

In the more advanced cases where a great deal of damage has already developed or where large ulcers already exist, healing may take place only very slowly and with great difficulty. It should be apparent, however, that only a program based upon a sound nutritional approach and natural fortifying and rehabilitating care can yield beneficial and lasting results.

## Need For Vitamin and Mineral-Rich Raw Foods

Raw fruits and vegetables are essential for sound and vigorous health. They supply the essential vitamins, minerals, and enzymes, and in addition provide the best type of protein, as well as the most readily digestible carbohydrates. They are the only complete and living foods, and are correctly considered by the more progressive nutritionists as the true "building stones" of health.

It should be clear why, during the active stage of these diseases, raw foods are not well tolerated. These foods contain a great deal of the roughage or coarse substances irritating to the inflamed or ulcerated areas of the stomach.

Nonetheless, even though these valuable foods must at first be omitted, we must still make sure to use foods which provide not only the easily digestible proteins and carbohydrates but also an abundance of the valuable vitamins, minerals, and enzymes. Fruits and vegetables provide an ample supply of these essential food elements but to obtain maximum benefits we must make sure that these foods are carefully prepared. They should be steamed in their own juices and should never be fried or overcooked. Furthermore, the liquid of these foods should never be poured off. Salt or other irritating spices and condiments should never be used, even by healthy persons. A waterless steamer for the preparation of these foods is usually most suitable. It will not only preserve their natural flavors but also most of the vitamins and minerals which less careful cooking would waste or destroy.

When raw fruits and raw vegetables are not well tolerated, raw fruit and vegetable juices can often be used to supplement the diet. The juices of carrot and sweet apple, or carrot, celery, and sweet apple, or carrot, parsley and sweet apple, or carrot, crisp green cabbage, and sweet apple, make ideal combinations and will go a long way in supplying the valuable essential vitamins, minerals, and enzymes. Freshly squeezed grape or apple juice is also a great value.

The vegetable and fruit juices should, whenever possible, be made in the home immediately before using. One of the best investments in health is a juicer, which may be obtained at any health or specialty food store.

Only ripe, fresh fruits and carefully selected fresh vegetables are recommended for this purpose and, whenever possible, only those that have been grown under ideal organic methods should be used, since they are most valuable from the standpoint of health and nutrition.

In severe ulcer cases, the raw vegetable juices are not always well tolerated at first. Where this is the case, we have no alternative but rely on the raw skimmed milk diet for relief. In these cases milk is virtually a specific. It absorbs the excess acid in the stomach and soothes the irritated and inflamed tissues.

Many persons with a history of ulcers continue with the soft, bland diet even after the ulcers have completely healed. This is a grave error, since by omitting the vitamin and mineral-rich raw fruits and vegetables they fail to get many of the essential food elements necessary for superb, vigorous health.

### Milk Sometimes Not Well Tolerated

While milk is virtually a specific in most ulcer cases, we are occasionally confronted by a case in which milk is not well tolerated. We remember one woman who developed severe stomach pains every time she tried to take milk. This patient was suffering from an allergy to this food, which she apparently developed from the antacid remedies she had taken over a period of many years. The usual soft, bland diet, five days a week, and a mixed vegetable broth diet on the other two days of the week, plus the use of the other health restorative measures recommended in these cases, brought about a complete recovery.

### Stomach Obstructions

#### Pylorospasm—Pyloric Stenosis

At the junction between the stomach and the small intestine is found the pylorus, or pyloric canal. This is a valve-like mechanism that controls the opening through which the totally and partly digested food passes. In advanced cases of inflammation or ulcers of the stomach, this part sometimes becomes blocked or obstructed. In the simpler cases the obstruction may be caused by muscular spasms, in which case it can usually be easily corrected. This condition is known as pylorospasm.

In more serious cases blockage may be caused by scars and adhesions, and in these cases the condition usually presents a much more difficult problem.

We have pointed out that when the inflammation or ulcers are of long standing, the tissues of the stomach become hardened and thickened, and scars often form. When these changes take place in the pyloric region, the opening through which the food passes becomes constricted and the tissues lose much of their resiliency and are, therefore, unable to stretch and contract normally. When this condition develops, we have what is known as a pyloric stenosis or pyloric obstruction.

When the opening is partially blocked, the passage of food is delayed and this often causes a great deal of distress. These cases are sometimes mistaken for ulcers or even cancer of the stomach, and are sometimes mistakenly operated upon when all that is required is adherence to a soft, bland diet, the use of small quantities of food, and a well-regulated program of living.

Neglect or improper care in these cases may ultimately lead to complete obstruction. Where this happens, surgery may be unavoidable. However, before surgery is resorted to, it is essential that we determine whether the obstruction is complete and of a permanent nature or whether it is merely partial or temporary owing to inflammation or a muscular spasm induced by an irritation of the nerves.

Where surgery is unavoidable, it is well to bear in mind that this is usually in the nature of an emergency and does not protect the patient against the development of new scars and a new obstruction. To protect against a recurrence, a carefully regulated program of living and the use of bland, easily digestible and assimilable foods are essential.

## Can Ulcers Be Avoided

We have mentioned that doctors as well as laymen often blame ulcers on nervous tension, and disregard or minimize all other precipitating factors. This is as irrational as placing the blame for an increase in chronic and degenerative diseases on aging and not on our careless and haphazard mode of living, where it really belongs.

We have quoted Dr. Sara M. Jordan, who pointed out that placing the blame solely or primarily on tension or emotional stress is a gross fallacy. Dr. Jordan does not believe that ulcers are unavoidable, and suggests that those who are predisposed to the development of this disease and wish to avoid it take stock of their habits and make certain that they check the following:

1. Are you tense, overtired, or worried?

2. Are you getting enough sleep?

3. Are you putting enough relaxation into every day and every weekend?

4. Are you taking a more or less prolonged diversion from work—a real vacation—once or twice a year?

5. How are your eating habits; do you choose the right food for your digestive tract to handle easily?

6. Are you indulging too much in those socially pleasant poisons—alcohol and tobacco?[1]

You will note that Dr. Jordan stresses the importance of the right kind of food and also recognizes the harm done by alcohol and tobacco. We are sure that every intelligent doctor will go along with her fine reasoning. Our hats off to this sterling lady who on many occasions has stressed the importance of human values and sound living principles.

## A Change in Fundamentals Imperative

We have mentioned that some ulcers may heal even when the tendency to ulcers is not eradicated, and that as long as this tendency exists, recurrences are always possible.

Ulcers cause a great deal of suffering and we know that those who are afflicted with this ailment would be willing to pay almost anything to obtain help, but unless they realize that they must follow a hygienic, well-balanced way of life and must obtain proper care—they will get

[1] *Today's Health*, June, 1959.

nowhere. To regain health, all ulcer-causing influences must be eliminated and all impaired bodily functions must be rebuilt.

## Do Ulcers Develop into Cancer?

Some sufferers from inflammation or ulcers of the stomach are greatly disturbed. They are worried not merely because of the pains they suffer or because they are unable to eat the foods they like, but because they are haunted by the fear that they may be developing cancer or are already suffering from it.

Pains naturally frighten people, and when the suffering persists it is easy to see how fears about this dangerous affliction can easily arise. In long-standing cases of inflammation or ulcers of the stomach, these fears often overshadow the actual disease and take a great deal out of the patient. There is no reason why inflammation or ulcers of the stomach should persist or why they should ultimately develop into a more serious ailment except where neglect or improper care and unwholesome living habits interfere with recovery and rebuilding. Aside from all this, however, it should be of help to point out that the presence of pain is not an indication of cancer; as a matter of fact, its presence in most instances actually argues against it.

Boyd[2] points out that ulcers usually give a long history of pain, while cancer in the stomach most often develops insidiously without any pain. However, where cancer of the stomach is accompanied by pain, the pains usually show up immediately after eating and are not lessened by food, while in ulcers of the stomach, food induces relief and the pains, as a rule, recur about two hours after the meal.

An examination of the gastric juices also helps to determine whether the pains are due to ulcers or cancer. In ulcers of the stomach, we usually have an excess of hydrochloric acid, while in cancer of the stomach the quantity of acid is either greatly diminished or it is totally absent.

At this point, we wish to mention that while there is a wide divergence of opinion among authorities on how often ulcers turn to cancer, the weight of opinion is that this happens only on rare occasions. Boyd points out that while

[2] Boyd, *Pathology of Internal Diseases.*

"the workers at Mayo Clinic hold that many simple ulcers become malignant ... Ewing, Dibble, and others consider that not more than 5 per cent of ulcers become malignant." In explaining why this difference of opinion exists, Boyd states:

The difference of opinion depends on different interpretations of the microscopic appearance. To one pathologist, the presence of isolated epithelial cells and atypical tubules in the neighborhood of an ulcer spells carcinoma (cancer) while to another they are the result of distortion produced by the contracting fibrous tissue or merely part of the regenerative process.[3]

In other words, the distortions seen under the microscope in these cases, which are diagnosed as cancer, are in reality but the changes that set in when an inflammation or ulcer heals.

Boyd elaborates on this question in his *Pathology for the Physician* by pointing out that while cancer is sometimes found in ulcer cases, it is present in most instances because an existing cancerous lesion has become ulcerated, and not because an ulcer turned to cancer.

It should also be apparent that while an ulcer condition is sometimes followed by cancer, this is not necessarily because ulcers develop into cancer but because when unhealthy habits of living that lead to the development of ulcers are continued, further deterioration is inevitable, and in those with a predisposition to cancer, this disease may ultimately show up.

Dr. Stanley L. Robbins confirmed that ulcers change into cancer only rarely, when in a paper read at the Symposium on Gastric Ulcers at the 108th Annual Meeting of the American Medical Association, June 10, 1959, he called attention to the fact that studies conducted at the Mallory Institute of Pathology during the years 1943 to 1949 proved that "transformation from a benign to a malignant lesion was calculated to take place in less than 1% of peptic ulcers."

"The possibility that a benign peptic ulcer may become malignant has, I believe, been overemphasized," Dr. Rob-

[3] *Ibid.*

bins continued further. He stated that while cancer sometimes shows up in patients who have suffered from benign conditions for years, there is no precluding the possibility that the benign peptic ulcer "healed, only to be followed after some period by a malignancy arising in an entirely different site."[4]

### A Case History! Dr. I.S.

The case of Dr. I.S. illustrates what the program outlined here can do in cases of ulcers of the stomach:

About 20 years ago, I suffered an attack of indigestion accompanied by the vomiting of blood and bloody stools.

Subsequently this was diagnosed as peptic ulcer. A soft bland diet and an antacid were recommended. Because the relief was only temporary, another M.D. was consulted. His diagnosis was subacute appendicitis, for which he advised immediate operation. A G.I. X-ray series was taken, which supposedly confirmed this.

Before the operation I decided to consult another M.D. who, after another G.I. X-ray series, diagnosed Duodenal Ulcer. The standard milk and cream diet was recommended and after several months, the only change was a tremendous gain of weight and extreme lethargy.

At this time another M.D. was consulted, another G.I. series was taken. His diagnosis was terminal (distal) ileitis, for which he advised operation.

I consulted another M.D. who diagnosed Duodenal Ulcer, Severe Allergy, Arthritis of the upper back and shoulders, and Hypo-thyroidism, for all of which, assorted drugs were prescribed. Also an allergy-testing regimen was instituted.

This entire treatment was followed religiously for 1 year, doing more harm than good.

As a last resort, in desperation, I consulted a physician who treated these cases with simple natural methods.

After a short time under his care all pain disappeared and very gradually I began to feel better.

[4] "Contributions of the Pathologist To Present-Day Concepts of Gastric Ulcer," *Journal of the American Medical Association,* December 12, 1959.

## A Friend in Need

The story of how this patient ultimately found his way to natural methods should be of interest. You will notice that he had been ailing for many years and was treated at different times for various ailments, without any apparent results. His wife as well as the other members of his family were greatly worried, and not knowing where to turn for help were seriously considering placing him in some institution.

Quite by accident, they met their family dentist who, when told of their plans, urged them to give him one more chance before taking this drastic step, explaining to them that nature often helps where doctors seem most hopeless.

"How long did it take before you realized that you were on the right track?" the patient was once asked by a friend who knew how seriously ill he was.

"The improvement during the first two or three weeks was so striking that by then we knew that we were doing the right thing," Dr. I.S. replied.

One or two or even several case histories are not necessarily conclusive. However, when you can tell of hundreds of cases that responded similarly to these simple natural methods, then you know that you have at your disposal an approach that cannot be excelled.

## Worry, Fear, and Indecision No Help

Fear and worry do not solve anything. If you are suffering from inflammation or ulcers of the stomach, make sure that you strive for complete recovery, and remember that this can be accomplished only when a rational health-building program is persistently followed.

At this point, it would be well to keep in mind the admonitions expressed in a popular Swedish proverb:

Fear less, hope more; eat less, chew more; whine less, breathe more; talk less, say more; hate less, love more; and all good things will be yours.

## 5

## CONSTIPATION: A MOST COMMON DISORDER

Constipation is one of the most common disorders of man and if neglected or improperly treated can give rise to many serious complications.

In this disorder, the muscles of the large intestine have become weak and flabby, or have become irritated and spastic, and as a result are unable to function properly and expel the waste matter from the colon. When the muscles of the colon are in a healthy condition, they contract and relax in slow wavelike motions and propel the fecal residue towards the rectum, whence it is expelled. The time it takes to expel the residue of a meal varies, depending upon the amount and type of food eaten, the quantity that has been consumed, how well the food has been masticated, and whether the body is sufficiently rested and possesses the strength to function normally. Ordinarily, the length of time required between the consumption of a meal and the elimination of its residue should not be more than eighteen to twenty-four hours, or even less.

Those who move their bowels daily often assume that their bowels are functioning normally, but this is not necessarily the case. Many persons may have a daily bowel movement and yet suffer from constipation or sluggishness and delay. When the muscles of the colon are tired or flabby, they do not possess the power to propel the waste material onward, or they push it forward only very slowly and sluggishly. In such cases, the residue is usually retained in the colon much longer than would normally be the case, sometimes as long as 48 to 72 hours, or even longer. The regular intake of food also helps to push the waste material forward, and since food is taken in daily, this in many cases helps to maintain a daily evacuation, even when the colon does not possess the power to function normally.

In some cases, the bowels move daily and yet some material is retained in the colon. The retained material becomes dry and hard and often leads to an impaction. In many cases, some of the dried-up material adheres to the walls of the colon, clinging to the walls for years even though the bowels move daily. Elimination takes place in the center of the canal, while the old encrusted material continues to stick to the walls and is not dislodged. This hardened material can be loosened and eliminated only when a carefully planned program, embodying the use of wholesome natural foods and the type of care that we describe in the succeeding pages, is followed over an extended period of time.

### Healthy Infants Move Bowels After Each Feeding

Healthy infants move their bowels several times a day, usually after each feeding. Adults, too, would move their bowels after each meal, or at least twice daily, if the colon had the strength and health to function normally. When the bowels move only once a day, intestinal sluggishness is definitely indicated, while those who move their bowels only once every two or three days are badly constipated. These persons should not be complacent about it even though they are free of pain or discomfort, since by neglecting to correct the condition they are opening the door to all kinds of disturbances.

### Two Types of Constipation

When the muscles of the colon are flabby and weakened, they are unable to contract and relax properly. In such cases we are confronted with an atonic type of constipation. When the muscles become irritated and contracted, the condition is known as spastic constipation.

At times the colon may be flabby in some parts and spastic in others. In some cases the same part of the colon may be flabby and sluggish at one time and spastic and irritated at another time.

Constipation causes many discomforts, and is the forerunner of a great many diseases. It leads to the accumulation of gas, upsets digestion, interferes with the general circulation, and brings on irritability and nervous tension. It exerts pressure on the various organs in the abdomen and often affects the functions of the heart and the lungs. It impairs the functions of the liver and gallbladder and often precedes as well as contributes to their breakdown.

Colitis, hemorrhoids, fissures, fistulas, varicose veins, hernias, diverticuloses (pouches or pockets formed in the intestines), and prolapse of various internal organs are frequently caused by constipation.

Palpitation, nausea, headaches, bad taste, coated tongue, foul breath, muddy complexion, and dizziness can often be traced to it.

## Disorders of Colon often Followed by Unnecessary Surgery

Cases of long-standing or spastic constipation are often diagnosed as appendicitis or some other serious digestive disorder, and these cases are sometimes mistakenly operated upon with serious consequences to the patient.

Drs. Karl Albert Dresen and Guy L. Kratzer of the Proctology Department of the Hospital at Allentown, Pa., refer to this when, after stating that "an increasingly large number of patients suffer from the various manifestations of fecal impaction . . . [which] . . . can mimic other diseases by producing symptoms suggesting diarrhea, tumor, or urinary calculi," they point out that "proper management of the condition will prevent much suffering, many laparotomies [abdominal operations] and even colostomies [an operation which connects the colon with the abdominal wall and creates an artificial anus through which the waste is expelled]."[1]

Drs. Elmer W. Heffernon, William A. Millhoun, and Sidney W. Rosen of the Lahey Clinic stress the dangers that often follow when a spastic or irritable colon, mistakenly diagnosed as peptic ulcer, ulcerative colitis, enteritis diverticulitis, pancreatitis, hiatal hernia, and biliary tract [gallbladder] disease is needlessly operated upon. "All too often unnecessary laparotomies are performed," they emphasize and then insist that "multiple abdominal operations may have been performed with only temporary or no benefit to the patient."[2]

[1] *J.A.M.A.*, June 6, 1959.
[2] *J.A.M.A.*, June 6, 1959.

Others who refer to these mistakes and the needless operations that often follow are Kanter and Kasich. After discussing the condition known as an irritable or unstable colon, they write, "They (these cases) largely make up the group of unfortunates, known to every physician, who are operated upon because of a mistaken diagnosis and who spend the remainder of their lives looking for a surgeon who will repair the damage caused by the first operation. Surgery, instead of curing these patients, actually does harm, because an unstable colon is more frequent among those who have had operations."[3]

## Constipation Can Be Corrected

In most cases, this disorder can be corrected with little difficulty. Meals of raw, natural and carefully prepared foods, good eating habits, thorough chewing, control in the intake of food, moderate exercises, sufficient rest and sleep, and other sound health-building measures, help to strengthen the muscles of the colon and restore normal functioning.

In the more moderate cases, results are often attained in a very short time; in some cases, within a few weeks. In the more difficult or chronic cases, a great deal more time and patience may be required before the tone and vigor of the muscles are rebuilt and before the bowels can commence functioning normally again. However, whether the case is of a mild or severe nature, only a sound health-building program can provide permanent and lasting results.

## Scientific Fasting of Great Benefit

A scientifically conducted fast rests the organs and gives them a chance to rebuild. Whenever possible, start the program with a short fast. A more prolonged fast may be of great help in some cases, but this should be carried out only under careful supervision.

Those who find it difficult to follow a complete fast may start with a fruit juice diet or, as an alternative, a raw fruit diet for one or two days or even longer, and then

[3] Kanter and Kasich, *Handbook of Digestive Diseases.*

follow with one of the diets outlined below. A glass of freshly pressed orange juice, apple juice, grapefruit, or grape juice, or any kind of fresh raw fruit may be taken every two hours, or less often if the sufferer is not hungry. This applies, of course, only to cases uncomplicated by a condition in which the use of raw fruits or fruit juices is contraindicated.

Following the short fast or the fruit juice diet, a diet composed of simple, natural foods is recommended. The diet in these cases is usually determined by several factors. Weight, habit, hunger, as well as other health problems, have to be considered.

Those who are overweight should start with raw fruit during the day and take a protein or starch meal at night. Only one kind of fruit should be taken at a time, every two or three hours, or less often if the patient is not hungry. The evening meal should be composed of a large raw vegetable salad, baked potatoes, yams, sweet potatoes, corn on the cob as a starch, or a favorite protein, one or two steamed vegetables, and fruit for dessert. We recommend stewed fruits such as baked apple, applesauce, stewed peaches, or apricots with the carbohydrate meal, and raw fruit or berries with the protein meal.

Those who are underweight or who find the above menu insufficient may resort to two or three regular meals. The diet then may be composed of the following or an equivalent:

BREAKFAST    1. One kind of raw fruit or one kind of raw fruit and one kind of stewed fruit, such as baked apple, applesauce, stewed prunes, stewed peaches, or stewed pears;    2. Milk and water, skimmed raw milk, buttermilk, or yoghurt; Or, if a more substantial breakfast is desired:
1. A raw or stewed fruit (of those listed above);    2. Very ripe banana, or natural brown rice or wild rice, or buckwheat groats, or whole wheat melba toast;    3. Raw skimmed milk or buttermilk or yoghurt or any of the mild herb teas, such as alfalfa, mint, alfa mint, chamomile, sage, or rose hips tea (sweetened with honey).

NOON    1. A raw vegetable salad;    2. Potatoes, yams, or sweet potatoes (baked, steamed, or boiled in jacket), or corn on cob, or one or two slices of whole wheat melba toast, eaten dry, or a serving of natural brown rice;    3. One or two steamed vegetables, or freshly prepared vegetable soup. (Never use canned soups, and make sure not to add salt or butter);    4. Stewed or soaked fruit of those mentioned above for dessert.

DINNER    1. One large helping of raw vegetables; 2. One or two steamed vegetables;    3. Any one of your favorite protein foods;    4. And, if still hungry, raw or stewed fruit or berries for dessert.

## Special Diet in Spastic Constipation

The program outlined above is suitable for the ordinary type of constipation. Sufferers from spastic constipation, especially those who suffer pain after eating, may at first require a soft bland diet. In these cases, the soft bland diet suggested for a severely inflamed stomach, for ulcers of the stomach, or ulcerative colitis is indicated. Raw fruits and vegetables are added only after the acute symptoms have cleared up, or when the related disease which made raw foods unsuitable has been brought under control. The raw foods should be introduced in small amounts and should at first be used only in finely grated or chopped form, the same as in the other diseases.

A fruit juice diet, where permissible, about every three or four days, or at least one day a week, is often of great help in these cases.

Sufferers from constipation should eliminate pastries, cakes, sweets, ice cream, malteds, all soft drinks, all spices and condiments, all refined and processed foods, all rich foods, as well as all fried foods. They should never use coffee, tea, or chocolate, and when taking milk, buttermilk, or any liquid food, they must make sure to sip it slowly or take it with a spoon. They must eat moderately, since overeating often leads to digestive upsets and weakens the muscles of the colon.

Furthermore, they must make sure to eat slowly, to chew their food thoroughly, to eat only when hungry, and to omit food when emotionally upset or under tension.

The diets we have outlined above are merely samples of

the types of meals suitable in these cases. Discuss your diet with the doctor who is in charge of your case, but make sure that he has a thorough understanding of the principles of sound nutrition and is conversant with sound hygienic methods.

## For Interim Help

For interim help, cleansing enemas of lukewarm water are recommended. They should be used, as we have explained in a previous chapter, at first daily for the first three or four days, then every second day, and finally every third day. From then on they should be continued every third or fourth day until the bowels begin to function at least twice daily.

An effort must be made to establish habitual regularity in all cases. This can be accomplished by trying to move the bowels after each meal. Try to evacuate after each meal but make sure not to strain. Try for at least 8 to 10 minutes. Also make it a habit to try immediately upon arising and before retiring. In the more obstinate cases, patience will be required. However, if you persist the lazy and weakened intestinal muscles will ultimately become strengthened, and normal functioning will become a regular routine.

Do not ever suppress nature's call. When the delicate nerve endings re-awaken and start transmitting the signals indicative of the body's readiness for evacuation, never disregard them, if you wish to attain results.

It is also well to bear in mind that the squatting position helps to relax the rectal muscles and encourages bowel action. While modern toilet facilities do not lend themselves to this position, the use of a foot stool on which to rest your feet can compensate for this deficiency.

*A Case History:* MRS. SOPHIE R.

Laxatives are not only useless; they actually aggravate the condition and often contribute to the onset of new and more complicated diseases.

Mrs. R.'s case illustrates the futility of depending upon

laxatives instead of resorting to natural, corrective measures. We shall let her son relate the story of her experiences:

My mother, Mrs. Sophie R., aged 61, had been in very poor health ever since her change of life. She has had several ailments, one of which was constipation, the other high blood pressure. She was dependent on laxatives for bowel movements and was always under a doctor's care. Though many types of medicines and cures were tried, none would help her condition.

Then, she noticed blood while urinating. This was brought to the attention of the family doctor. He examined her and advised tests to be taken, to determine if a cancer existed. The tests proved that she had a noncancerous cyst on her womb, but the doctor advised her to have it removed.

The operation was performed. My mother was left weak and very run down. She lost a lot of weight and could not put any on. A period of nine months elapsed and it was suggested that she take a vacation to build up her health. My father took her to Europe to visit relatives she hadn't seen in a long while.

On her arrival she came down with diarrhea and terrible pains in her stomach, and ran a high fever. The following day she had terrible spasms in her stomach. Her condition was such that my father took her to a leading specialist. His diagnosis was that she had colitis. He advised her to stay in bed and take pills. Her condition did not improve and so she was taken to another doctor in another town and received the same diagnosis. The pains continued with no relief. It was then decided she return home and she did.

On her arrival my dad took her to another specialist. He took X-rays and concluded she had a case of colitis and a bad nervous condition. He prescribed medicine and said time would heal everything.

With this we decided a change of doctor was necessary. My mother heard of a doctor who treated his patients without drugs and thought she would try his system. At first we were a bit leery, but in just a few weeks time a definite change came over my mother. The spasms in her stomach were less and she began to put on weight. After about a month of treatments, she was moving her bowels regularly without any laxatives, she seemed a great deal stronger, and was able to do her own housework again.

We are deeply grateful for all that was done for her; as she is indeed a new person.

Elaborating on this case, an examination revealed that Mrs. R. suffered from long-standing constipation, spasticity of the colon, inflammation of the gallbladder, polyarthritis, and high blood pressure (182/96).

We recommend the care of this case by using at first a diet of soft, bland, alkaline foods, to which later small amounts of finely grated raw vegetables and fruits were added. Enemas, hot baths, moderate exercises, and plenty of rest and sleep were some of the other measures we recommended. This program carried on over a period of about six months not only corrected the constipation but also overcame the gall-bladder inflammation, restored the blood pressure to normal, and eliminated all arthritis symptoms.

## Laxatives Cause Untold Harm

Laxatives are irritants and when they are taken into the system ultimately cause a great deal of harm. They induce bowel movements by irritating the colon. To get rid of the irritant, the tissues pour out a great deal of fluid and this helps to flush out the colon.

The irritating effect of these remedies, however, ultimately causes a further weakening of the colon and more drastic remedies are then required to obtain relief.

It should not require much reasoning to show why the use of these remedies ultimately leads to more serious intestinal disorders.

## Do Our Intestines Need Lubricating Oils?

Millions of people take mineral oil for relief of constipation in the belief that it will pass through the body in its original state and serve as an intestinal lubricant.

When an edible oil is taken into the stomach and passes

through the digestive system undigested, it only indicates that the digestive organs are not functioning well. The digestible portion of anything taken into the stomach must be digested or something is wrong. Normally, only that portion of a food which is indigestible should pass through undigested. Mineral oil, not being a food, passes into the colon undigested.

However, while it induces bowel action, it impairs the health of the colon since it removes not only the waste material but also essential vitamins and minerals. Also, when taken over an extended period of time, it deposits a film of oil on the mucous membrane of the digestive tract and thus ultimately slows down the functioning of the intestinal muscles even more.

When the colon is in a healthy condition, it manufactures its own lubricating fluid and no substance introduced from without can take its place.

Generally, talk of lubrication arises because of the impactions and the accumulation of hard, dry stools. The best way to correct these conditions is to include an ample supply of raw fruits and vegetables in the diet, since they provide ample fluids and bulk, and act favorably on the colon. These cases also require an abundance of rest and sleep. A regulated program of exercises and wholesome outdoor activities will help to rebuild the tone and vigor of the abdominal organs, including the muscles of the colon.

### Is Water Drinking Essential?

Where the stool is hard and dry, a lot of water drinking is often advised. Many persons, including physicians, still believe that we must drink eight glasses of water daily to stay well. Remember that the accumulated stool becomes dry not for lack of fluid but because the residue in the colon is retained for too long a time and too much fluid has been extracted out of it.

We have no objection to the use of one or two cups of hot water flavored with lemon juice or teakettle tea (1/4 milk to 3/4 hot water) upon arising, since this tends to flush the system and often induces a bowel movement. However, we are opposed to the forced drinking of water, since this only waterlogs the tissues. Water should be taken only when one is thirsty, just as food should be taken only when one is hungry.

Some are partial to the use of coffee or tea after a meal since this induces a bowel movement in some cases. These beverages are entirely out of the question for those who are really interested in restoring normal bowel functioning. Both coffee and tea, with their high tannic acid content, have an astringent effect on the bowels and will aggravate rather than correct constipation, although the temporary effect may be to induce a bowel movement.

It is claimed that a cigarette after a meal will induce a bowel movement. Perhaps, but in the long run it will have the same harmful effect as a laxative.

## How About Laxative Foods?

So-called laxative foods act upon the bowels primarily because of their fibrous content; their bulk acts upon the walls of the colon and stimulates bowel action. We are in favor of fibrous foods, and a diet that includes liberal amounts of raw fruits and raw vegetables provides the roughage needed to maintain peristaltic action and normal bowel functioning. However, we wish to stress that we approve of these foods not primarily because of their bulk or because they tend on occasion to induce bowel action, but because they are good foods. We must differentiate between bowel movements that take place normally because the colon functions naturally, and bowel functions that are induced merely because bulky foods such as figs, prunes or other foods containing roughage temporarily stimulate the bowels to act.

We have no objection to these foods as foods. But if they are taken because of their laxative qualities, they will ultimately prove a disappointment for they soon lose their laxative effect and the patient is as badly off as before. To overcome constipation we need not a temporary stimulus to induce bowel action but must strengthen and rebuild the tone and functioning of the colon.

## What About Agar-Agar and Psyllium Seed Products

Remedies containing agar-agar or those manufactured from psyllium seeds or other water-retaining substances are often used to relieve constipation. These remedies act upon the colon because of their bulk and because they absorb a great deal of water, which is then carried into the large intestine.

We do not object too strenuously when these remedies are used to meet a temporary need, but must stress the fact that while they provide relief, they will not correct the underlying weaknesses, which can be done only through the use of good foods, corrective exercises, and a rational way of living.

These remedies, especially those composed of psyllium seeds, sometimes cause an impaction in the colon and actually defeat the purpose for which they are taken.

## Are Enemas Harmful?

Some object to the use of enemas. It is interesting to point out that this opposition is often found among persons who see nothing wrong in the use of laxatives and cathartics, and often actually recommend them.

Enemas can be harmful when used excessively, habitually, carelessly, or at the wrong time. However, when used in accordance with the indications or needs of the case, they may be lifesaving. We have already emphasized that enemas should be used only as a temporary measure and that they should be discontinued as soon as the need for them has passed. Enemas are not a cure for constipation, but when used for relief they are infinitely more helpful than the artificial laxatives and cathartics, or any of the other measures that induce bowel action artificially by stimulation or irritation.

We know that there are many remedies on the market that provide relief, but ask the person who has been using them, flitting from one remedy to another, and you will soon discover that the results were only temporary and sporadic, and that in the long run the condition only grew worse.

Constipation need not be a lifelong ailment. Proper food properly combined, good eating habits, moderate exercises, and a well-regulated way of living will help overcome even the most obstinate type of constipation. However, patience and steadfastness are imperative if lasting results are to be attained.

## 6

# ULCERATIVE COLITIS: A LIFE-THREATENING DISEASE

One of the most painful and dangerous diseases is ulcerative colitis. Colitis is an inflammation of the large intestine. When the irritation which has given rise to the inflammation persists, patches of the colon become deprived of their supply of oxygen, and when this happens ulcers develop. This condition is known as ulcerative colitis.

In ulcerative colitis, the bowel movements are usually painful, loose, watery, and frequent; in some cases as often as 20 to 30 times a day, often with considerable amounts of pus, mucus, and blood.

Recurrent cramps and severe pains in the abdomen, rapid emaciation, severe anemia, and extreme debility, are some of the symptoms that accompany this disease.

In this disease, some ulcers may be large, while others may be very small, even pinpoint in size. Some ulcers affect only the surface tissues, while others penetrate into the deeper tissues and, as in ulcers of the stomach, may lead to perforation. When small ulcers fail to heal, they increase in size and those which are close to one another often join and form large ulcers.

The walls of the colon became hardened and thickened in some areas, friable in others. Some parts may become badly damaged and undergo a great deal of degeneration, with sloughing off of tissue, while other parts may be badly inflamed but show little or no breakdown.

Polyps (small stemlike tumors or growths) may develop and there may be extensive scarring that will cause a considerable degree of distortion and shrinking.

To relieve the anemia, blood transfusions are often recommended, and surgery is sometimes considered necessary to cut away (resect) the badly ulcerated or hardened parts of the colon.

Where this type of surgery is performed, an artificial opening has to be created through which the waste from the colon can be expelled. In cases where only part of the colon is removed, the opening is produced by connecting the abdominal wall with the remaining portion of the colon. This type of operation is known as a colostomy. Where the entire colon is removed, the opening is created by connecting the abdominal wall with the ileum (the lower portion of the small intestine) and this is known as an ileostomy.

This disease, as with a rule, takes a long time to develop and, like ulcers of the stomach, is usually the outgrowth of irritants and toxins that affect the surface as well as the deep tissues of the colon. Emotional disturbances, nutritional abuses, dietary deficiencies, and parasitic infestation are all potential contributory factors in this disease.

This disease, as ulcers of the stomach, usually starts as a simple inflammation. The early inflammatory stages are sometimes accompanied by cramps and diarrhea or a frequent desire to move the bowels. More often the colon will simply be sore and irritated and present the characteristic signs of a spastic colon. In some cases, diarrhea will alternate with constipation.

In the early stages this ailment can, as a rule, be easily corrected. Dr. Richard C. Cabot, Professor of Clinical Medicine, Harvard University Medical School, discussing the acute or early type of colitis in *A Layman's Handbook of Medicine*, points out that *"the important remedies are rest, warmth and starvation* (our emphasis)."

Total abstention from food or, where this is not feasible or desirable, abstention from solid food for a few days, a few lukewarm water enemas to clean out the bowels, and plenty of sleep, rest, and warmth are of great help in all acute digestive disorders, and usually provide a fine start in the care of the early or acute case of colitis.

Where a liquid diet is used, apple juice or the freshly prepared hot vegetable broth is to be preferred. Citrus fruit juices may be too irritating in these cases and, therefore, should be avoided.

After the acute condition is brought under control, a careful program of living and sound hygienic measures must be instituted to rebuild the weakened and damaged tissues and guard against the development of the more serious type of the disease.

If the disease has already reached a more advanced stage, a more intensive program is required. Our greatest difficulties, however, are where extensive ulceration exists. In such cases, we usually have a great deal of debility and weakness, and much patience is often required before the condition can be brought under control.

It should be apparent why Cabot suggested "starvation"; in other words, abstention from food, as most helpful in an early or sudden attack of acute colitis. When the colon is acutely inflamed, even small portions of food may cause irritation and increase the inflammation. When we abstain from food, or omit solid foods, we give the inflamed and irritated tissues a chance to rest and heal.

This is the reason it is best that these cases start with one or even several days of controlled fasting, and why this, as in all other acute digestive disorders, should then be followed with a soft, bland, nonfibrous diet.

### Soft, Bland Foods

Where the patient is greatly debilitated and weakened, complete or total abstention from food may not be advisable. In these cases, small meals of soft, bland foods are then recommended from the very beginning.

The following is an outline of a diet that has proved successful in these cases:

BREAKFAST    1. Stewed or baked apple, applesauce, or finely grated raw apple. Omit all sweetening. Delicious or Golden Delicious apples are best;    2. Very ripe, raw, baked, broiled, or steamed bananas, or ripe baked plantains.

LUNCH    1. Yam, sweet potatoes, or Irish potatoes, baked, steamed, or broiled in jacket—to be eaten without skin;    2. One or two steamed vegetables;    3. If still hungry, a baked apple for dessert.

No salt or butter should be used with the vegetables. We consider the root vegetables such as carrots, parsnips, turnips, and such vegetables as squash and eggplant as the best to start with, but later the tender string beans, young tender okra, and the young green peas may be added. As the condition improves, other vegetables may be used. In very severe cases, the vegetables may have to be puréed to eliminate irritating fibers.

DINNER    The same kind of meal as at noontime; the vegetables should be varied to avoid monotony.

Where available, the ripe fresh papaya, the better grade of ripe mango, or moderate portions of avocado are recommended for cases of ulceration. Small quantities of the juice or such bland vegetables as carrots, celery, parsley, or cabbage are often tolerated well in these cases. Dr. Jacob M. Leavitt, who helped to edit this volume, and to whom we are deeply indebted for his interest, has impressed us with the fact that cabbage contains natural thiouracil, which is very beneficial in cases of thyroid overactivity.

The juice of apples or grapes may also be used when tolerated, either separately or in combination with vegetable juices. The juice of the pomegranate is also of great value.

This diet should be followed until the pain has been eliminated or greatly lessened. By then, the stools should begin to be well formed, the need to move the bowels frequently should have considerably diminished, and the discharge of blood and mucus should either have ceased completely or be materially lessened.

### Other Foods Added Gradually

Once this stage has been reached, other wholesome, nourishing foods may then be gradually added. By this time, the following changes are permissible.

BREAKFAST    1. Stewed or baked apple, or applesauce or raw grated apples;    2. Very ripe, raw or baked banana, natural brown or wild rice, buckwheat groats, or steel-cut groats.

LUNCH    1. One or two steamed vegetables;    2. Small portions of your favorite protein;    3. Unsweetened applesauce, baked apple, or stewed pears or peaches for dessert.

DINNER    1. One or two steamed vegetables;    2. Potatoes, yams or sweet potatoes, baked, boiled or steamed, prepared in the jacket;    3. Unsweetened applesauce, baked apple, stewed pears or peaches for dessert.

Between meals, raw finely grated and peeled or baked apple, or applesauce, or very ripe or baked banana, or sweet grapes (minus skins and seeds) may be used.

If a warm liquid is desired between meals, one of the bland herb teas such as alfalfa tea, chamomile tea, linden flower tea, sage tea, or a cup of hot freshly made vegetable broth may be taken.

Also small quantities of raw vegetable juices may be taken between meals whenever they can be handled without difficulty.

To make the juices, use, whenever possible, vegetables and fruits which have not been sprayed, and clean or scrub them thoroughly.

## Other Care Essential

The warm cleansing enemas, the relaxing hot baths, an abundance of rest and sleep, as well as good hygienic nursing care, are essential. However, in using these measures, certain precautions must not be overlooked.

We recommend warm cleansing enemas daily during the first two or three days to make sure that any residue that has accumulated in the colon or may cling to its walls and cause irritation be flushed out. However, it is important that *only small quantities of water* be used, usually no more than about 2 or 3 glasses at a time.

After that, the enemas should be discontinued or used only when needed to relieve extreme discomfort.

The question is often brought up why enemas should be needed at all in these cases since the bowels move frequently anyhow.

To clear up this question, it is well to bear in mind that we are dealing with a condition in which the tissues are highly irritated and inflamed, and that any fermenting or putrifying material stagnating in the colon only increases the irritation. It is best therefore that, whenever possible, the intestinal canal be washed out. Also stagnant waste matter that clings to the walls will act as an irritant and should be loosened and eliminated. However, since the tissues are inflamed and ulcerated, it is essential that the enemas be taken cautiously, and that only small quantities of water be used. Furthermore, we must make sure not to exert too much force or pressure.

## *Enema An Emergency Measure*

It is well to reiterate that the enema must at all times be regarded as an emergency measure, and must not become a habit. It is of great help when actually needed but should be discontinued as soon as the purpose for which it is used has been accomplished.

The enemas, when properly used, not only clean out the accumulated wastes but also relieve the pressure caused by the gases and the accumulated waste material on adjacent organs. This helps to restore better circulation to the abdominal organs and enables them to function more normally. However, when used injudiciously or excessively they may wash away the natural secretions and cause added irritation.

The warm baths are helpful because they are relaxing and tend to relieve the recurrent spastic pains. Hot, moist compresses applied over the abdomen are also of great help for this purpose.

The patient must be trained to eat slowly and to take only small quantities of food at a time. Colitis sufferers are as a rule very irritable and restless and everything must be done to induce relaxation and emotional control.

Those who suffer from cold feet, and this is a common symptom, should use a hot water bottle or an electric pad or resort to hot foot baths to increase the circulation to their feet. One or two tablespoons of dry mustard or a handful of epsom salt may be added to the water for greater effectiveness.

Those who are severely debilitated and weakened and who are extremely anemic may have to stay in bed until thay have regained sufficient vitality to enable them to become more active. These patients especially need a great deal of rest and sleep to rebuild their health and vitality. The spastic pains and frequent loose bowel movements are very exhausting and often deprive the patient of strength.

When the patient grows stronger, exercises are recommended. At the beginning, only the mildest types of exercise are suggested, usually not more than a few deep breathing exercises and gentle leg movements. As strength increases, the frequency and the type of exercises should be increased, and the patient should be encouraged to get out of bed and start walking around the house.

### Patience Required

In the more aggravated cases, it may take several weeks before definite improvement is noted. However, as time goes on the pains will gradually lessen, the bowels will begin to move less frequently, the stools will become well formed, and the mucus, pus, and blood in the stools will diminish and ultimately disappear.

At this stage, small quantities of finely grated raw vegetables such as carrots, turnips, cucumbers, etc., as well as some of the tender fresh raw fruits may be added to the diet. Then, we slowly add other raw fruits and vegetables, as soon as we find that they can be handled without discomfort.

### On the Question of Milk

We have mentioned that ulcerative colitis is in many ways similar to ulcers of the stomach and that sufferers from this disease, as well as those who suffer from ulcers of the stomach, require a soft, bland, nonfibrous diet.

There is, however, one very striking difference in the diet of these two ailments. We have seen that milk is often of great value in ulcers of the stomach; the same is not the case in ulcerative colitis. In this disease, milk in any form is usually not well tolerated and should, therefore, be excluded from the diet. It is also known that milk is a good culture medium for bacterial growth and hence not a suitable food for those who suffer from inflamed intestines or any form of allergy.

### Risks of Neglect Great

Ulcerative colitis is usually accompanied by a great deal of discomfort and pain, and often leads to many dangerous complications. In some of these cases doctors recommend surgery for the removal of part of or even the whole colon.

You will remember that a colostomy or ileostomy is an operation in which the colon or ileum is connected with the abdominal wall to create an artificial opening through which the waste of the body is eliminated. Where part or all of the colon has been removed, this deformity remains a permanent condition.

It is pitiful to think how many of these operations could be prevented if real, sound care were employed in time. It should be apparent that surgery does not remove the cause of the disease, and at most provides but temporary relief, leaving the patient permanently damaged. To obtain results, the causative factors must be removed and the damaged tissues must be given a chance to heal, and this can, in the vast majority of cases, be accomplished only through the use of a carefully regulated diet and sound hygienic care. Irrespective of the amount of damage, these are the only methods that can promise complete and lasting results.

## Allergy in Ulcerative Colitis

As stated in the previous chapter, certain cases of constipation are sometimes mistaken for appendicitis or other digestive disturbances and are occasionally unnecessarily operated upon. Similar mistakes occur in cases of ulcerative colitis.

Dr. Karpen[1] describes a case of allergic colitis mistakenly diagnosed as appendicitis and operated upon, and then points out that only after the operation was it discovered that the appendix was normal in every detail, and that the trouble was in the colon.

Continuing the discussion of colitis resulting from allergy, Dr. Karpen refers to Andresen, who describes three stages of allergic reactions: "a mild reaction commonly called 'mucous colitis' or 'irritable colon'; a more severe reaction which he terms 'colon spasm' or 'colitis'; and a very severe reaction simulating intestinal obstruction,

[1] "Acute Allergic Colitis Presenting the Clinical Picture of Acute Appendicitis," *J.A.M.A.*, April 11, 1959.

acute inflammation, or perforation." Karpen hints that operations may have to be accepted as a routine, and quotes Ratner to the effect that these allergic reactions could be very severe and "amenable only to operation."

At this point, it is well to emphasize that blaming an allergy for an acute attack of colitis, or for that matter any other digestive disorder, does not in reality explain anything, since the hypersensitivity that exists in an allergic condition does not develop out of nowhere. We must never overlook the fact that sufferers from allergy are in poor health and that the condition is often an outgrowth of years of abuses that have weakened the tissues and made them excessively sensitive to certain foods or substances taken into the system or that come in contact with the body.

To overcome this condition the damaged or weakened tissues must be strengthened and rehabilitated, and this can be accomplished only through the use of a well-balanced nutritional program, correct eating habits, corrective exercises, plenty of rest and sleep, emotional control, fresh air and sunshine, and other sound health-building measures.

Another fact we must not overlook in connection with this is that while it is true, as Dr. Karpen states, that the "mortality and morbidity from appendectomy have been reduced to extremely low levels," the colon, following such an operation, is left even more sensitive and unstable. It is well to return to the statement of Kanter and Kasich quoted in the previous chapter, in which they point out that "they [the cases mistakenly operated upon] largely made up the group of unfortunates known to every physician because of a mistaken diagnosis, who spend the remainder of their lives looking for a surgeon who will repair the damage caused by the first operation."

*A Case History:* RALPH L.

The case history of Ralph L. will illustrate how a very difficult case of ulcerative colitis can be made to respond to treatment when sound health-building measures are employed. We shall allow Ralph L. to tell his own story.

I was always considered a "skinny kid." My mother was always concerned about my weight but when the doctor said that is how it is and always will be, it put her fears to rest.

However, when at the age of 14 I actually began to lose weight and have intestinal pains, once again I was marched down to the local doctor, who proclaimed that there was nothing wrong with me that a high-calorie diet couldn't cure. When the loss in weight continued and the pains grew worse, I was taken to a prominent diagnostician who informed my family that I was suffering from ulcerative mucous colitis and would require immediate hospital care. Thus commenced six miserable months during which I was in the hospital almost constantly, had 13 blood transfusions, was given as many as 30 different drugs and treatments, and all to no avail.

My weight, at the age of 15, was 60 pounds, my stools were bloody and frequent, and my psychological state was worse. My parents were desperate. It was apparent that orthodox treatment was getting me nowhere. Through a friend my folks heard of the results obtained by a doctor who employed only natural methods in his treatment, and decided to take the supreme risk of placing me under the care of this doctor.

I was taken home from the hospital in an extremely weak condition. As soon as I arrived home, the doctor was there to see me. My drugs were thrown away. My diet was changed to just the opposite of the one I was receiving in the hospital. I was given sunbaths on the roof and mild manipulations to stimulate the circulation, for I could not walk except with severe pain because I had been confined to a hospital bed for over six months. Psychologically my state was still poor. I was not convinced that this was the right way, particularly since I liked many foods that were forbidden to me.

You can imagine the change in my attitude when after a single week the immediate symptoms of my condition had disappeared. Naturally I was still very weak and thin but the critical phase had passed and I realized that we had finally reached the right road. From that time on there was constant improvement until I considered myself completely cured.

At the age of 18 I was drafted into the Army. Because

of my colitis history, I was given a very thorough physical examination. No trace of the colitis could be found. I was taken into general service and spent three years in the armed forces both at home and abroad.

I am now 34 years old, have my own CPA practice, and am married, with one child. My weight is about 160 (too much, I fear). I never have had a recurrence of the colitis.

*Another Case History:* ALFRED T.

The story of Alfred T. is another one which illustrates what can be accomplished when simple, natural methods are used. Here is how his mother sums up their experiences:

When our son was 16 years old he was stricken with a very severe case of colitis. The doctor labeled it "Shiga" colitis (named after Dr. Shiga, a Japanese, who discovered it among his patients in the Orient). We were told that it is a very virulent form of colitis. We immediately took him to a specialist recommended by our family doctor. That was the beginning of a pilgrimage to doctors and specialists, 12 in all, which lasted a year. Specialist A advised hospitalization for research and treatment. He remained in the hospital several weeks. When Specialist A dismissed him he reassured us that our son's improvement would follow. But after a few days he felt worse than before he entered the hospital. We took him back to Specialist A. After X-rays, Specialist A informed us that more of the colon had become infected, and that it would be necessary to cut out the infected part of same. We refused to have our son go through with the operation. We kept on taking our son from one specialist to another but with no success. He was going downhill rapidly by now. He was losing weight rapidly, diarrhea became more pronounced and his circulation was poor. Added to this, he started to run a temperature. He would be normal in the morning but it would rise to 101° or 102° by evening. About this time we heard of a renowned specialist who was considered the very best authority on colitis of his time. Specialist B recommended hospitalization. When our son entered the hospital he only weighed 91 pounds. Specialist B wanted to fatten him up. He was fed large portions of meat twice a day. At the end of 2 months he was discharged from the hospital. Although he had gained 14 pounds he was feeling miserable. He was always hungry but the pain after eating was so severe that he was afraid to eat. The diarrhea was as bad as ever. We went back to Specialist B. He was honest with us and admitted that our son's case baffled him, that he "had tried his bag of tricks" but they didn't work. He did say that he would like to try a new experiment, which would consist of injecting the fluid of our son's sickness into white mice in order to derive a serum that could be used on our son. He estimated the preparing would take about six weeks. Just about this time we heard of a physician who worked only with natural methods, and who was getting excellent results with his colitis patients. My husband was skeptical since this doctor was not practicing orthodox medical methods, but he agreed to hear what he had to say. We were quite impressed by his explanation of the disease and method of healing by natural methods. Since we were getting nowhere by the orthodox medical methods, we decided to give this method a try. When our son started treatment, he weighed 104 lbs. Not only was he sick physically but his morale was low. When our son was under his care for about 3 weeks we received a phone call from Specialist B telling us that the serum was ready and to bring our son over to start the experiment. We were in quite a dilemma. We weren't sure whether this new method would be able to heal our son and we wanted to play it safe. So we inquired from Specialist B how long the serum would keep. When he told us it would be good for 6 months, we decided to continue. Although our son had been treated only 3 weeks, we already saw one noticeable improvement, i.e., his temperature became normal and continued to be normal. To conclude, at the end of five months, our son had completely recovered. He had gained 60 lbs. That was 21 years ago. He has stayed well ever since. He is now an athlete and enjoys many outdoor sports. Needless to say, we feel very grateful for it all.

## Healthy Stomach Destroys Bacilli and Parasites

You will remember that among the influences contributing to the development of colitis we mentioned parasitic infestations. In connection with this, it is well to point out that bacilli or parasites usually get into the colon only when the stomach is not able to function normally and, therefore, cannot destroy them. W. D. Foethout and W. W. Tuttle make this point clear in their *Textbook of Physiology*, when, discussing the action of the hydrochloric acid upon germs, they emphasize that "it is perhaps for the best of the animal economy that almost at the very beginning of the alimentary canal we have a fluid that is inimical to the life, growth and activity of these germs," and then explain that bacteria such as the germs of tuberculosis, dysentery, and typhoid pass from the stomach into the intestines, but that this happens "especially when the activity of the stomach is below normal."

This fact only illustrates anew how harmful are the antacid or alkaline remedies, or any of the other remedies that impede or interfere with the normal secretions of the stomach, to the health and welfare of the digestive system as a whole, and why they must be avoided.

Continuing somewhat further the subject of bacteria or parasites, it is well to point out that none of us is immune from swallowing vast numbers of bacteria or bacilli, since they surround us everywhere and many are taken in with food and drink. However, as long as the stomach continues to function normally, it secretes the hydrochloric acid and other digestive enzymes that normally act upon the bacteria, bacilli, or parasites in the same way as upon the food we eat.

However, even in cases where the stomach is unable to destroy them, and where because of this some of them reach the alimentary canal alive, they still need not become harmful, since under normal conditions the alimentary tract possesses the power to keep them in check and establish a harmless relationship with them. This relationship is known as a state of symbiosis. We must never overlook the fact that only when the colon is unable to establish this symbiotic relationship can bacteria, bacilli, or parasites gain the upper hand.

## Eternal Vigilance Needed

Those who have recovered from ulcerative colitis must continue to follow a careful program of living if they wish to continue to stay well; a return to their former debilitating habits will, in most instances, bring about a return of the original condition, often in a more complicated form.

We remember the case of Anthony F., who was about 19 or 20 years old when we first saw him. He was pale, haggard, wan, and greatly emaciated, almost skin and bones. He suffered intense abdominal pains and was forced to move his bowels sometimes as often as 20 to 30 times a day, expelling loose watery stools tinged with blood, mucus, and pus. A blood test revealed an extreme anemia; the hemoglobin content of his blood was sometimes as low as 30 per cent, a condition that often exists in severe cases of ulcerative colitis.

We followed the usual procedure outlined above but, because of his extreme illness, it took some weeks before there were signs of improvement and altogether about eight or nine months before a complete recovery set in.

About two years later we were called to see Anthony again. After his recovery, he first adhered to the program outlined for him. However, as time went on he gradually became careless and returned to the same unwholesome habits of living that he followed in the past, such as the use of wrong foods, smoking, drinking, late hours, and various other kinds of dissipation.

Again we resorted to the program that helped him originally, and within a few months Anthony was again in good health. By this time, however, he had learned his lesson. When we saw him some years later and asked him whether he was taking care of himself, he replied that he had paid too high a price for his health and never intended to become careless again.

## Diverticulitis

Sufferers from spastic colitis or irritated or spastic colon sometimes develop pouches or pockets in the large intestine. These pouches or pockets are known as diverticuli and the condition is known as diverticulosis. When these pouches or pockets become inflamed, the condition is known as diverticulitis. In the acute stage, this condition is marked by pain, nausea, sometimes by vomiting and fever; while the chronic stage presents the typical symptoms of a localized colitis.

These cases are sometimes operated upon, but it should be evident that this procedure does not solve the problem since diverticuli often appear in great numbers and the removal of some diverticuli or the relief of one attack does not prevent a recurrence. As a matter of fact, this is exactly what happens. Kantor and Kasich state that in "acute exacerbation the whole intestinal wall gradually becomes thickened and indurated."

## The Story of a Colectomy

We must never overlook the fact that when the colon is removed in part or in toto the patient is left crippled for life. Needless to say, the psychological and physical scars left by such an operation can never be completely erased.

We are thinking of the case of Mrs. G., who underwent a colectomy—an operation in which the whole colon was removed. As a result, she was left with a permanent ileostomy.

Following the operation, Mrs. G. was advised to adhere to the standard soft diet that is usually prescribed in these cases. This diet is, of course, highly deficient, and sooner or later is bound to show its effect. This is what happened to Mrs. G. Needless to say, she became badly frightened. Her food began to pass through before it was fully digested, and her evacuations became loose, watery, and very messy, reminding her of the condition existing before the operation was performed. She appeared badly undernourished, suffered from anemia and sleeplessness, became extremely nervous and irritable, showed extreme signs of fatigue, and was psychologically in a very bad state. A change was imperative if the patient was to avoid a complete collapse. Of course, in cases of this kind the results, at best, can be only of a limited nature. The excised colon cannot be put back and the ileostomy remains a psychological problem for life.

The care in this instance started with a change to a soft, bland diet, similar to the one outlined in previous chapters. For breakfast, she was permitted at first baked apple or stewed peaches, and ripe raw or baked banana, while ripe raw mango, ripe raw peeled peaches, or raw or stewed apple, with natural brown rice or buckwheat groats, or a slice of wholewheat melba toast, were added later.

For lunch, she was allowed steamed vegetables, such as carrots, squash, eggplant, turnips, parsnips, and potatoes, baked or boiled in the jacket (eaten without the skin). Finely grated raw cucumber, raw zucchini, and carrots were added later, when the symptoms had subsided.

For dinner, one or two steamed vegetables (of those mentioned above) with four ounces of an easily digestible protein were recommended at first, while the finely grated raw cucumber, zucchini, carrot, and tomato were added later.

For proteins, we suggested the easily digestible soft, bland cheeses and, when the patient began to ask for it, small portions of chicken, lean fish, and lean meat were permitted.

It should not be necessary to mention that at the onset Mrs. G. was not sure whether her body could handle some of these foods and was, therefore, very apprehensive about incorporating them into her diet. She was afraid that they might actually aggravate her condition, and therefore followed the suggestions made to her only very reluctantly. It did not take long, however, before she began to notice a marked improvement in her condition. Her stools became more firm and regular, she began to sleep better, and she began to feel stronger in every way.

"This is some change for me," Mrs. G. remarked. "Just think of it! I can eat peaches, mangoes, raw grated cucumber, tomatoes—foods I could not touch for years, and I feel only the better for it."

Mrs. G. is married, has two grown children, leads an active social life, and devotes one day a week to work as a volunteer in a hospital. Formerly, every little effort left her limp and worn out, and the day at the hospital used to take all the strength out of her. "Now I can do a full day's work at the hospital and at the end of the day feel as strong as ever," Mrs. G. jubilantly exclaimed recently.

## Ileitis

Ileitis or regional enteritis is a condition similar to colitis. The only difference is that while colitis generally involves the large intestine, ileitis involves the lower portion of the small intestine, the ileum.

We have seen that the small intestine is divided anatomically into three parts. The upper part, which connects with the stomach, is known as the duodenum; the middle as the jejunum; and the lower part, which connects with the large intestine, as the ileum. It is this part of the small intestine that is inflamed and damaged in ileitis. However, the damage and the inflammation are not always limited to this part only, and often extend into the large intestine.

This ailment was much in the news when President Eisenhower was operated upon for it.

### A Case History: BOBBY H.

To illustrate how these cases often can be helped without surgery, we will narrate the history of a young man who was successfully treated for this condition at about the same time that the President was operated upon for it.

Bobby H., 22 years old, had been suffering from intestinal disorders since childhood, and in giving his history he said that he didn't remember a day in his life that had been entirely free from pain and distress.

His mother, who accompanied him to our office, was frantic. "Do you think he can be helped?" she kept asking, again and again, when her son was out of hearing. "Doctors said that he was suffering from terminal ileitis and that he must have an ileostomy." The word "terminal" in medical terminology has an ominous sound, since it is often used to indicate that a disease has reached an advanced stage and that the case is practically hopeless. When used in connection with ileitis, however, it merely implies that the illness affects the terminal or distal end of the ileum. In Bobby's case the lower portion of the ileum was involved, but the condition was not limited to this part only; it also extended into the large intestine.

With some effort and repeated assurance that Bobby

could get well without surgery, the mother was finally calmed down. The same program recommended in the more advanced cases of spastic colitis was instituted for him, and he followed it carefully for about six months. By that time, Bobby was completely well again.

He is now married, has a two-year-old baby girl, and both he and Marilyn, his charming wife, are very happy.

We talked with Bobby two or three years after his recovery, and he told us that some months after he got well he visited the doctor who took care of him before he subjected himself to our care and treatment. This doctor took a series of X-rays which disclosed that the scar tissues had become much softer and smoother, and that Bobby's condition as a whole showed a vast degree of improvement.

Not all cases of ileitis or ulcerative colitis are alike. Cases vary, and some are more resistant to treatment than others. It should be apparent, however, that even in severely advanced cases recovery is often possible, when the regimen outlined in this chapter is carefully followed.

## 7

## YOUR LIVER AND YOUR DIGESTION

*Is Life Worth Living? Depends On How The Liver Treats His Liver.*

—ANONYMOUS

Do you know that a vigorous, normally functioning liver is one of our best protections against disease?

The reason for this should be readily apparent. The liver is one of our most essential organs. It plays a vital role in the digestion and assimilation of food, as well as in the elimination and/or detoxification or neutralization of the toxins of the body.

Some of the functions of the liver illustrate the role it plays in the maintenance of our health and well-being! It manufactures the bile essential for the digestion of fats. When the liver is unable to secrete enough bile the fats are not completely digested, and this can lead to many serious ailments. Fats not fully digested tend to deposit a film of fat on other foods, and they too become more difficult to digest.

This explains in part why we recommend that no butter be used with potatoes or bread and why it is advisable that in cooking the use of fat be greatly restricted or even completely eliminated.

The bile also prevents putrefaction in the colon and by accelerating peristaltic action helps to regulate bowel functioning.

Another function of the liver is further to modify the digested protein foods and prepare them for assimilation by the cells and tissues of the body.

The liver also completes the break-up of the starches and sugars, and stores the final product, in the form of glycogen, for future use, releasing it only when the body requires it for fuel and energy. When the body is deficient in sugar, the liver (under certain conditions) can convert protein and fat into sugar.

The liver also acts as a vast reservoir for vitamins, minerals, and enzymes, *and even manufactures some of them when the needs of the body are great.* It converts the carotene of carrots and other yellow vegetables into vitamin A and stores many of the other vitamins and minerals for use when needed.

*Finally, one of the most essential tasks of the liver is to neutralize and render harmless the many irritating substances and toxins that accumulate in the body as a result of the metabolic processes, or are taken into the system with our food and drink or in the form of chemicals and drugs.*

Whenever the body encounters difficulty in handling such foods as rich, concentrated cheeses, meats, or fats, it usually is because the efficiency of the liver has become impaired.

That a failure or impairment in the functions of the liver can lead to serious damage and undermine the functions of the digestive system is well known. The late Dr. Max Gerson in *A Cancer Therapy* quoted Kasper Blond, who stated that "the whole syndrome of metabolic disorders which we call oesophagitis [inflammation of the oesophagus], gastritis, duodenitis [inflammation of the duodenum], gastric and duodenal ulcer, cholecystitis [gallbladder inflammation], pancreatitis [inflammation of the pancreas], proctitis [inflammation of the rectum], and others, are considered only stages of a dynamic process, *starting with liver failure and portal-hypertension* [hardening of the blood vessels which provide the liver with its circulation], and resulting in cirrhosis [hardening] of the liver tissue, and sometimes in cancer."

Diabetes, heart disease, kidney damage, circulatory disorders, and blood diseases are only a few of the many other afflictions that show up when the liver is unable to function properly.

### How the Liver Becomes Damaged

Injury or destruction to the liver cells is usually brought on by various poisons or irritants that circulate in the bloodstream; nutritional deficiencies and interferences in circulation are other contributory factors.

Dr. Boyd describes the effect of toxins on the cells of the liver in the following words: "The cells of the liver are bathed in the blood brought by the portal vein from the gastrointestinal tract, blood which may contain toxins known or unknown. The result of such toxic action may be the death of some or many of the cells of a liver lobule, it may be of one or many of the lobules themselves."[1]

What are the toxins carried to the liver that have a destructive effect upon its cells? Dr. Boyd leaves no doubt as to what they are when he states: "Among the numerous agents, most diverse in character, which may cause degeneration and necrosis of the liver cells may be mentioned chemicals, both organic and inorganic, certain drugs and tarlike substances, foreign proteins and products of protein decomposition, bacterial toxins, infections and exposure to radiation."[2]

Let us analyze this statement. Boyd begins by mentioning "chemicals, both organic and inorganic." We emphasize in other parts of this encyclopedia how harmful the chemicals used in the growing and processing of foods can be. His warning only confirms how important it is that we use care in the selection of the foods we eat.

Dr. Boyd then mentions "certain drugs and tarlike substances." Few persons are aware that aspirin, Anacin, Pyramidon, phenacetin, and the sulfa drugs are coal-tar products. It is well to realize that the only reason the harmful effect of these drugs is not always immediately evident is because the liver is doing its best to neutralize them and render them harmless. If, however, the liver becomes worn out or damaged, then there will be trouble.

In another part of his book, Boyd lists chloroform, phosphorus, mercury, arsenic, and other drugs which, singly or in combination, will damage the liver. It is essential to point out that all drugs have to be detoxified if the body is to be protected against their harmful effects, and that all of them tend to undermine the health and efficiency of the liver.

Boyd is only one of many who stress that drugs can cause a great deal of liver damage. Dr. Fenton Schaffner of the Department of Medicine and Pathology, Mount

[1] Boyd, *Pathology of Internal Disease.*
[2] *Ibid.*

Sinai Hospital, in a report presented before the Section on Gastroenterology and Proctology at the 109th annual meeting of the American Medical Association, pointed out that "jaundice induced by drugs may be the result of hepatocellular damage [damage to the liver cells], cholestasis [stoppage of bile flow], or hemolysis [breakdown of the blood]."

"As therapeutics progressed from Galenicals[3] to complex chemicals which profoundly affect many biochemical reactions in the body, iatrogenic [physician-induced] diseases have become more numerous. The liver, because of its central role in metabolism and excretion of many drugs, is a frequent target of an untoward and unexpected action of a drug," Dr. Schaffner said. He made it clear that the various forms of drug jaundice are not readily distinguishable from other liver diseases, and that like them the disorders usually commence with anorexia (lack of appetite), malaise (weakness) and fever. "The distaste for tobacco, skin inflammation with intense itching, and simultaneous involvement of other organs such as the heart, kidney, bone marrow, and colon," are also often present.

A highly significant point stressed by Dr. Schaffner is that the liver reaction occurring from the use of a drug is sometimes delayed, and may not show up "until after the patient has been taking it for weeks, or even up to a month after its administration has been discontinued."[4]

It is interesting to mention at this point that medicine is not unaware that a healthy body builds its own immunity to infection. The great tragedy is that in actual practice this point is in most instances overlooked or disregarded. Osler states in his *Practice of Medicine* that *"the human individual in normal health is practically immune to natural infection, and that only when the body is in a depleted condition can an infection develop."*

Louis Pasteur, too, was evidently aware of this, since, according to Rene Dubos, he pointed out in his writings

[3] Medicines prepared according to the formulas of the celebrated Greek physician, Galen, who was born A.D. 130 and gained great fame as a practitioner. It is interesting to note that these medicines were prepared primarily from organic ingredients and, therefore, did not possess the toxic qualities of present-day drugs.

[4] "Iatrogenic Jaundice," *J.A.M.A.*, November 26, 1960.

"that the response of the infected individual was determined by his hereditary endowment, his state of nutrition, his environment including the climate, and even his mental state," and in the course of his studies on the disease of the silkworm known as *flacherie*, "came to the conclusion, startling for the time, that the microorganisms present in such large numbers in the intestinal tract of the silkworms were *'more an effect than a cause of the disease.'* "[5]

It seems from the above that our approach to the treatment of disease by means of antibacterial remedies, in other words, such remedies as the sulfa drugs and the antibiotics, whose primary purpose is to destroy or inhibit the action of the different microorganisms instead of eradicating the cause, is way off its track and bound to fail. This fact is slowly, painfully becoming evident. By using the antibiotics or other antibacterial remedies, we create a false sense of security and often lay the foundation for a great many serious complications.

Albert G. Maisel in *Today's Health,* a monthly publication of the American Medical Association, warns that "no antibiotic yet developed is completely free from a tendency to produce, as a side effect, a toxic reaction," and then explains that *antibiotics disrupt the delicate germ balance in the body, encourage the development of resistant bacteria, and may evoke allergic reactions ranging from hives to sudden death.*[6]

In dealing with some of the problems that have resulted from the use of the various antibacterial agents, Dr. Maxwell Finland, Dr. Wilfred F. Jones, and Mildred W. Barnes of the Boston City Hospital and the Department of Medicine, Harvard Medical School, point to the large outbreaks of infectious diseases in nurseries and maternity wards and "high incidence of infections in originally clean surgical wounds and as complications of debilitating diseases, *events which have resulted in considerable morbidity and appreciable mortality within hospitals.*"

After enumerating the various types of bacteria that have become resistant to these remedies and the infections that "respond poorly to treatment with these drugs and

[5] Rene Dubos, *Mirage of Health.*
[6] "Warning Flag for Wonder Drugs," in *Today's Health,* October, 1959.

are the cause of an increasing number of deaths," the authors continue with the following significant statement: "Few, if any, of the numerous reports have dealt with the changes in the frequency with which serious and fatal infections with these and other bacteria are being encountered in the same hospitals since the advent of modern chemotherapeutic drugs."[7]

We agree fully with Dr. J. Wendel Macleod, Dean of Medicine, University of Saskatchewan, who rightly complains that "large sections of our people clamor excessively for X-ray examinations, chemical tests, and surgical procedures" and concludes, "confidence in the healing power of nature has been displaced by undue dependence upon the popular drugs of the moment."[8]

## The Dangers of Radiation

With reference to the question of "exposure to radiation," this danger is unfortunately not always within our control. If the new schemes for the preservation of foods by means of radiation should become an actuality, this threat would increase. We need not point out that the reckless and promiscuous use of X-rays adds immensely to this danger.

## Other Harmful Influences

Boyd points out further that dietary deficiencies and a high fat intake can undermine the health of the liver. The function of the liver becomes impaired when it becomes overwhelmed by toxins or when, owing to malnutrition or inadequate nutrition, it fails to obtain the necessary nutrient elements, or when an interference in circulation deprives its cells of the oxygen they need.

Boyd states that when the liver cells fail to get the oxygen they need "efficient carbohydrate metabolism cannot take place and the cells become infiltrated with fat which replaces the normal glycogen." He says, too, that an interference in the supply of oxygen to the liver cells may lead

[7] Occurrence of Serious Bacterial Infections Since Introduction of Anti-Bacterial Agents," *J.A.M.A.*, August 29, 1959.
[8] *The New York Times*, September 2, 1959.

to cirrhosis (hardening) or necrosis (death) of the liver cells.

## Diseases of the Liver

One of the most common diseases of the liver is infectious hepatitis or inflammation of the liver. This disease is usually accompanied by headaches, nausea, malaise, and often a slight fever and jaundice.

This disease may result in the destruction of many liver cells, but it is well to bear in mind that good care along nutritional and hygienic lines often clears up the condition in a relatively short time and protects the liver against permanent damage.

When great areas of the liver become destroyed, some very serious liver disorders may develop.

Some of the more serious liver disorders that may ultimately appear are:

### Fatty Degeneration or Infiltration of the Liver

This disease develops when the liver is unable to break up fat and as a result becomes infiltrated with droplets or globules of it. In this disease the destroyed liver cells become replaced by fatty tissue. The liver usually becomes considerably enlarged and yet, because the liver cells have so light that it can float on water. This condition is often been replaced by fat, is very much lighter in weight, often found in diabetes, pernicious anemia, and chronic alcoholism.

### Cirrhosis of the Liver

In this disease, the liver becomes hardened and infiltrated with scar tissue. The damaged parts of the liver at first become greatly enlarged, but later begin to shrivel up and atrophy. At this stage, the liver is usually very hard and small, sometimes as small as half its natural size. When the liver is enlarged, the condition is known as hypertrophic cirrhosis, while when the liver shrivels up and wastes away, it is known as atrophic cirrhosis.

*Abscesses and cancer* are other serious liver diseases.

In these diseases, jaundice is one of the most outstanding symptoms. Jaundice develops when the bile cannot be emptied into the colon and is absorbed instead into the bloodstream, causing a discoloration of the skin and mucous membrane.

## Recovery Depends upon Degree of Damage

The question of recovery in these degenerative diseases depends to a great extent upon how far the damage has progressed, as well as upon the recuperative or healing powers of the individual case.

The liver does possess vast recuperative powers. Even when large parts of it have already been destroyed, it can often still rebuild itself and regain a fair degree of efficiency. Another point worth remembering is that even when great parts of the liver are already destroyed, the remaining portions will continue to carry on all the necessary functions, although on a less efficient scale. From all this, it should be apparent that the liver possesses vast reserves and can often show dramatic recovery. Nonetheless, in view of its importance to the body's economy, it should be evident that we are not very wise when we expose this vital organ to reckless abuses.

## Biliousness

At this point, a discussion of the disorder sometimes referred to as biliousness is in order. This disorder was at one time regarded as a disorder of the liver, but is now considered to be an outgrowth of constipation. It shows up when there is an increase in the secretion and a backing up of bile.

Constipation, loss of appetite, coated tongue, bad taste in the mouth, headache, dizziness, nausea and, occasionally, extreme pain in the pit of the stomach, with vomiting and fever, usually accompany it.

### How Bilious Attacks Should be Treated

To begin with, all food must be stopped. When nausea or vomiting is present, even water should be withheld since anything taken by mouth only increases the nausea or the urge to retch. When these symptoms persist, an effort to induce vomiting artificially is often helpful. This can be accomplished by pushing the finger down the throat to force vomiting, or may be brought on by swallowing down quickly two tablespoonfuls of ordinary table salt dissolved in a glass of lukewarm water. Two glasses of plain cold water should be swallowed quickly immediately after the salt solution has been taken.

This solution sometimes washes down the irritating material and provides relief in this way, but in the majority of cases it will cause an emptying of the stomach by vomiting.

Nausea is sometimes relieved by hot water flavored with lemon juice. Sucking on a piece of lemon is also helpful in some cases, since it tends to accelerate both vomiting and bowel action.

Hot applications over the abdomen and heat applied between the shoulder blades does much to relieve abdominal pains.

Warm cleansing enemas, hot baths, and plenty of rest and sleep are essential in these cases. The feet must be kept warm.

### What To Do After Acute Symptoms Have Subsided

After the acute symptoms have subsided, small quantities of easily digestible bland foods may be introduced. To start with, we recommend small quantities of raw or stewed fruits for breakfast, and small meals composed of grated raw and plain steamed vegetables for the noon and evening meals. This is followed a few days later with one of the simpler diets that we have outlined in our previous chapters, with the addition of an easily digestible protein to one meal and a baked potato or other easily digestible bulky starch food, such as brown rice or buckwheat groats, to the other.

The meals should in all cases be made up of simple bland foods, carefully combined. The fewer the combinations at a meal, the better.

Fat foods (butter, cream, eggs, and the fat meats and fish), spices (pepper, salt, mustard, and vinegar), stimulants of every kind (coffee, tea, chocolate, and alcohol), and processed and refined foods must be strictly excluded.

The use of a grapefruit or grapefruit juice diet for several days before introducing solid food is highly recommended in these cases. The use of a juice diet for one or two days a week regularly during the corrective phase of a liver disorder is often of great value.

## A Positive Health Program

Don't wait until your liver becomes damaged before adopting a positive health program. Stop abusing it and it will serve you well through life. Treat it right and you will have no reason for regret. The basic health rules outlined in previous chapters should be observed. In addition, these specifics refer particularly to cases of liver disorder:

We recommend that bread be omitted or, at best, be used sparingly, and only in place of another starch food. Only whole wheat bread should be used and only when well toasted. It should be eaten dry and should be thoroughly chewed. No butter or jam should ever be added to it.

All processed or hydrogenated fats should be avoided. The natural oils such as cold-pressed virgin olive soil, soy bean oil, peanut oil, corn oil, sesame oil, or sunflower oil may be used, but even these fats must be used sparingly. These oils may be used in combination with lemon juice as a dressing on the raw vegetable salads. Even the natural oils have to be used sparingly because all fats have to be resaponified by the bile, and this places an added burden on the liver.

Alcohol and tobacco are injurious to the liver, as well as to the heart and nervous system, and those who use them often pay a great price for it.

All refined and processed foods must be eliminated, since most packaged foods contain chemical preservatives and additives injurious to the liver.

Sufferers from diseases of the liver must make sure to eat sparingly and to chew their food thoroughly. They must never eat unless really hungry.

If ill, obtain help but make sure that the doctor who is in charge of your case has a thorough understanding of hygienic principles and knows how to apply them. We must always strive to restore normal body functioning and this can only be accomplished by following sound health-building procedures. Sedatives, tranquilizers, or any of the other remedies that suppress or mask the symptoms of disease, only throw an added burden upon the liver and ultimately cause damage to it.

A diet of freshly pressed pure fruit or vegetable juices one or two days a week is of tremendous help. Freshly squeezed grapefruit, apple or carrot juice, or unsweetened grape juice, or fresh pomegranate juice in season may be used.

## Difficulty in Determining Liver Damage

Why is it so difficult to detect the earlier stages of liver damage, since a vast number of laboratory tests are now used to determine whether or not the liver is functioning properly?

Unfortunately, these tests are not always exact and in many instances fail to reveal the true picture of the diseased condition. The *Journal of the American Medical Association*, February 11, 1956, in reply to a question by a doctor on the interpretation of these tests, writes: "Many of the so-called liver function tests measure 'function' of the liver only indirectly; many are empirical, the exact basis for their relation to disease of the liver being unknown; most are nonspecific, being frequently positive in disease of tissues other than the liver, and the majority are insufficiently sensitive, liver disease sometimes being present with a normal test." The reply further points out that "following vital hepatitis, the liver biopsy may return to normal and yet disturbances in some of these tests may remain. Rarely will the sulfobromophtalein, serum bilirubin, or alkalinephosphatase levels be elevated in this circumstance. The cephalin flocculation level usually returns to normal soon after the patient is clinically well, but sometimes remains elevated for some weeks or months. The thymol turbidity may remain abnormal in exceptional cases for as long as a year or more after an acute episode. Likewise the serum globulin level may sometimes be elevated for prolonged periods of time, although the albumin level usually returns to normal relatively rapidly." The article continues: "A diagnosis of the liver disease or of its absence, or of a kind of liver disease, can rarely be made by any one or group of these tests. Many patients with chronic stabilized cirrhosis, for example, may have a normal cephalinflocculation test, thymol turbidity test, serum bilirubin level, alkaline phosphatase level, cholesterol level and cholesterol esters, and prothrombin time," the reply points out.

Fenton Schaffner, previously quoted, in referring to some of the tests performed to check liver function, pointed out that "while complete recovery is the rule following cholestatic jaundice (jaundice brought on by an obstruction in the flow of bile) within three to four weeks, hyperbilirubinemia may persist for months and abnormalities in the results of other hepatic (liver) tests such as serum alkaline phosphatase or leucine aminopeptidase activity may be abnormal for years."

A well-known New York physician, reporting on a patient suffering from diabetes, widespread osteoarthritis, thyrotoxicosis (toxic goiter) and well-established neuropathy (nerve damage), made it clear that impaired liver function may exist even when tests fail to show it. "The tests for liver function as yet show no marked liver damage, although the presence of diabetes is presumptive evidence of liver dysfunction. This is confirmed by the rapid sedimentation rate," he stated.

We quote these statements because they confirm what we have stated on many occasions, namely, that since the liver is one of our major lines of defense, it is called into play in practically all diseases and, as a result, is in most instances functionally or even structurally impaired, even when clinical symptoms or any of the established liver tests are unable to verify it. Possessing an extremely large margin of safety, the liver may appear perfectly normal even when subjected to great stress or undergoing a great deal of damage.

This is why we emphasize that, to maintain the liver in a healthy condition or to restore it to health, our main need is not more tests but a careful and healthful way of living.

# 8

## YOUR GALLBLADDER AND YOUR DIGESTION

The gallbladder is a small pear-shaped organ attached to the undersurface of the liver. Its function is to store the bile, which is secreted by the liver, and empty it into the small intestine whenever it is needed.

Since the gallbladder serves merely as a storage place for the bile, it is not nearly as important an organ as the liver, which produces the bile.

Yet, unlike the liver, in which a great deal of inflammation and deterioration can often exist for long periods of time without any apparent discomfort, an inflammation of the gallbladder is usually accompanied by a great deal of pain and suffering.

In a diseased gallbladder many destructive changes can take place. An inflamed gallbladder usually becomes distended and swollen, and tiny hemorrhages and ulcers often develop.

As the inflammation continues, the walls of the gallbladder become thickened and filled with scar tissue, and its power to contract and empty the bile diminishes and ultimately may be lost completely.

An inflammation of the gallbladder may occur as an outcome of disturbances in the gallbladder proper, or may develop as a result of disturbances in the bile duct or in any other organ close to the gallbladder or the duct and can cause interference in the drainage of the bile.

When the bile becomes stagnant in the gallbladder, it gradually begins to change. The solid elements begin to crystallize and gravel and stones begin to form. The liquid portion too undergoes disintegration, changing to substances that vary from a bile-stained loose fluid to thick pus.

## Bile Duct Obstruction

Many factors lead to an obstruction in the bile duct. The duct may become obstructed when long-standing irritation causes its tissues to harden, destroying its ability to stretch and relax. It also becomes obstructed when, following a previous inflammation, scars or adhesions have formed. Particles of mucus that get into the bile duct as well as pressure from adjacent organs that have become inflamed or enlarged also cause pressure on the duct and interfere with the outflow of bile.

Stones in the gallbladder may also obstruct the duct and cause an interference with drainage. In a case of this kind, however, the presence of a previous inflammation that has given rise to the formation of stones may be assumed.

Long-standing irritation of the gallbladder by toxins carried to it by the bloodstream is another factor that plays a part in the onset of inflammation of the gallbladder and/or bile duct, and leads to the formation of stones. These toxins are present in the bloodstream either because the liver has been unable to destroy them or render them harmless, or because the kidneys or other eliminative organs have not been able to expel them.

A frequent cause of gallbladder inflammation is a derangement in the chemical makeup of the bile or a high concentration of cholesterol. These chemical disturbances are usually the outgrowth of faulty nutrition and incorrect living habits and are often brought on by an impairment in the metabolism of the body. A high concentration of cholesterol in the gallbladder often goes hand in hand with a high cholesterol content in the blood.

## Gallbladder Disease Related to Other Diseases

From the facts stated above, we should realize that a gallbladder disease does not stand alone but is usually related to or the outgrowth of other disorders. Investigation will disclose that sufferers from this disease are often afflicted by a variety of other digestive disorders. Most of them are constipated. Others suffer from gastritis. In the great majority of cases the liver is involved.

Drs. James J. Foster and Donald L. Knudson, from the

Department of Medicine and Radiology, Marquette University School of Medicine, in the *Journal of the American Medical Association*, September 20, 1958, pointed out that cholelithiasis, hiatus hernia, and diverticulitis (the presence of gallstones, a break in the muscles of the diaphragm, and inflammation of pouches or sacs in the colon), are often found as a triad, and that constipation is a predisposing factor. They stress the fact that straining at stool and the increased intra-abdominal and intracolonic pressure can give rise to these three associated diseases. They also refer to Goldman and Ivey, who point out that the distension of the colon that accompanies constipation "can initiate reflex stimuli to inhibit free bile flow, the corollary being that such biliary stasis can contribute to gallstone formation."

We are certain that an investigation in the history of gallbladder sufferers would disclose that in most cases these disorders began with some simple digestive upset that could easily have been overcome and that the more serious disorders developed merely because the earlier upsets were either improperly treated or completely neglected.

## Composition of Stones Varies

Since the chemical imbalance in the bile is not always the same, the stones that develop in each case are not always of the same type. Some stones may be formed only of a concentration of cholesterol, others only of calcium or of some of the other solids, while others may be a composition of the different solids of which the bile is composed.

This is the reason why stones do not always show up equally well on the X-ray plate, and why soft stones made up primarily of cholesterol often do not show up at all, even when fully formed.

The size of the stones also varies considerably. Some may be very small, even of the pinpoint variety, while others may be very large. In some cases, the gallbladder may contain a great many stones of various sizes.

## Inflammation Without Pain

While an acute gallbladder attack is usually accompanied by severe pains, a low-grade gallbladder inflammation may sometimes exist without causing any distress or pain. This is especially true in persons who are not overly sensitive. In some cases, the duct may be only partially obstructed and while the bile does not flow freely, it empties sufficiently to keep the patient fairly comfortable. On the other hand, an acute gallbladder attack may sometimes be misinterpreted as a simple attack of indigestion or other acute stomach or intestinal disorder.

## Acute Gallbladder Symptoms

An acute gallbladder attack usually comes on with dramatic suddennness and is, as a rule, excruciatingly painful. It is usually accompanied by severe colic and the attack may last for hours, occasionally even as long as a day or two. Fever and some jaundice are often associated with these attacks.

An acute gallbladder attack may sometimes be mistaken for ulcers of the stomach. Certain differences, however, help distinguish one from the other. Acute ulcer pains are usually relieved by food, especially milk, while in an acute gallbladder attack the intake of food does not lessen the pain in any degree. An acute gallbladder attack also comes on spasmodically in the form of colic and usually radiates to the back, while acute ulcer pains are, as a rule, localized and constant.

A spastic colon or spastic colitis may also produce reflex pains in the gallbladder region, but these pains are generally less intense than the pains in an acute gallbladder attack.

During a heart attack, pains often radiate into the gallbladder region, and these cases may sometimes be mistakenly operated upon for gallbladder trouble with grave consequences to the patient.

Similar mistakes are also made in inflammation or ulcers of the stomach, or spastic colitis. Sufferers from these diseases are sometimes operated upon for gallbladder disease and only after the operation has been performed is the mistake discovered. The gallbladder is found either entirely clear, or even when involved, as in the cases where stones are present, is nevertheless not the cause of the attack, since the pains originated elsewhere.

### Pains Usually Caused by Inflammation

Pains in the gallbladder are, in most instances, caused not by stones but by inflammation. Stones may be present in the gallbladder for years and not cause any pains. Stones cause pain only when they get into the duct and interfere with the flow of the bile.

When the inflammation of the gallbladder subsides, the pains usually cease, even though the stones are still in the gallbladder.

When the gallbladder begins to function normally again, it discharges not only the fluids that have become locked up in the gallbladder, but also the gravel and those stones which are small enough to pass through the duct.

However, when a stone gets into the duct it often sets up a new irritation, causing a blockage all over again, and this often gives rise to a new gallbladder attack.

When stones or gravel pass through the duct, they empty into the small intestine and are eventually eliminated through the bowels.

Even when an acute gallbladder inflammation has cleared up and drainage has been re-established, the gallbladder is often left considerably weakened, and unless the underlying causes are eliminated, renewed attacks and the formation of new stones are to be expected.

### All Functions Must Be Rehabilitated

To rebuild the gallbladder, we must not only eliminate the gallbladder inflammation, but must also restore the functions of all others organs related to it or which affect its functioning. Disorders of the digestive system must be eliminated. Excess weight must be reduced, constipation must be corrected, the nerves must be strengthened and rebuilt, and the circulation must be restored to normal.

## Care During an Acute Gallbladder Attack

An acute gallbladder attack may occasionally be brought on when a stone gets into the duct and interferes with the free flow of the bile. In these cases, measures must be employed to relax the duct in order to give the stone a chance to pass through. Medically, opiates are used for this purpose.

However, since opiates have a disturbing and often harmful effect upon the body, we recommend the use of simple, natural methods which, when properly applied, accomplish the same ends, but leave no bad after-effects.

As soon as an acute attack sets in, it is imperative that all food be discontinued and that only hot water be taken, plain or flavored with a few drops of lemon or lime juice. This will help to flush the system. We recommend the use of frequent enemas to clean out the bowels and hot baths to induce relaxation. Hot, moist compresses applied over the gallbladder region are often of great help.

These measures must be continued until the acute attack has been completely subdued. It is true that opiates usually provide relief more rapidly, but since they leave the body considerably weakened and subject to recurrent attacks, we prefer to rely upon this simple natural approach. In addition, the measures suggested help to lay the foundation for improved health.

After the acute attack has subsided, the abdomen may continue to be sore and sensitive, but this will diminish with each passing day and will usually disappear within a week.

Following the clearing up of the acute attack, the simple, health-building program recommended in the previous chapters for the other digestive disorders will help to rebuild the health of the patient and ultimately bring about complete recovery.

After recovery, a sound living regimen must be continued, since the same abuses that have caused the inflammation and favored the formation of gravel and stones in the first place can readily bring about a recurrence of the condition.

### Thousands Saved from Needless Surgery

This type of care has been instrumental in saving thousands of gallbladder sufferers from needless surgery. However, to attain lasting results it is imperative that this program be carried out consistently in accordance with the particular needs of the case. Sufferers from this disease should, whenever possible, be under the care of a physician, but should make sure that the physician who is taking care of them has a complete grasp of sound physiological principles and knows how to apply them in accordance with the requirements of the individual case.

### Can Stones Dissolve or Disintegrate?

The question often arises whether gallstones can be dissolved. Most doctors usually answer this question in the negative, but then how many follow the program we are outlining here, or apply it consistently enough to effect or attain the desired results?

We have emphasized repeatedly that, when this procedure is followed consistently, the metabolic functions of the body are gradually restored to normal and that stones often dissolve or disintegrate. Those formed of the softer substances, such as cholesterol, usually disappear more rapidly, but even those formed of the harder substances will often break down, although much more time may be required before results are attained.

It is interesting to mention that stones occasionally dissolve even where the patient's living habits have not been altered to any marked degree, which illustrates that even under adverse conditions the body's reparative forces are sometimes powerful enough to bring about recovery. On the other hand, where the patient's living habits are carefully adjusted, results of a most dramatic nature are often attained.

Dr. Joseph F. Linsman, Associate Clinical Professor of Radiology, College of Medical Evangelists, and Dr. Eliot Corday, Assistant Clinical Professor of Medicine, University of California, reporting in the *Journal of the American Medical Association*, describe the case of a physician in whom an examination of the gallbladder by X-rays on October 12, 1954, revealed the presence in the gallbladder of "10 rounded negative shadows, measuring 7 to 9 mm. in diameter, with an appearance characteristic of gallstones," but that a recheck on October 16, 1958, revealed that the stones had completely disappeared.

The authors further cite the case of a twenty-three-year-old woman who suffered attacks of biliary (gallbladder) colic during her pregnancy and in whom X-rays *taken two weeks after the delivery* "revealed numerous, clearly delineated radiolucent calculi (stones) which measured 2 to 3 mm. in size," but who showed no stones in the gallbladder and the bile ducts when operated upon seven weeks later.

They further refer to a case reported by Kommerell and Wolpers in which X-rays disclosed twenty-one small stones (measuring up to 5 or 6 mm. in diameter), and three larger ones (measuring about 10 mm. in diameter). *X-ray studies repeated yearly in this case "revealed that the stones became gradually smaller but no fewer,"* and ultimately completely disappeared. The authors emphasize that the stones in these cases could not have passed out "by migration," since they disappeared without any colic or jaundice.

In a later issue of *The Journal* (January 23, 1960), when a correspondent questioned the findings of the authors, Dr. Linsman stressed the fact that the case they observed was subjected to exhaustive studies, including "at least twenty exposures made with the patient in varying degrees of rotation in prone, supine, and upright positions before and after the administration of a fatty meal"; that a careful recheck was made following the receipt of the letter; and that at both times "there was no sign of abnormality of the gallbladder which showed normal opacification (shadows) and no evidence of stones."

Dr. Linsman further stated that he would be happy to make all the X-rays available to those who challenged his findings so that they might be convinced "that the gallstones actually disappeared."

Now, what brought about the disappearance of these stones? We can do no better than quote the authors who state that "since one of the causes of nonopaque gallstones is related to disordered cholesterol metabolism, one conjectures whether further alteration of the cholesterol metabolism in our patient may have had something to do with the disappearance of his gallstones."[1]

What is of added interest in this report is the fact that the stones that disappeared were clearly visible on the X-ray plates and were, therefore, most likely of the harder type of stones.


### Surgery Seldom Necessary

We are aware that where a case has been badly neglected, where the gallbladder has become filled with stones, or has become gangrenous, surgery may be necessary. The fact that a case may occasionally reach such an advanced stage, however, must not blind us to the fact that, in the vast majority of cases, conservative, nonsurgical, hygienic measures can be most successful, and can eliminate all need for surgery.

A physician who is conversant with natural methods and who possesses the necessary skill and experience will recognize when a case has reached the stage where surgery is unavoidable. In such rare or occasional cases, surgery is constructive and life-saving. A fact to remember is that only when we have reached the stage where conservative (nonsurgical) measures can no longer be of help is surgery advisable, and not otherwise.

*A Case History:* MRS. ANNA A.

To illustrate how a carefully regulated dietary regimen and sound hygienic measures work in these cases, we wish to present the case history of Mrs. Anna A. We shall let Mrs. A. tell her own story.

Shortly after my daughter was born I began to experience pains in the region of my gallbladder. At first the feeling was one of discomfort and, though annoying, didn't worry me much. However, as time went on, the attacks became more severe and more frequent.

My family physician prescribed some medication for me

[1] "Spontaneous Disappearance of Gallstones," *J.A.M.A.*, October 24, 1959.

and told me to avoid spicy and fatty foods. He also suggested I take a dose of epsom salts once a week.

Although I followed his advice, I still continued to get attacks which left me feeling limp and weak. It was just as though a red-hot band had been drawn tightly around me. The pains usually radiated from back to the front under my ribs.

I recall the time I felt such an attack coming on while I was driving my car, and I had to pull over to the side of the road, for the terrific pain left me weak and helpless.

I had been suffering these painful attacks for several years and they kept getting worse and more frequent, until one night I awoke in such agony that I literally crawled on the floor. Our doctor gave me morphine shots but the pain was so excruciating that it seemed as though nothing was of any help. I suffered torture for several days, and then was told that I had large gallstones blocking the duct and that only surgery could give me any relief. I was told that surgery was necessary *immediately* and it would be folly and dangerous to postpone it.

When my sister who lives in another city was called and told about this, she immediately visited me, called Dr. W. for an appointment, and insisted that I accompany her to his office.

Although she already had convinced me that only Dr. W.'s method of treatment could help me back to health again, *without* surgery, convincing my husband was not so easy. He was determined that his "doctor knows best." However, my sister was just as determined that surgery was *not* the best method, for she had completely overcome a gallbladder condition *plus* arthritis by following Dr. W.'s advice.

Fortunately my husband finally (though reluctantly, I might add) agreed with her that you can always resort to surgery, so "let's give nature a chance first."

Under this natural way of regaining my health, I lost a number of unhealthy pounds (I was quite heavy), and after several months, I felt better than I had felt for many, many years. My husband's fears that I would suffer painful attacks without being able to use medication (as Dr. W. frowns on medication of any kind) proved to be unfounded, for not *once* during the period I was under Dr. W.'s guidance did I have an attack.

My troubles are now a thing of the past. And best of all, I learned to eat right, and consequently live right.

When Mrs. A. placed herself under this care, she was forty-five years old. We are pleased to note that she made right living a lifetime habit—a wise decision, for only when we continue to adhere to a sound program of living can we be sure of protecting ourselves against a recurrence of the pathological condition.

*Another Case:* PAUL C., *Age Eighty*

Paul C. at the age of eighty also has an interesting story to tell:

January 7, 1941 was the day I was emancipated from the surgeon's scalpel. I was sixty then. Four years before I had had my first experience with the knife, undergoing an appendectomy. A year afterward I was operated on again—for an inguinal hernia on the right side. Subsequently my medico-surgeon was candidly looking ahead to removal of my gallbladder which had been "kicking up a row."

I felt miserable and looked it because every weekend a splitting headache drove me to the usual ache suppressor. A friend noting my misery asked what was bothering me. I explained, whereupon she said, "Why don't you turn to the natural method? It can help you." She suggested a doctor who practiced along these lines.

The following Monday after school hours [the writer was then an assistant principal of a leading school in New York City], I visited this doctor. After examining me, he informed me that he could help me, provided I would cooperate. After three weeks of treatment and following directives regarding foods, early and definite improvement was felt and no more weekend headaches disturbed me.

After three months, my health was restored without any medication of any kind. I still have my gallbladder, which does not annoy me, moreover, at age eighty I am actively employed at least four hours a day and feel well as long as I continue to observe directions regarding food. I eat to live and enjoy my food. No other way will do. This way is a way of life; it's healthy living.

You will note from Paul's report that he is adhering to his healthy way of living. When we met Paul recently, he made it a point to remind us that when he started his care in 1941, he was promised that if he would adhere faithfully to the program outlined for him he would have at least another twenty healthy years of life. This promise has already become a reality. From the way Paul looks even at his advanced age, we are confident that he is good for at least twenty years more. No wonder Paul regards January 7, 1941, as his emancipation day.

These case histories demonstrate conclusively that the health-building measures should be the measures of first choice, and that surgery should come into consideration only in those rare cases where the disease has progressed to the point where sound hygienic nonsurgical procedures can no longer provide the help that is needed.

### Health Cannot Be Switched On and Off

The efficacy of this approach and the faith that it engenders in patients who follow it are often actually their undoing. They feel that if for some reason or other their health should break down, they have nothing to fear since they can always return to the care that has helped them in the past. What they often fail to realize is that health cannot be turned on and off like a switch, that each time illness recurs more damage is likely to develop, and that ultimately the damage may become so great that complete recovery may be unattainable.

## 9

## YOUR NERVES AND YOUR DIGESTION

In an earlier part of this section, we pointed out that doctors as well as laymen often stress the role of the nerves in the onset of digestive disorders.

That emotional upsets and nervous tension contribute to the onset of these diseases is not questioned. It is well known that the nerves play a vital role in all bodily functions, and the digestive system is no exception.

However, we differ emphatically from those who place major or exclusive blame on the nervous system and disregard or minimize all other influences.

A basic factor frequently disregarded is that poor nutrition and unwholesome living habits have a depleting and enervating effect on the nervous system and that this, in turn, affects the functions of the digestive system as well as the rest of the body.

We must never forget that, while weakened or debilitated nerves impair the functions of the digestive organs, the intake of poor food and deleterious living habits undermine the health of the nerves.

That faulty diets undermine the health of the nerves is well known. The *Journal of the American Medical Association*, July 25, 1959, in reply to a query by a physician on the X-ray characteristics found in the gastrointestinal tract in patients with malnutrition, avitaminosis, and starvation, states that the conditions found in these cases are grouped under the term of "malabsorption syndrome" and that *"these conditions in some patients produce, or at least are associated with, a disorder of motor function in the small intestine manifested by hypotonicity and slow transit time."*

While these medical terms may seem incomprehensible to the average layman, they simply explain in professional jargon that malnutrition or starvation impairs the health of the nerves that control the functioning and tone of the small intestine.

"In advanced nutritional disorders, gas distention of the intestine may simulate ileus," the reply states, and continues, "variability of the effects on the intestine seems to depend in part on the severity and duration of the nutritional disorder and on the *kind* and *amount* of dietary treatment in the past."

Among the effects produced by "these disorders of motor function," the answer mentions delayed functioning, general weakness, tissue distention, and reduction or obliteration of the mucosal folds, "leaving the inner surface of the intestine smooth." It concludes that while with proper treatment these disorders often disappear, "they are irreversible in some advanced cases." Stating it more clearly, long-standing deficiencies brought about by improper diet may cause so much damage to the tissues and nerves of the digestive system that complete restoration may no longer be possible.

This merely points out anew the influence of sound nutrition on the function of the digestive organs. This also explains why the use of remedies that camouflage the symptoms of the disease have no lasting value and ultimately lead only to more damage. The final breakdown may be delayed, but when it eventually comes the damage may be beyond repair.

The solution for sufferers from these disorders does not lie in the use of the so-called tranquilizers, energizing drugs, sedatives, or any of the other symptom-relieving drugs, but upon a way of life that nourishes and rehabilitates the whole organism, including the nervous system.

## A Program That Rehabilitates and Fortifies the Nerves

In other words, all the functions of the body are closely interrelated. Since healthy nerves depend upon a healthy body, all the functions of the body must be restored to normal if the digestive system is to be restored to a healthy condition. This involves the correction not only of the weaknesses or disorders that are obvious or discernible, but also of those that are insidious or not easily detectable.

The following program will prove of great value in fortifying and rehabilitating the nervous system, as well as the other organs and tissues of the body.

1. Begin by following a well-balanced diet. Make sure that your meals consist primarily of wholesome, natural foods, and provide an adequate supply of easily digestible proteins and carbohydrates, as well as an abundance of fresh fruits and vegetables.

All denatured and processed foods such as the white flour and white sugar products, the refined cereals, the rich, concentrated fat foods such as butter, cream, the fat meats and fish and the hydrogenated or processed fats, all condiments and highly spiced foods, the concentrated sweets, as well as the stimulants such as coffee, tea, chocolate, and alcohol must be strictly excluded.

2. Make sure to overcome faulty eating habits. Food should be eaten slowly and should be well chewed. We should eat only when hungry and should be careful not to overeat.

3. Corrective exercises are of great help. A moderate amount of deep breathing, as well as the leg and sitting-up exercises, carried out regularly every morning and evening or at least once a day, and other healthful physical activities such as hikes, walking, etc., have an invigorating effect upon the body and strengthen the nervous system.

4. Plenty of rest and sleep is imperative. It is well to remember that healing and repair are carried on most effectively during periods of rest and sleep.

5. Regular rest periods do much to rebuild and strengthen the muscular body as well as the nervous system. A nap after the noon meal and rest periods whenever possible or when tired do much to safeguard our health.

6. Poise, calmness, and self-control are essential. Learn to relax and maintain your composure even under stress or irritation. Stop being sorry for yourself and learn to live with others. Develop self-confidence. Also remember that fear solves nothing and only adds to your problems.

7. Hot baths taken daily before retiring relax the nervous system and induce better sleep. However, where a bath before retiring is not practical or where it has a stimulating or exciting effect, it should be taken in the morning, but should be followed by a period of rest.

8. Make sure to have regular bowel evacuations. We stress the need for two or three evacuations daily when

two or three meals are eaten. Never delay when the urge to evacuate asserts itself. Where chronic constipation or bowel sluggishness exists, some time may be required before regularity is established. Patience is essential before results are attained. Enemas should be used for relief when necessary.

9. A hobby or some absorbing interest can be of great help. It relaxes the nervous system and adds to the joys of living. After health has been rebuilt and a constructive way of living has become an enjoyable procedure, a devotion to a useful purpose only helps to make life more interesting. We must never forget that we add to our pleasures of living to the extent that we give to others.

Remember that health is one of our most cherished possessions. The wise are careful not to waste it. However, when because of neglect or unforeseen or uncontrollable circumstances a condition of ill health has arisen, the wise know that they must not seek solace in transient relief, but must attack the problem by uprooting the underlying causes and by promoting rehabilitation through the use of sound rebuilding measures.

In connection with this, we would like to mention that Dr. Jacob M. Leavitt, to whom we referred in an earlier part of this book, in a clever play of words emphasized the fact that while health is a most precious gift, it can boomerang into "Gift," the German equivalent of poison or toxin, when neglected or abused.

## 10

## HEART ATTACKS AND INDIGESTION

Many readers have no doubt heard of individuals who thought that they suffered from an attack of indigestion and found out later that it was actually a heart attack. Such occurrences are common, but what is of interest is that such mistakes are made not only by laymen but also by doctors.

Boyd points out that the symptoms that occur in these attacks "may stimulate such acute abdominal conditions as perforated gastric or duodenal ulcer, gallstone colic, or acute pancreatitis," and further states that unless the possibility of a heart attack is kept in mind "it is easy to see how the abdomen may be opened with unfortunate consequences."

On the other hand, a digestive upset or an acute gallbladder attack may sometimes be mistaken for a heart attack. When these attacks subside, those involved, laymen as well as doctors, often continue under the illusion that the patient suffered a heart attack and recovered from it.

Digestive upsets often cause pressure against the heart and this in turn interferes with its functions and impedes the circulation. They contribute to a weakening or flabbiness of the heart muscle, and often lead to a dilatation or enlargement of the heart.

It is true that faulty eating and harmful living habits can cause certain heart symptoms such as palpitation, heart irregularity, weakness, or pain around the heart. It is essential to remember that these symptoms do not always indicate that the heart is damaged, since they can also be caused by weakened or debilitated nerves or digestive upsets.

These symptoms, even when not the result of a heart condition, must nevertheless be regarded as a warning, since if permitted to continue over an extended period of time they can ultimately lead to a permanent impairment of the heart. When a patient who suffers from certain distressing symptoms in the region of the heart is reassured that he is in good condition, he must still not be complacent about it, since a failure to correct the ailment responsible for these symptoms can ultimately damage the heart or bring on some other serious ailment.

We know of many persons who had a thorough checkup and were assured that the heart was in good condition, and yet a short time later succumbed to a heart attack. President Eisenhower is a case in point. It is well known that the President had periodic checkups and was subjected to one of these checkups only a short time before his heart attack. Even the most thorough examination cannot provide the assurance that is derived from a program of living that helps to conserve the vitality and health of the body as a whole. However, such a program must not be merely a temporary phase but should be continued through life.

## Hardening of the Arteries and Indigestion

Sufferers from hardening of the arteries often complain of heaviness or fullness in the stomach or other digestive discomforts. This is especially true in cases where the abdominal arteries are involved.

We must realize that disorders of the heart as well as of the circulatory system are the outgrowth of a disturbed metabolism, and that if the distressing digestive symptoms which accompany these disorders are to be prevented, careful nutrition and rational living habits become essential.

It is well known that doctors as a group show a higher mortality rate from diseases of the circulatory system than the lay population. Dr. Charles E. McArthur deals with this problem in an article in the *Journal of the American Medical Association* and emphasizes the fact that the medical profession is greatly concerned about it. He points out, however, that the problem is not insurmountable since the elimination of concentrated carbohydrates (sugars and starches) from the diet and the substitution of simple foods can do much to change the picture.

"Much is said about the high fat content of our diets, but little has been said about the evil caused in our foods or about their possible relationship to hypercholesteremia or hyperlipidemia," Dr. McArthur trenchantly states, and then proceeds to point out that he had suspected for some time "that the concentrated carbohydrates of our present-day diet might be one of the factors in atherosclerosis." He continues further by saying that when he placed patients suffering from this disease "on a diet of lean meats and vegetable salad, using a vegetable oil such as corn to make the salad dressing," he invariably attained excellent results.

To clarify this further, we wish to call attention to the fact that cakes, pastries, malteds, ice cream, sweets, puddings, the refined cereals, and all white flour and white sugar products are among the highly concentrated carbohydrate foods. While we deal in this book primarily with the diseases of the digestive system, it is interesting to note that the detrimental effects of these foods in other diseases are gradually beginning to be recognized; we hope that ere long doctors of all schools of healing will emphasize how harmful they are and discourage their use.

## Digestive Disorders and the Circulation

From what we stated above, it should be clear that an impairment in digestion also leads to an impairment in circulation. We have seen that pressure of gas impairs the circulation in the abdomen, and it should be evident that this interferes not only with the blood supply to the digestive organs, but also to all the organs of the body, including the heart. Digestive disorders deplete the energies of the body, and this too leads to a slowing down of the circulation.

Sufferers from digestive disorders are often disturbed by cold, clammy hands and feet or other circulatory disorders, and the cause of these disturbances should not be too difficult to recognize.

All these facts only illustrate anew the importance of following a program that rehabilitates and rebuilds the body as a whole, rather than attempting to treat disease symptomatically. The functions of the digestive system as well as those of the heart, the blood vessels, the kidneys, and all other parts of the body are closely interrelated and must function harmoniously if good health is to be attained.

We referred in our first chapter to a recent study by the Society of Actuaries (life insurance statisticians) which re-iterated a fact long known in insurance and progressive health circles, namely, that the ideal weight for a long and healthy life is actually fifteen to twenty pounds below the so-called standard weight, and that even a relatively small increase in weight contributes to an increase in mortality from heart and blood vessel diseases.

This report also discloses that even a relatively small elevation in blood pressure leads to a shortening of life; while an elevation in blood pressure, no matter how slight, in combination with a small increase in weight, only adds to the damage and causes a material increase in the death rate from these diseases.

"I can offer no obvious explanation of the mechanism whereby moderate overweight in combination with blood pressure of only the slightest upward departure from normal produces a mortality experience nearly twice the expected," stated Dr. John J. Hutchinson, Medical Director of the New York Life Insurance Company, in his comment on these findings.

The reason should be obvious. Even a moderate increase in weight, as well as a slight elevation in blood pressure, adds to the burden of the heart, while the two together greatly multiply the strain.

Continuing further on the subject of heart and blood vessel diseases, we are glad to note that the trend toward a more regulated and healthful way of living as a protection against these diseases is now becoming much more evident.

"The middle-aged man who is lean, takes exercise, avoids too much fat in his diet, does not smoke, and keeps his blood pressure down, apparently has a good chance of avoiding a heart attack," were the views expressed at the American Public Health Association's eighty-seventh annual meeting, according to Murray Illson's special report to *The New York Times.*

"The rare physician who emphasized these facts as long as thirty to forty years ago and who, because of this, was called an ignoramus or, by those less charitable, even a charlatan, finds himself amply vindicated," remarked a physician recently.

## 11

## OXYGEN: THE BREATH OF LIFE

What do you think would happen to a person who was deprived of air? He would become asphyxiated, wouldn't he?

This is exactly what happens to the individual cells, the countless billions of cells in the body, when they are deprived of the oxygen they need.

We can live without food for many days or even weeks at a time, but without oxygen life is impossible for more than a few minutes. This applies not only to the body as a whole but to each individual cell.

Each cell must receive the oxygen it needs or it will deteriorate and die. Oxygen starvation leads to the formation of ulcers or causes tissue disintegration, while a disturbance in the supply of oxygen to the tissues gives rise to many serious disorders.

The lungs and the circulatory system are functioning every moment of our life to keep the cells of the body constantly supplied with oxygen. The lungs inhale clean, fresh air, which is then pumped by the heart into the vast arterial network for general distribution to all parts of the body.

The cells of the body receive the oxygen from the blood in exchange for the impurities which they give off to be carried back to the lungs for elimination.

It should be evident from all this that circulation plays a vital part in the maintenance of health not merely of the digestive system but of the whole body.

Many factors contribute to a healthy circulation. Wholesome nourishing food, plenty of rest and sleep, normal physical activities, as well as the proper mental attitude, keep our body and mind in good condition and help to maintain a healthy bloodstream. A well-planned program of physical exercises can also be of great benefit. Properly planned exercises help to remove underlying interferences, strengthen weakened or damaged organs, rebuild muscular tone, and promote more thorough elimination.

Where the patient is greatly debilitated, only the mildest type of exercises should be indulged in at first, since when carried to excess they lead to an increase in fatigue and actually hamper what we are trying to accomplish.

## Never Exercise at the Expense of Rest

We must always bear in mind that when the body is worn out, its first and most indispensable need is rest. Only after the body has become rested and strengthened are exercises indicated. We should start with the mildest exercises at first and add the more strenuous types only as the body gains in strength and vitality. We must also remember that exercises must never be carried beyond the point of fatigue.

Never be impatient, but let your doctor advise you when you are ready to start exercising and when the exercises should be increased. Expert supervision at such times is of great help.

The following are some of the exercises we have used with excellent results in digestive disorders.

DEEP-BREATHING EXERCISES    1. Lie flat on the back with arms stretched out at your sides, palms downward. Keep mouth closed and inhale deeply and slowly through both nostrils; then exhale slowly, also through the nostrils. Relax and repeat.    2. Keep mouth closed and inhale through the right nostril, keeping the left nostril closed with your thumb, then exhale slowly through the left nostril while keeping the right nostril closed.    3. Repeat the same exercise through left nostril, inhaling through the left and exhaling through the right nostril.

Those who are weak and debilitated should not do these exercises more than two or three times morning and night; but should increase the number as they gain in strength and vitality, gradually increasing the number up to ten times.

LEG-RAISING EXERCISES    1. Lie flat on the back, legs stretched out. Relax completely. Raise right leg slowly as far as you can reach while keeping the left leg fully stretched out, then lower until you touch floor. Relax and repeat.    2. Repeat the same exercise with the left leg.    3. Repeat the same exercise with both legs together.

Those who are greatly debilitated should begin with Nos. 1 and 2, and add No. 3 only as they grow stronger. Begin by doing them two or three times, morning and night, and gradually increase up to ten times.

SITTING-UP EXERCISES    1. Lie flat on the back and relax. Stretch hands over head, then raise body in sitting position, trying to touch toes with finger tips. Keep knees stretched while doing it.    2. Repeat this exercise, inhaling as you assume the reclining position, and exhaling while raising the body in sitting position.

ABDOMINAL MUSCLE EXERCISES    Lie flat on the back and relax. Then pull in abdomen, as far as possible, then push out as far as you can.

ADVANCED LEG EXERCISES    1. Assume reclining position as in the first leg exercises. Raise right leg as high as you can, keeping knee straight; then move leg as far to the left as possible, then stretch as far to the right as possible; then bring back to center and lower slowly until you touch the floor.    2. Repeat this exercise with left leg, stretching over first to right side, then to left side, then back to center, then lower slowly to floor.    3. Repeat with both legs.

KNEE-CHINNING EXERCISES    1. Lie flat on back, legs stretched, hands clasped behind head. Raise head and pull up right knee, trying to touch chin with knee.    2. Repeat with left knee.    3. Repeat with both knees.

STRETCHING EXERCISES    1. Stand upright with arms stretched over your head. Bend forward, trying to touch your toes with your finger tips, then straighten up and repeat.    2. Stand upright with legs spread far apart; then swing your body slowly to the right side, trying to touch right toes with left finger tips. Straighten up and then swing body slowly to the left side, trying to touch left toes with right finger tips. Repeat two or three times and then gradually increase number.      3. Stand upright with legs far apart. Reach with left hand to left side, trying to touch floor; then reach with right hand to right side. Repeat two or three times and then gradually increase the number.

## 12

# SYMPTOM-RELIEVING DRUGS LEAD TO MORE DISEASE

*No Nocere (It Must Not Harm) First Law in Medicine*

We cannot stress too strongly the fact that palliative or symptom-relieving drugs used in the treatment of digestive disorders only add to the severity of these disorders. This is not only our observation but also the observation of many leading authorities.

If you turn back to the statement of Dr. Gordon McHardy in the first chapter of this section, you will note how severe the damage can be. What is most striking in connection with this, however, is the fact that the harm is not caused by drugs of a severely irritating or caustic nature but by the ordinary kind of drugs used in common practice. These drugs are harmful even when used in small or medicinal doses and their harmful effects often show up most unexpectedly.

Dealing with the subject of penicillin, Dr. Howard I. Weinstein, a research director of the Food and Drug Administration, has pointed out that "about 3,000 or 4,000 persons in the United States suffer serious reactions to penicillin each year," and that of these "300 to 400 die."[1] Needless to say, these figures are most likely an understatement, for many serious reactions and/or deaths brought on by penicillin are blamed on the disease itself rather than on the penicillin used in its treatment.

Discussing penicillin further, we find Stephen M. Spencer quoting Dr. Henry Welsh, Director of the Food and Drug Administration Division of Antibiotics, to the effect that the fatalities that occur from this drug are not due to its indiscriminate use by physicians, but to a "mysterious and violent response of the body known as anaphylactic shock." He mentions that "the symptoms of anaphylaxis include a tingling of the tongue, a dryness of the

[1] *New York World Telegram and The Sun,* November 6, 1959.

mouth, heavy sweating, palpitation, dizziness, feeling of oppression, a tightness in the chest, extreme weakness, and finally collapse."[2]

A report cited in the *Journal of the American Medical Association* records the observations by Muir and Cossar who found that, of a group of 106 patients hospitalized for gastroduodenal hemorrhage, 54 per cent had taken aspirin within 48 hours of their first hemorrhage, compared with 15 per cent of a control series hospitalized for miscellaneous conditions.

On the basis of these findings, the authors then "conclude that aspirin was a dangerous drug, particularly for those in whom it caused gastric pain and in those with a known peptic ulcer."[3]

*Time,* October 27, 1958, quotes Dr. Jesse D. Rising of the University of Kansas who, in *Postgraduate Medicine*, describes many of the dangerous side effects resulting from drugs in common use today. Dr. Rising points out that Thorazine can cause severe liver damage, the cortisone-type hormones can cause peptic ulcers to the point of perforation, that diuretic Diamox can cause enough upset to a congested liver to lead to hepatic coma, and that the antibiotics can lead to an inflammation of the intestine which may turn into "a deadly disease."

We can well understand why Dr. Rising, who does not advocate the abandonment of the use of drugs, nevertheless concludes by stating that the thoughtful physician "will not lightly prescribe [them, and] will exert every effort to understand ... the harmful effects that may result from their use."

Thousands of drugs are constantly being prescribed for all kinds of real and imaginary ills and new drugs are constantly being added to the list. While in many cases the liver and other detoxifying organs are able to destroy these drugs or render them harmless, in a great many others they have a pronounced toxic effect upon the body; their long-term effects are unpredictable.

Drs. Bernhard B. Brodie, W. Robert Jondorf, and Roger P. Maickel of the National Heart Institute's Laboratory of Chemical Pharmacology, United States Public Health Ser-

2 *Saturday Evening Post,* May 23, 1959.
3 *J.A.M.A.,* June 13, 1959.

vice, warned in a recent report that it may be dangerous to administer such commonly used drugs as barbiturates, the analgesics, aminopyrine and phenacetin, the laxative phenolphthalein, and other similar drugs to expectant mothers and newborn infants, since their studies have revealed that "newborn mammals lack the ability to change drugs into inactive products."

"That newborn mammals are unable to metabolize these compounds is of obvious importance in considering the use of drugs in childbirth and for newborn infants," these experts state.[4]

## A Sound Approach to Disease

The average person reading all this is bound to wonder: If drugs are dangerous, what are we to do in case of disease? What can we do to overcome a fever or a cold or an upset stomach? How can we get rid of pains, a cough, or cramps?

The answer is not as difficult as it seems. We simply must return to what a well-known doctor once described as Hippocratic medicine. Our approach at all times must be based upon the principles enunciated by Hippocrates, namely, *Vis medicatrix naturae*. We must never forget that the power of healing is an inherent quality of the organism, and that this power manifests itself even when in our ignorance we place obstacles in its way.

We could benefit immensely if we would eliminate all the obstacles to, and interferences with, the body's healing processes, and resorted to those measures which promote rehabilitation and repair.

We cannot emphasize too strongly the fact that this is accomplished not when suppressive drugs are used, but when the underlying causes of the disease are eradicated and rational health-building measures are employed.

One of the primary laws in medicine is *no nocere*, it must not harm. It should be obvious that any approach violating this law defeats our purpose.

[4] *The New York Times,* Science Section, May 17, 1959.

## 13

## THE CURSE OF CHEMICAL POLLUTANTS AND ADDITIVES

Chemicals and additives used in the raising and processing of food contribute to the onset of disease.

It should be apparent why this is the case. These foreign substances do not add anything of value to the food but are irritating and often toxic to the bodily tissues. They can be used without any apparent ill effect merely because the liver and other detoxifying and eliminating organs are able to neutralize them or dispose of them. But what happens when the efficiency of the liver or any of the other detoxifying or eliminating organs becomes impaired?

While medical literature rarely touches upon the hazards inherent in the use of these chemicals, these facts are becoming increasingly more known as is evidenced by the following quotations:

*Organic Gardening and Farming,* a monthly publication devoted to organo-culture, in the July 1959 issue quotes the following from the *American Journal of Digestive Diseases:* "Without exception, every one of the chlorinated cyclic hydrocarbon insecticides is a liver poison. This is true of the entire series from the solvent monochloro-benzene and the mothicide paradichlorobenzene to DDT and the chlorinated naphthalenes Aldrin and Dieldrin. The chlorinated naphthalenes were shown to produce hepatitis."[1]

Turning to *Reader's Digest,* the following statement by Robert S. Strother should prove significant: "Doctors are increasingly troubled by the possibility that DDT and its much more poisonous descendants may be responsible for the rise of leukemia, hepatitis, Hodgkin's disease and other degenerative diseases."[2]

[1] "The Case Against Poison Spray," *Organic Gardening and Farming,* July, 1959.
[2] "Backfire in the War Against Insects," *Reader's Digest.*

## The Danger to Animals

Scientists everywhere are being aroused to the dangers inherent to animals as well as man in these chemicals. Dr. George Wallace, Professor of Zoology, Michigan State University, stated at a Convention of the National Audubon Society that: "If pest eradication programs now under way or envisioned are carried out, we shall have been witnesses, within a single decade to a greater extermination of animal life than in all the previous years of man's history on earth."

Dr. John L. George, a biologist of the United States Fish and Wildlife Service, confirms this when, in his discussion of the current program for the eradication of the imported fire ant, he states that "pesticidal applications may have adverse effects upon wildlife," and then continues by saying that "Sand fly control in Florida resulted in heavy loss of aquatic life, while operations for control of forest insects in New Brunswick and the Yellowstone resulted in extensive damage to fish."

Summing up the views expressed at this Convention, the *New York Herald Tribune* commented somberly: "It was generally agreed among the speakers at this Convention that applications of such insecticides as DDT, Dieldrin and Heptachlor can and do destroy animal life other than the target pest; sometimes it has been shown this destruction is considerable." The newspaper continues by saying that while "proponents of the insecticides contend that the *surviving creatures will soon repopulate sprayed areas, opponents ask if it is not also true ... that the insecticides may kill off natural enemies of the pests.*"

Allen D. Cruickshank, ornithologist, author, and artist, writing in the *Audubon Field Notes*, confirms that there were heavy bird losses in the East in 1958 when he states that "uncontrolled use of powerful insecticides, herbicides, and fungicides may well be, and probably is, the destructive force. ... *Unless the use of these poisons is soon controlled by strict State and Federal laws, they certainly will have disastrous effects on the bird life of the entire nation,*" Dr. Cruickshank continues.

B. W. Bierers, V.M.D., and C. L. Vickers, D.V.M., in

the *Journal of the American Veterinary Medical Association*, May 15, 1959, describe the harmful effect of fungicide-treated and fumigated grains fed to egg-laying hens, and show that corn treated with the fungicide tetramethylthiuran disulfide (TMTD) resulted in the production of soft-shelled and misshapen eggs and that grains fumigated with ethylene dibramide (EDB), widely used to fumigate grains for the control of weevils "resulted in a gradual diminution in egg size and, in extreme cases, in complete cessation of egg production." They concluded that corn containing TMTD when "fed to laying hens may have a disastrous effect on egg production even when such grains are heavily diluted with nontreated corn."[3]

The *Connecticut Wildlife Conservation Bulletin*, March-April 1958, published by the Connecticut State Board of Fisheries and Game, refers to a statement of the National Audubon Society that warns "that all use of highly toxic modern insecticides, fungicides, and so-called pesticides by governmental agencies, farmers, and other land owners, including gardeners, *carries with it a much higher potential of harm to human beings and wildlife than is generally recognized.*"

*The New York Times*, January 8, 1958, dealing editorially with the government campaign to put out the fire ant, states: "It is rank folly for the government to embark on an insect-control program of this scope without knowing precisely what damage the pesticide itself will do to both human and animal life, especially over a long period"; and then concludes by saying, "Some of the money Congress is now spending on this control program would be put to better use on projects studying just what the spread of toxic chemicals from the air will do to bird and animal life and reproduction, and to human health."[4]

The great tragedy is that in most instances these chemicals affect the body slowly, imperceptibly, and that, as a result, the great majority of people are not aware of their insidious effects. They continue blissful in their ignorance and when struck by ill health do not realize that these

[3] *J.A.M.A.*, August 29, 1959.
[4] "Putting Out the Fire Ant," *The New York Times*, January 8, 1958.

dangerous chemicals may have contributed to their breakdown.

## Why Only Cranberries?

Most persons undoubtedly remember the uproar emanating from the cranberry industry when the Department of Health, Education, and Welfare prohibited the sale of cranberries when some of them were found to contain aminotriazole, a chemical known to have cancer-producing effects.

*The New York Times*, in an editorial dealing with this question, pointed out that "tough as Secretary Flemming's announcement was on the cranberry industry, it called attention in the most dramatic way to the dangers inherent in the promiscuous use of toxic chemicals in American agriculture," and then continues by saying that "cranberries make up but an infinitesimal fraction of the foods produced in this country, which are touched in some degree by chemical insecticides, pesticides, additives, preservatives, etc., that do everything from changing the conditions of growth to changing the color of the finished product. It is a shocking thing that their use is permitted while we are still in ignorance of the long-range damage they may do," the editorial continues, and then states that "the size of the problem is suggested by the fact that since 1950 the volume of pesticides for agricultural control purposes has jumped six to seven times ... it is estimated that more than a billion pounds of chemical poisons are now being used annually on American farms.

"Experiments have already shown that serious harm is done by use of some of these chemicals to wildlife, and the fact is that nobody really knows yet just how harmful they may in the long run be to human life," the editorial concludes.

It should be evident that the hope that we can continue to use poisonous sprays without paying a penalty for it is a delusion, since the same poisons that kill the bugs can also kill us.

Following the cranberry episode, another additive used in the food industry, stilbestrol, a hormone used to force the growth of cattle and poultry, came into discussion. This hormone is injected in cattle and fowl to force a gain in weight. Since this hormone is also used as a treatment during the menopause, it would be well that physicians who persist in prescribing it bear in mind the statement presented at the Symposium on Medicated Feeds, 1956, by Granville Knight, W. Coda Martin, Rigaberto Iglesias, and William E. Smith, in which they pointed out that the "administration of estrogens, among which diethylstilbestrol is one of the most potent, has been responsible for a wide range of pathologic changes in human beings and in animals." They stated further that this remedy can induce polyps, fibroids, and cancers of the uterus, cancers of the cervix, cancers of the breast, hyperplasia of prostatic stroma and of endometrium, tumors of the testicle and hypophysis, and leukemias in mice, rats, and guinea pigs.[5]

As is usual in such matters, there were some who disagreed with this statement. Dr. Franz Gersner, Director of Endocrinology Research of Colorado A. & M., in questioning the view expressed by these authorities, called attention to the fact "that an appreciable amount of estrogens or their precursors are contained in green leafy vegetables and forage, such as lettuce, subterranean clover and alfalfa, and in grains such as soybeans, corn, and their by-products," and that "cereal grass pastures which are in the young, succulent stage of growth" are especially rich in them.

What Dr. Gersner seems to overlook is that there is quite a difference between the action of hormones that are an integral part of the food we eat and hormones isolated or extracted for use to stimulate or alter body metabolism. The hormones that are an integral part of the food we eat are utilized by the body to maintain normal metabolic functioning, while when taken as a specific or isolated element to alter or stimulate body metabolism, as is done when stilbestrol is used to increase the growth of cattle or poultry, or when used in the treatment of the menopause, has the effect of disrupting normal bodily functioning and can lead to an infinite number of serious disorders. Needless to say that when these hormones are of a synthetic nature, they are even more likely to be harmful.

The reason we do not succumb to the toxins or irritants

[5] In a paper entitled "Possible Cancer Hazards Presented by Feeding Diethystilbestrol in Cattle."

taken into the system or generated in the body as part of the metabolic processes is because the liver, the kidneys, the glands, as well as all other protective organs of the body, continue to counteract these poisons and in this way protect us against their harmful effects.

It should be apparent that to obtain the greatest amount of protection the body must at all times be kept in an optimum state of health, since only then can we be sure that our protective and defensive organs can do an effective job of detoxification and elimination and protect us against the harmful effects of these chemicals. This can only be done by following the way of life outlined in the pages of this encyclopedia.

At the same time, it is essential that we do not sit idly by and permit these evil practices to continue, since there is a limit to the burden that can be placed upon the protective mechanisms and the risk is ever present. Those who can possibly do so should try to obtain foods grown without chemical additives and in the most natural way, while nobody—and we mean nobody—should ever use the lifeless, denatured, and processed foods that crowd the shelves of our food markets. At the same time, we should also do all we possibly can to promote changes or modifications in agriculture and food manufacturing that will eliminate or at least lessen the prevailing dangerous practices. In the present artificial situation, eternal vigilance is imperative if we are to obtain at least a certain degree of protection.

## 14

## A RÉSUMÉ OF FACTS WORTH KNOWING

Prove all things; hold fast that which is good.
                                    I Thessalonians 5:21

As you have wound your way through the pages of this section, you have found a clear pattern unfolding itself. It discloses how faulty nutrition, unhealthy living habits, and emotional stresses lay the foundation for these disorders and how a change to wholesome natural foods and sound health-building measures promotes healing as well as the rebuilding of physical vigor and emotional stability.

Since the causes that lead to the onset of these diseases are basically alike, the changes that must be made to correct them are, therefore, to a great degree similar.

The differences depend primarily upon the characteristic variations that exist in the particular disease as well as in the individual case. We have seen that where the tissues are highly sensitive and sore or ulcerated, only soft, bland, nonirritating foods must be used at first, since the raw foods can be highly irritating. However, even then we insist that the diet provide all the essential food elements including the valuable vitamins, minerals, and enzymes.

This program takes you away from mere symptom-relieving measures and leads you in the direction of sound body and health rebuilding.

At this point, it is well to mention that while a disorder may express itself only in one organ, and while the suffering or discomforts may show up only in one part of the body, other organs or parts of the body are usually involved, although perhaps not to the same degree.

A complete diagnostic survey will disclose that sufferers from inflammation or ulcers of the stomach or gallbladder disease also often suffer from constipation; that gallbladder and liver disease often go together; and that the nerves play a vital part in practically all these diseases. This explains why, in our attempt to bring about correction, the care must not be limited merely to one organ but calls for a rehabilitation of the whole body.

## The Importance of Choosing the Right Doctor

While everybody will agree that it is important to choose the right doctor, the average individual does not always know whether the doctor who is in charge of the case is really acquainted with the procedures that provide permanent results and are most effective from the health-building point of view.

To make sure that you have chosen wisely, make sure that the doctor you have selected is not only acquainted with what ails you, but also understands how these ailments develop, as well as what adjustments have to be made if the condition is to be overcome or brought under control.

We must always bear in mind that all healing emanates from within the organism and is accomplished only when the recuperative powers within the body are helped in their effort to bring about recovery.

The experienced doctor understands how diseases originate and knows how they can be eradicated. He recognizes the need for wholesome nourishing foods, is aware of the importance of rest, sleep, and relaxation; and realizes that only a well-planned program of hygienic care can provide permanent results.

Furthermore, he makes certain that the patient acquires a complete grasp not only of what he must do to recover, but also how he must continue, to prevent a recurrence of ill health.

We are well aware that, in periods of stress or suffering, people usually turn to their doctor in the hope that he may be able to suggest some specific remedy to relieve their discomforts or pains.

The experienced doctor, however, knows that while certain remedies can temporarily relieve the distressing symptoms, they have no corrective value and, in the long run, only aggravate the damage.

Our aim should be to strive for complete recovery and this can only be achieved when a thorough health-building program as outlined here is followed.

The doctor who follows such a program is the only one who can provide real help, since he understands what must be done, and encourages his patient to make the necessary adjustments.

Many doctors are aware that wholesome food and careful living habits are essential if the functions of the digestive organs are to be rebuilt, but unfortunately either do not possess the necessary time or experience to encourage the patient to make the necessary changes or are unable to inspire him with sufficient confidence to follow through until full recovery is attained.

We must always remember that the mere knowledge of what is right is not enough and, furthermore, we must always bear in mind that to obtain the desired results, the correct thing must be done at the right time and in the right way.

### Health Within Your Reach

Everything has a beginning and so do digestive disorders. Most of these disorders begin almost imperceptibly, but keep building up, and when not checked in time or corrected, ultimately sprout into full-blown diseases. It is the story of the little acorn growing into a mighty oak, except that in this case it isn't the oak growing, but a weed that threatens the life-blood of the whole body.

We have pointed out that many of these cases are incorrectly diagnosed, and that this often leads to needless surgery with grave consequences to the patient. It is important to mention at this point that these mistakes are in most instances not the result of mere guesswork but are due to an incorrect interpretation of the findings, following intensive internal and external examinations.

We do not wish to imply that these work-ups serve no useful purpose. As a matter of fact they are often of great value, since when skillfully performed and properly evaluated they help eliminate fear and enable the doctor and the patient to plan a program most suitable in the particular case.

To arrive at the proper conclusions, however, the physician who performs these tests must not only possess the necessary proficiency to make a correct diagnosis, but must also possess the experience necessary to enable him to interpret the findings in line with what sound recuperative measures can accomplish to relieve the complaint.

## Present a Copy of This Volume to Your Doctor

Many doctors are under the impression that the patient is not happy unless something is prescribed for his ailment and, therefore, often write a prescription even when they think it is not needed. Some will use what is known in medical terminology as a placebo or a make-believe drug, while others will prescribe a remedy medically indicated in the case.

Let your doctor know that you are not interested in getting a prescription and that you want him to take care of you the natural way.

Even if your doctor is of the conventional medical school, he may be progressive enough to realize that a much better job can be done without medicine, and maybe happy to work along with you in this way. Remember that doctors are the children of Hippocrates, the father of medicine, who long ago proclaimed the curative powers of nature, and just a little prodding from you may bring your doctor back to the priceless heritage left to him many years ago by this great teacher.

If your doctor belongs to one of the newer professions that have developed in the last half century in response to a need, should he be naturopath, chiropractor, or osteopath, you should have even less difficulty, because these professions have come into existence as a revolt against the failure of the old school to follow the fundamental teachings of Hippocrates. Their approach is based on the philosophy that nature cures, and that the doctor must work with the vital powers of the body if he is to help the patient.

Always remember that the progressive doctor continues to learn new things all the time. There was a time when doctors minimized the importance of nutrition or disregarded it altogether, but, like Topsy's Eva, the value of nutrition has grown apace in recent years. Today, most doctors realize the need of excluding salt in certain diseases, many recognize the importance of eliminating the "hard" and processed fats, others stress the need of eating less, while many are becoming aware of the fact that the refined and processed foods, the so-called "empty" calories, are harmful.

Also, while hundreds of new drugs are being turned out yearly by the drug industry, doctors are becoming increasingly aware of their dangerous side-effects and their hazards to life.

In short, many doctors are getting ready for a re-evaluation of their *modus operandi* and of the great benefits that can be derived from a return to the fundamental principles of Hippocratic teachings.

## 15

## CONCLUSION

We are told that we are the richest and best fed nation in the world, and yet even the most superficial investigation will disclose that we have more sufferers from chronic and degenerative diseases than almost any other country in the world. Millions of our people suffer from headaches, sinus trouble, asthma, and other catarrhal diseases, while the number of sufferers from heart disease, high blood pressure, kidney trouble, arthritis, diabetes, and cancer is constantly on the increase. Diagnostic surveys will disclose that a great many of these victims also suffer from digestive disorders, and that these disorders either precede the more serious ailments or develop in conjunction with them. Furthermore, a few moments' thought should make us realize that they are usually closely interrelated.

### Why We Have Failed

The reason for our failure to establish a standard of health commensurate with the many advantages at our disposal should be apparent. Many persons are entirely unaware that the type of food we eat and our habits of living have anything to do with our state of health, while others are reluctant to make the changes suggested to them and hope that they can obtain help through the use of some drugs. Irrespective of whether you belong in the first or second category, it is well that you realize that a failure to uproot the underlying causes of disease will, in the long run, lead only to more disease and greater suffering.

### A Re-Evaluation Needed

It should be apparent that a re-evaluation in our management of disease is urgently needed and that the sooner this is brought about, the sooner will we discover the real path to health.

As far as the functions of the digestive organs are concerned, even though you receive only faint warnings that something is wrong, why wait until a more serious condition develops? Why not protect yourself by obtaining the guidance that you need to help you make the changes that are necessary to prevent further breakdown?

In the early stages these diseases can, in most instances, be easily overcome. A change to natural foods, good eating habits, and sound hygienic care will help restore the functions of the digestive system with little or no difficulty.

In the more severe or more chronic cases, more intensive care and patience may naturally be required, but even then it is well to realize that only by following a program based upon sound hygienic principles can lasting and effective results be attained.

Furthermore, this program if followed faithfully and consistently will protect the body against many of the other diseases from which individuals commonly suffer, and establish the foundation for vibrant health throughout life.

"The clean tongue, the clear head, and the bright eye are birthrights of each day," Dr. Osler once stated. These birthrights are yours to have, but the only way you can acquire them is when you follow a way of life that enables the body to maintain vital, vigorous health.

The knowledge about the digestive system and its disorders contained in this section can be your key to healthier digestion and a happier life. So too, by coming to understand the true causes of respiratory disorders, whether the common cold or acute pneumonia, will you be in a better position to protect yourself from their onset.

This valuable information is presented in the next section, as is a discussion of diabetes, a life-destroying disease, for which proper care and treatment is essential.

Section Two:

# DISEASES OF THE
# RESPIRATORY SYSTEM

## 1

# THE COMMON COLD

When we talk of the diseases of the respiratory system, the first disorder that comes to mind is the common cold. There is an old adage, often repeated facetiously, that a cold gets well without treatment in a week and with treatment in seven days.

This may sound like a mere aphorism but, in reality, it reveals much that is true about this common ailment. It says, first, that no remedy exists for it; second, that it is a self-limiting disease. In other words, if left alone and not complicated through neglect or wrong treatment, a "cold" will usually run its course and disappear.

When discussing this common disorder, a number of questions need clarification. The most obvious are: (1) What is a cold? (2) How is it caused? (3) What role do germs or viruses play in its development?

## How a Cold Develops

The answer to the first question should be obvious. A cold develops when the mucous membrane of the nasal passages and/or the other organs of the respiratory system have become inflamed and irritated by toxic waste products that have accumulated in the system, and must be eliminated.

To be in good health, the body must at all times discard its toxic waste products. Normally, the body throws off these toxins through the kidneys, the lungs, the skin, and the intestines. However, when it becomes overworked or exhausted or when it becomes overloaded with too many of these toxic by-products, the organs of elimination are unable to cope with all the work, and an excess accumulates in the system.

In a cold we have a running nose with a discharge of mucus; it is often accompanied by a cough, sometimes by fever, and the patient is usually greatly debilitated. These are merely the symptoms that show up when the toxins that could not be eliminated in the regular way are being eliminated through the nasal passages and/or the other respiratory organs.

In other words, the catarrhal symptoms that show up during a cold are merely a clearing process, or an attempt on the part of the organism to throw off toxins which, if retained in the system, would be inimical or dangerous to life.

Saying it differently, a cold is the tail end or end result of what is generally called an "infection," but is, in reality, an upset in body chemistry. A cold, therefore, actually serves a constructive purpose for it is the body's way of rectifying this imbalance.

To overcome a cold in the most effective way our aim, therefore, should be to aid the body to throw off its toxic waste products as rapidly as possible and to restore all its organs to normal functioning.

Turning to the second question, it should be evident that what we have said in clarification of the first question actually embraces, in part, the answer to the second. Anything that impairs or interferes with the normal eliminative functions of the body or causes an excess of toxins to accumulate in the system creates a chemical imbalance in the organism and contributes to the development of a cold.

Overfatigue is one factor. When the body becomes overtired, it cannot function efficiently; this slows up the function of the eliminative organs and ultimately builds a toxic condition that may result in a cold.

Chilling is another factor. When the body becomes chilled, the elimination through the skin is checked or retarded and the functions of the other eliminative organs also slow up. When this happens, the mucous membrane of the nasal passages and the other organs of the respiratory system are often called upon to compensate for the failure of the regular organs of elimination.

In connection with this, we wish to say that the same amount of exposure does not affect everybody alike. The weak or run-down person often becomes chilled easily and will develop a cold or other acute respiratory disorder, while the healthy person, one who possesses enough reserve power to make the necessary adjustments, will come through the same amount of exposure with little or no difficulty.

Overeating, the use of excessive quantities of rich and highly concentrate foods, as well as exposure to other distressing or irritating influences, impair the normal workings of the body, and may contribute to the development of a cold or other respiratory disorder.

## The Role of Germs or Viruses

The third question, "What role do viruses play in the development of a cold?" calls to mind the famous Shakespearean saying: "Full of sound and fury, signifying nothing."

To begin with, it is well to know that germs, per se, are not our enemies. Scientists know that micro-organisms (germs and viruses) and their host (the living body) normally live in harmony with one another. This harmonious relationship, known as the symbiosis of the body, exists as long as the body is in a healthy condition. It becomes upset when the body becomes weakened or toxic, and thereby loses the power to maintain the status quo.

In other words, the body and the micro-organisms that live in it keep each other in balance or live in harmony with one another, as long as the body is in a healthy condition.

Rene Dubos, a leading research scientist associated with the Rockefeller Foundation for Medical Research, refers to this relationship when he points out that all kinds of "bacteria such as tubercle bacilli, streptococci or staphylococci, many types of viruses potentially capable of producing influenza, intestinal disorders, and various forms of paralysis," as well as "all kinds of protozoa and worms," live in harmony, with the human body that is their host, and that an upset generally takes place only when something has gone wrong with the internal chemistry of the body.[1]

Once these facts are fully understood, the confusions and uncertainties that surround the simple cold are easily dispelled, and the measures that can help overcome it become obvious. We come to understand that a cold is the

[1] Rene Dubos, *The Mirage of Health.*

outgrowth of abuses that have interfered with the body's normal functioning and have disrupted the normal chemistry of the body, thereby creating the need for a vicarious type of elimination that will restore the normal balance or equilibrium of the organism.

This can easily be done. We simply must plan a program of care that promotes the elimination of toxins and restores the weakened or depleted organs to normal functioning capacity.

## Effective Care for Colds

The following is a plan that accomplishes this in the most effective way possible. We start by eliminating all solid food. We do this to cut down the work of the digestive organs and provide them with a period of rest. This also lessens the load on the eliminative organs, and gives them a chance to catch up with their work. Orange juice, grapefruit juice, apple juice, grape juice, hot lemonade sweetened gently with honey, or hot vegetable broth is permitted, but no solid food.

Then we suggest warm cleansing enemas to promote increased bowel elimination, and one or even two hot epsom salt baths a day to bring about increased elimination through the skin and kidneys.

Complete rest is wise. Complete bed rest is essential when a cold is accompanied by fever, but is of value even when fever is not present.

This is a most effective program for sufferers from this simple ailment, and usually helps them to overcome the disorder within a very short period of time.

After the cold has been conquered, the adoption of a well-regulated diet composed of wholesome natural foods and the adherence to sound health-building measures will strengthen the body and establish an optimum state of health.

## 2

## INFLUENZA

In the discussion of influenza, as in that of the simple cold, there is a great deal of talk of germs and viruses. However, from previous discussion it should be evident that the primary cause of this ailment is to be found in lowered bodily resistance and a disturbance of the body chemistry. We must never forget that germs are always with us, but that they multiply and become virulent only when the body has become greatly debilitated or has broken down as a result of stress, abuse, or deficiencies of various sorts.

Boyd, dealing with the question of infection in influenza, shows how little this point is understood when he explains that "some of the major questions regarding the disease still remain unanswered," and then emphasizes that "we are not certain how the infection is transmitted from one person to another, nor what is the exact nature of the disease."

He then refers to two remarkable experiments that were carried out in the United States where "every effort was made to convey the disease from patients to a large number of healthy volunteers who had never had influenza. The patient coughed in the faces of the volunteers, infected sputum was painted over the nasopharynx, blood was injected, but not a single volunteer developed the disease."

### Influenza: A Simple Disease

Influenza, too, is a simple disease and usually responds easily to proper care. Boyd quotes MacCallum to the effect that "no one ever died of influenza pure and simple." These cases become more serious when they develop into a severe acute bronchitis, bronchopneumonia, or some other complicating disorder. However, the use of the simple natural measures suggested in this volume will usually protect the patient against these complications and help promote rapid recovery.

Discussing the increased fatalities that occur during great epidemics, Boyd mentions that the "causal agent" at such times "takes on heightened virulence as surely it must ... after passage through countless bodies." However, it should be evident from earlier discussion that lowered body resistance, not germs or viruses, is the primary factor in this disease.

Furthermore, whenever a case of influenza ends in chronic damage or mortality, it well behooves those concerned to question whether the unfortunate results could not have been prevented if the measures advocated here had been employed.

When, not so very long ago, the American people were urged to submit to mass vaccination against the Asian flu, Dr. Thomas G. Ward, Associate Professor of the University of Notre Dame's Llobund Laboratories, who directed tests of the new vaccine for the U.S. Public Health Service, stated that he would not take the vaccine himself. He argued that Asian flu was a mild sickness and that he would rather build up immunity to the virus through exposure to a mild illness than accept the limited protection of the vaccine.

## How to Treat Influenza

At that time, we presented the following program as a most effective means of protecting the body against not only the Asian variety, but all types of influenza:[1]

1. Complete rest in bed until full recovery has taken place.

2. The elimination of all foods except diluted fruit juices or hot water flavored with lemon juice. Diluted orange, grapefruit, apple, pineapple, or grape juice is very pleasant.

3. The use of warm water cleansing enemas for the first

[1] Epidemics of influenza have come to be known under different names, such as Spanish influenza and Asian influenza, but it is well to bear in mind that all types of influenza are merely variations of the same type of disease and therefore require essentially the same type of care.

few days. The enemas should gradually be discontinued, as normal bowel action is restored and the acute condition is brought under control.

4. The use of hot epsom salt baths once or even twice a day; the patient to return to bed immediately after the hot bath, and cover well to induce perspiration.

5. The patient's room must be kept well ventilated and free of noise, and all excitement must be avoided.

6. The application of cold compresses (not ice) to the forehead to keep the head cool, and a hot water bottle or heating pad to the feet to keep them warm, are of great help. The Greek saying, "Keep your head cool, your stomach right, and your feet warm, and you will need no doctor" is particularly apt.

While we quote this proverb, we do not wish to imply that those who suffer from this disorder should not obtain competent professional care. Each case is an individual problem and should, therefore, receive careful attention. It is essential, however, that the doctor in charge of the case possess a thorough understanding of the body's recuperative powers and is thoroughly versed in sound physiologic practices.

After the acute stage has been brought under control, a wholesome, natural diet, plus a hygienic plan of living will strengthen and rebuild the body and protect it against future attacks.

# 3

## PNEUMONIA

Before entering into a full discussion of pneumonia, we must emphasize that many misconceptions exist in the public mind with regard to the success of modern-day treatment of this disease.

We have come to believe that pneumonia can be overcome with modern antibiotic therapy in a matter of a very few days, sometimes even in a day or two. However, this is not really true. No real case of pneumonia is completely overcome unless the massive inflammation that exists in this disease is completely eliminated. The antibiotics often suppress fever and the other symptoms of this disease, but this does not necessarily mean that the disease has really been overcome.

In pneumonia there is an extensive, massive inflammation of the lung with a severe degree of toxemia or poisoning, and fever.

At the onset of the disease the affected part or parts of the lung become inflamed and congested and start pouring out a thick sticky substance that fills up the soft spongelike air spaces in the lung. This sticky substance causes the affected part or parts of the lung to solidify and take on the appearance of a solid organ like the liver. However, because the solidified parts of the lung are engorged with blood, the color at first is red.

In about four or five days, the red color changes to gray. By this time, the solidified substance that filled up the air spaces has become even harder, and the lung is heavier than ever. The color has changed from red to gray because by that time the red blood cells have already disintegrated, and therefore the infiltrated material has lost its fresh appearance.

In the final stage, the solidified material begins to soften and liquefy, and then becomes absorbed. The congestion then clears up and the lung returns to its normal state.

The most marked characteristics of pneumonia are difficult and rapid breathing and high fever. Extreme debility is usually present, and jaundice sometimes complicates the picture.

## Major Types of Pneumonia

This disease has been classifed into various types, but there are really only two major forms: bronchopneumonia and lobar pneumonia.

Bronchopneumonia develops gradually, and usually shows up as a complication of influenza, bronchitis, measles, whooping cough, or even the common cold. In this type, only patches or spots of the affected lung are involved.

Lobar pneumonia usually develops suddenly. Its onset is marked by chills, fever, coughing, chest pains, and shortness of breath. Nausea, vomiting, diarrhea, and headaches also often accompany this condition. This type of pneumonia differs from bronchopneumonia in that the inflammation will involve a whole section or sections at once, rather than just spots.

Recovery varies with the case. In some cases, health returns by a gradual clearing up of the symptoms. In lobar pneumonia, however, the change is often sudden and dramatic. The patient may seem to be in grave peril and yet within a few hours may have passed the critical stage and be on the road to recovery.

Various complications increase the dangers in pneumonia. In some cases, resolution of the solidified mass may be incomplete; in others, the lung tissue may break down; while in some, matter of a purulent or pussy nature may form. This latter is the condition known as empyema. Pericarditis, an inflammation and thickening of the covering of the heart, and otitis media, an inflammation of the middle ear, are some of the other serious complications that may develop.

Pleurisy is present in almost all cases of pneumonia, and will tend to intensify the patient's suffering.

To determine the type of treatment that is best in these cases, it is imperative that we investigate the results that were obtained with the different forms of treatment that have been used in the last fifty years, and compare them with the results that can be obtained when measures are employed that aim at promoting detoxification, the rebuilding of bodily resistance, and the restoration of the body to its normal state.

The treatment of pneumonia has gone through a transformation in the last fifty years. At the turn of the century, treatment in pneumonia was directed primarily to the control of symptoms. This was known as supportive treatment. Aside from the use of oxygen, which is a great need in some cases, the other remedies then prescribed included narcotics to induce sleep and make the patient comfortable, and medicines to reduce fever, relieve pain, ease the cough, and support the heart.

## Reason for High Mortality

Mortality was extremely high in those days, and we cannot help but refer back to the statement of Dr. Sherman who, in his discussion of asthma, points out that "drugs that reduce anxiety, relieve insomnia, and suppress coughing may be physiological luxuries,"[1] which the sufferer from asthma can ill afford. When Dr. Sherman warned that asthma patients who are treated with drugs that suppress coughing and the other symptoms of the disease may drown in their own secretions, he actually described what often happened in pneumonia when similar suppressive drugs were used.

With regard to the other drugs, it should be obvious that remedies that induced sleep and made the patient more comfortable and/or masked the other symptoms of the disease, actually suppressed the defensive mechanism of the body, and deprived the patient of the only weapon he had with which he might have hoped to overcome it. This explains why so many of these cases developed serious complications, and why the mortality in those years was so high.

[1] We quote extensively from Dr. Sherman's report in our discussion of asthma. Readers may turn to those pages for a more complete picture of his views.

## Effects of Serum Therapy and Antibiotics

The introduction of serum therapy eliminated the use of many of the suppressive drugs and brought about a reduction in mortality. The sulfa drugs followed, but they caused many toxic side effects, and were ultimately replaced by the antibiotics. Today, pneumonia is treated primarily with antibiotics, although some doctors use the sulfa drugs as well as antibiotics. There is no question that the replacement of mass medication with the antibiotics brought about a considerable reduction in mortality.

It is well to stress at this point that antibiotics have no curative effect. They inhibit bacterial action and thereby check some of the symptoms of the disease, but the congestion still exists and the disease is not overcome until the material that has filled in the air spaces and has become solidified is finally resolved and absorbed.

It is, therefore, important that we realize that although antibiotic therapy is an improvement over previous treatments, it also acts as a suppressant and thereby interferes with the defense mechanism of the body, and this is undoubtedly the reason why the mortality, although materially reduced, is still frightening.

Doctors are becoming increasingly aware that antibiotics interfere with the defense mechanism of the body. A noted New York physician, with whom we discussed this point, hinted as much when he told us that doctors have come to realize that in pneumonia a variety of micro-organisms may be involved, and, therefore, they do not always rush in with antibiotics. They first have all the laboratory work done, a procedure that often takes two to three days to complete, and, in the meantime, give the patient's body a chance to mobilize its own defenses.

Controlled experiments have demonstrated that patients with pneumonia who are given a chance to develop their own natural immunities are much more comfortable during their illness, do not develop as many complications, and usually recover much more rapidly. Those cases, on the other hand, in which antibiotics have been used from the very beginning of the disease are usually subject to relapses, often develop serious complications, and usually take much longer to get well.

This may explain why the mortality from pneumonia has again shown a frightening uptrend in recent years. Alexander Rihm, Jr., executive secretary of the State Air Pollution Control Board, recently reported that New York City's pneumonia death rate "had risen from 31.5 for each 100,000 of population in 1949 to 50.6 in 1959." Mr. Rihm presented these figures in connection with a discussion of air pollution, but since the death rate in places where the air pollution is less has increased to practically the same extent, it should be evident that other factors were responsible. "In the eleven upstate cities of New York in the same period the pneumonia death rate rose from 23.9 to 38.9 while in the "non-metropolitan areas of the state where air pollution is lightest, the increase was from 16.9 to 29.2."[2]

The hazards of antibiotic therapy have been recognized for a long time, and proof of these dangers has been mounting at a rapid rate. Rushing in with antibiotics or any other antibacterial drugs often complicates the situation since while these remedies inhibit or destroy the bacteria supposedly responsible for the disease, they also inhibit or destroy the favorable micro-organisms and, undoubtedly, other living entities necessary to the maintenance of life and health, such as the enzymes, and possibly even our own cell structures.

It has been known for some time that the antibiotics, by inhibiting or destroying the favorable intestinal bacteria, lay the foundation for a great many serious intestinal disorders. The fact that they interfere with the body's efforts to cope with the disease by building up its own natural immunity is but another of their many evil effects, and only increases the danger in these cases.

When sulfa drugs are used in addition to the antibiotics, the risks are only multiplied. No wonder this type of therapy in pneumonia, although less life-destroying than the previous treatments with mass medication, still produces a frightening mortality.

[2] *The New York Times,* June 13, 1961.

## *Mortality Need Not Be High*

Osler, whose *Principles and Practice of Medicine* was first published in the latter part of the last century, stated that the mortality in those years was between 20 and 40 per cent, but then called attention to the fact that the death rate in the German army in over 40,000 cases was only 3.6 per cent.

We consider this highly significant, since it proves that the mortality from this disease need not be high when those who suffer from it possess good recuperative powers.

Pneumonia is dangerous to the old because they are usually greatly debilitated; to the alcoholic because of the damage that alcohol has done to the body; and to those who live a fast life and dissipate their natural reserves. It is also dangerous when it shows up in connection with some other serious disease such as heart disease, or when it develops as a complication after surgery.

## Proper Care in Pneumonia Cases

It is imperative that we recognize that the less the defensive mechanism of the body is interfered with, the greater the chances for recovery.

Now, what methods of treatment will not interfere with the body's defense mechanism, and will provide successful results in these cases?

At the onset it is important that we realize that good nursing is most essential in the treatment of this disease.

The patient must be kept quiet and relaxed, both physically and mentally, must be kept warm and comfortable, and must be protected against overexertion.

The sickroom must be well ventilated and must be kept clean and quiet. Visitors should not be allowed to visit the patient during the active stage of the illness.

The patient should be supplied freely with fluids. Hot or cold water whenever desired, plain or flavored with lemon juice, and diluted fruit juices are soothing and refreshing. No solid food should be allowed during the acute phase of the disease.

Constipation must be controlled. Daily enemas are of great help for this purpose.

Where the patient is not too weak, hot baths twice a day, for a few minutes at a time, are of great help. Following the baths, the patients should be wrapped in cool or tepid wet packs. These packs improve circulation, promote elimination through the skin, and make the patient more comfortable. The packs are left on for one to one and a half hours. The patient is then sponged off with tepid or cool water and made comfortable.

Where the patient is too weak for the full baths, hot mustard foot baths may be used, and the moist packs should then be applied.

In some cases, the use of Antiphlogistine poultices in place of the wet packs will be of great value. These poultices, applied over the whole chest, are changed twice daily, and are left on for 12 hours at a time.

The edict that the feet be kept comfortably warm and the head cool should be remembered, for these measures will add to the patient's comfort and induce relaxation.

Tepid or cool spongings also help to make the patient more comfortable.

For greater comfort, the patient may be propped up in bed; his position should be changed frequently.

In severe cases, oxygen may be necessary, and is often of great help.

This program, adjusted to the individual case, is carried on until the congestion has been resolved and the patient is out of danger.

Patients with some influenzal or borderline types of pneumonia may recover within a very few days. A massive type of lobar pneumonia, however, has to run its full course of consolidation, hepatization, and resolution, before the illness is completely overcome. In some cases of bronchopneumonia only small patches or spots may be involved, and cases of influenza or acute bronchitis may sometimes be mistakenly diagnosed as pneumonia. While these cases may respond quickly, they do not represent the pattern that is to be expected in the more massive types of pneumonia.

Following recovery, a bland diet composed of the wholesome natural foods should be gradually introduced to rebuild the patient's health and vitality.

When started in time, this program will often retard the development of pneumonia, and where this is impossible will lessen its severity. It will also help to bring about recovery without complications.

Since types of pneumonia vary with individual cases, it should be evident that the care cannot be applied in a stereotyped fashion, but must be adjusted to the needs of the individual case. This is why we emphasize that a physician must be consulted, and that the one selected should possess a thorough grasp of sound physiological principles, be fully aware of the dangers of suppression, and have the necessary skill and experience in the application of the measures here outlined.

### *A Case History:* FRANK H.

A single case history does not usually tell much. However, in view of his age at the time of his latest attack of pneumonia, and in view of his previous experiences with the disease, the case history of Frank H. is of more than ordinary significance.

Frank was seventy-six years old when he suffered from his last attack of pneumonia. This attack took place in 1960, while his two previous attacks were in 1944 and in 1950.

During his latest attack, the patient was gravely ill. His physician found an active process all over his chest. Frank was hardly able to breathe, and he was extremely weak and wasted. He was so sick that, in view of his age, the physician thought that he might be suffering from lung cancer.

To establish a diagnosis, he insisted that the patient be taken to the hospital for X-rays and other tests, and also requested that the services of a specialist be engaged for a complete diagnostic check-up. The specialist reported:

The present illness apparently was of about one month's duration with cough, fever, chills, and sputum. As you know, Mr. H. has been reluctant to accept medication and apparently saw no physician for this illness.

When I saw him on March 1, he was sitting up in bed, coughing, hoarse almost to the point of being unable to speak, thin and dehydrated. His lungs revealed fine rales at both bases, the left more marked than the right. He was breathing with the accessory muscles of respiration. There was marked fixation of the diaphragm bilaterally. Indirect laryngoscopy revealed his cords to move well but there was great dehydration of the oropharynx, tongue, and trachea. Mucopus was also present in the fauces. . . .

It was my impression that Mr. H. had rather far advanced pulmonary emphysema with chronic bronchitis and superimposed acute infection, probably acute bronchitis, and possibly bronchopneumonia. I suggested antibiotic therapy, which would be more sensibly given of course after obtaining sputum cultures. However, his insistence on going home may have made this impossible. . . .

I think the possibility of tumor is relatively slight. . . .

Frank H. remained at home and was treated with natural methods. After he had fully recovered—he became again as active and alert as he had ever been—we talked to the physician who had seen him, and who exclaimed: "Really remarkable! I never thought he would make it!"

In conclusion, we wish to append part of a note which we received from Mrs. H.:

This last time Frank had pneumonia we got the surprise of our life for even with the patient now being seventy-six years of age, recovery was speedier than previously when many kinds of drugs, given orally and with injections, were used. This time no medication of any kind was given. Treatment was with massage, hot mustard foot baths, Antiphlogistine chest poultices, and, most important, rest, and the simplest of food. Several days it was water only, then fruit juices.

This was in March, and in June the patient was doing some light work in the garden each day, such as hoeing and weeding. In August he took a trip to Nova Scotia, doing all the driving there and back for 1800 miles, the return trip of 900 miles being done in three days. He has been following your regime for living, has improved steadily, has not had an ache, cold or pain since.

## Acute and Chronic Sinusitis

The sinuses are the hollow spaces or cavities in the bones

of the head that surround the base of the nose. These spaces warm and moisten the air as it is inhaled, and also act as resonating chambers in speech formation.

When the sinuses become irritated and inflamed, the passages become engorged and blocked. This causes pressure and pain, which is often accompanied by excruciating headaches.

In chronic sinusitis, the mucous membrane of the sinuses usually swells and thickens. Polyps often form and a great deal of scar tissue will ultimately develop. A constant postnasal drip is a prevalent symptom in these cases.

Sinus conditions often show up as part of a simple cold or in connection with influenza, pneumonia, or any of the other acute or chronic respiratory disorders, such as bronchitis and bronchial asthma.

### Care in Acute Sinusitis

In acute sinusitis the same care as in any other acute respiratory disease is usually indicated.

Abstinence from food for a few days, warm cleansing enemas, and plenty of rest and sleep hasten the elimination of irritating and toxic waste products, and restore the tissues to a healthy condition. For local relief of pain, the application of heat to the back of the head and cold moist compresses (*not ice*) over the forehead are recommended. In some cases the use of hot, moist compresses over the forehead has a more soothing effect, and is therefore to be recommended in preference to the cold compresses.

After the acute stage is overcome, a carefully regulated nutritional program and adherence to a sound program of living will rebuild the vitality of the patient and protect against recurrences.

# 4

## BRONCHITIS

When the inflammatory condition of an acute cold or acute sinus condition extends into the bronchial tubes, we have what is known as acute bronchitis. In this condition the trachea and bronchial tubes become inflamed and swollen, causing severe paroxysms of coughing, and often high fever. Large quantities of sticky, stringy mucus are usually expelled. There are cases, however, where the cough is dry and little or no mucus is brought up. In these cases, the paroxysms of coughing are usually more severe and more debilitating.

It is well to stress at this point that a cough is an effort on the part of the tissues to loosen up and expel irritating material, and that as such it must be regarded as part of the defensive mechanism of the body. It should not be suppressed.

To overcome the irritating and annoying cough the toxic or irritating substances must be eliminated, and the inflammation must be overcome. This can be accomplished most effectively when measures are employed that improve the circulation and increase the functions of the other organs of elimination, such as the kidneys, skin, and intestines. The program outlined previously for the acute cold, acute sinusitis, or influenza is therefore also applicable in acute bronchitis. It is well to point out though that an acute bronchial disorder may take somewhat longer to overcome than the simpler respiratory acute ailment, and that, therefore, more patience and perseverance may be required.

In conjunction with this ailment, we also wish to reiterate that since drugs or remedies that have a suppressive effect only interfere with the defensive efforts of the body, they should never be used, since they will only lay the foundation for a chronic bronchitis or other chronic chest disorder.

## Chronic Bronchitis

Sufferers from chronic bronchitis usually have histories of frequently recurring colds, acute bronchial attacks, or other acute respiratory diseases. The more advanced catarrhal disorders often begin with a simple cold, and might never develop if the earlier and simpler condition had been treated in accordance with sound physiological principles.

The treatment of chronic bronchitis involves essentially the same procedure as the treatment of any other chronic catarrhal condition. The circulation must be improved, the elimination of toxins must be promoted, and the general health of the body must be rebuilt. This requires a bland, nonirritating alkaline diet composed primarily of the raw and steamed vegetables, raw and stewed fruit, plus moderate amounts of proteins, and the use of easily digestible vegetable carbohydrates such as the root vegetables and/or the baked or boiled potatoes.

Fat foods, refined and processed flour and sugar products, refined cereals, coffee, tea, spices, and condiments must be eliminated. These foods cause an acid residue that is highly irritating and provide little or none of the needed protective elements. Dairy products too are inadvisable in these cases and should be avoided or greatly restricted.

Whenever possible, complete abstinence from food, or at least from solid food, for a limited period of time is highly advisable.

An abundance of rest and sleep, hot epsom salt baths, and deep breathing, as well as other moderate physical exercises, are of great help in these cases.

When a program of this kind is initiated, improvement in most instances begins almost at once. The discharge of mucus may first increase, but before long is greatly reduced; and ultimately dries up completely. The paroxysms of coughing gradually diminish in severity and, in time, are completely overcome.

In some cases this care may at first lead to the onset of one or even several colds. This is not an indication that the patient is getting worse, but that the acute condition that has been suppressed is reawakening and that the toxins and irritants that have accumulated in the tissues and caused the existing damage are breaking up and are being eliminated. These reactions are merely nature's effort to convert the chronic ailment into an acute state, and should therefore be welcomed, since this is the way the body usually overcomes its chronic ailments.

After the chronic bronchial condition has been overcome, the adoption of a sound nutritional program and a plan of living in accordance with the principles stressed in this encyclopedia, will rebuild the strength and health of the body and protect against future catarrhal ailments.

## The Need for Real Prevention

The well-informed physician knows that fever arises as an effort on the part of the organism to counteract or overcome irritating or toxic influences and, as such, serves a constructive purpose.

Doctors are also becoming increasingly aware that it is to the best interests of the patient that the body be given a chance to work out its own natural immunity and to overcome disease by means of its own natural defenses, rather than turn to the use of suppressive measures. Many doctors who use the antibiotics or other symptom-suppressive drugs are not very certain now whether this is really the most advisable procedure. They find themselves in the somewhat anomalous position of the man who holds onto the tail of a lion and can't decide to let go.

We must never forget that the suppression of acute diseases in the earlier years of life is often responsible for the chronic and degenerative diseases that show up in later life.

We seriously question whether our reliance on drug or antibiotic therapy has contributed anything of lasting value to health, but the fact that new and more menacing infectious diseases are appearing on the horizon is now well known, and it might be advisable to ask whether our present-day approach to the treatment of disease is not to a great extent responsible for this.

In thinking of our present-day concept in connection with the treatment of disease, we are reminded of Krylov's fable, in which he tells of a hermit who was taking a walk with his friend the bear, and when he became tired, laid down to rest and fell asleep. While sleeping, a fly descended on his nose and the bear tried to chase it away. The fly, however, continued to return and the bear, in his anger, picked up a stone and hurled it at the fly, killing the fly, but also crushing the skull of the hermit.

## 5

## BRONCHIAL ASTHMA

Bronchial asthma is an agonizing and often extremely serious ailment. The struggle for air and the labored breathing are highly distressing and make the life of the patient a torture.

Patients with this disease are overly sensitive and extremely nervous, and may be markedly exhausted. To watch them struggle for air when in an attack is often heartrending.

The difficulty in asthma exists because of an interference with the expulsion of the air from the lungs, and this interference usually takes place in the smaller branches of the bronchial tubes. Normally these bronchial tubes and their branches expand to permit the intake of air and contract to expel it. However, when they become inflamed and congested or go into spasm they close up. This blocks the expulsion of air and upsets the whole mechanism of inspiration and expiration.

In more advanced cases the affected branches of the bronchial tubes become thickened, the mucoid glands become enlarged, and scar tissue forms. This causes a permanent narrowing of the small pipes through which air is inhaled and exhaled. The increase in the production of mucus further obstructs the opening through which air is carried in and out of the lungs. Hardened plugs of mucus often add to the difficulty.

In very severe cases, or those of very long standing, the deterioration may reach a point where the bronchial tubes shrivel up and atrophy. At this point the power to function normally is severely and often permanently damaged. Then, parts of the lungs may become stretched by the air that is trapped in them. The stretching of the lungs brought on by the strain of bronchial attacks is known as bronchial emphysema.

We cannot emphasize too strongly the fact that if the simple colds or other acute respiratory diseases that precede bronchial asthma were treated along the lines outlined in this section, the asthma would in most cases not develop; this holds true even where special hereditary weaknesses have created a predisposition to the illness.

## The Dangers of Medication

That drugs have failed in the treatment of these cases is only too evident. Ephedrine, adrenalin, and other similar symptom-relieving remedies used in the past, and in more recent years cortisone, have not helped in these cases so far as correction is concerned. These remedies actually create a more chronic ailment and often endanger the life of the patient.

That the drugs used in the treatment of this disease are dangerous and sometimes even destructive to life is well known.

Dr. William B. Sherman of the Department of Medicine, Columbia University, Medical College of Physicians and Surgeons, discussing this subject at the 107th annual convention of the American Medical Convention was quite emphatic about this. Dr. Sherman started the discussion by pointing out that morphine, regarded as one of the most effective drugs in the treatment of the various respiratory disorders, such as asthma and emphysema, provides relief primarily by depressing the nervous centers, and then explained that "it is as dangerous as it is effective" and that "the more serious the condition of the patient, the greater is the danger."

"Several authors have suggested that it is the principal cause of death in asthma," Dr. Sherman concluded.

Since the dangers of morphine are fully recognized, many doctors hesitate to use it and instead turn to demerol, the barbiturates, chloral hydrate, alcohol, ether by rectum, and tranquilizers. However, while the baneful effects of these drugs, according to Dr. Sherman, are not as obvious, they, too, can cause serious damage.

Discussing demerol, Dr. Sherman pointed out that "in some cases, two or three doses of 50 mg. each in the course of a few hours have produced serious respiratory depression and, occasionally *apparently contributed to a fatal outcome*," and then emphasized that when used in acute attacks of short duration, "caution should be observed because of the danger of habituation (habit formation)."

Continuing, Dr. Sherman discussed the intravenous use of large doses of amytal and luminal in a heroic effort to break up the spasm in the bronchial tubes of the sufferer from these disorders, but then explained that while these remedies provide momentary relief, they can actually kill the patient since these cases suffer from a vast accumulation of mucus in the bronchial tubes, and in their anesthetized state can die from asphyxia. He reiterated this point by calling attention to the "possibility that the exhausted and sedated patient may be suffocated by his own secretions," and then concluded by saying that "like any drowning man, he cannot afford the luxury of sound sleep until the danger is removed."

Dr. Sherman repeated the same warning when discussing the effect of sedatives to suppress or inhibit a cough, stating that "while frequent cough may be distressing and ineffective and may aggravate the dyspnea (the difficult breathing), it is basically a protective mechanism" and, therefore, should not be suppressed.

Commenting on the anti-biotics, Dr. Sherman pointed out that these drugs, especially penicillin, can cause severe allergic reactions and may, therefore, be very hazardous to any sufferer from asthma. He also called attention to the fact that these patients may also "have violent allergic reactions to such simple drugs as aspirin."

From all this, it should be clear why Dr. Sherman stated that "measures which merely relieve the symptoms often do so at the expense of suppressing the already inadequate protective mechanism and may actually increase the danger of respiratory failure," in other words, sometimes even kill the patient, and why, in summing up he emphasized the fact that "drugs that reduce anxiety, relieve insomnia, and suppress coughing may be physiological luxuries" which these sufferers can ill afford.

Cortisone and its related drugs such as hydrocortisone, corticotropin, prednisone and prednisolone, are also often used in this disease. We suggest that our readers turn to the discussion on these drugs in our section on arthritis, and they will then realize that the sooner these drugs are eliminated the safer will it be for the patient. They do not rectify the disease, and are not only hazardous to the body generally, but also turn the disease into a more serious state.

The task that confronts us in these cases should therefore be clear. If this ailment is to be overcome or be brought under control, the first step is to eliminate the chronic bronchial congestion and rebuild the tissues so that they can perform their functions of inhaling pure air and exhaling impure air without difficulty.

To accomplish this, a complete rebuilding of the organs that are involved becomes imperative.

*A Case History:* THE MOTHER OF EMMA S.

That this can be done in the great majority of cases has been well established. To illustrate how effective this method can be, we wish to quote from the story Emma S. tells of how her mother suffered from this agonizing affliction, and how she regained her health.

Emma S. has written:

Of all miserable illnesses inflicted on the human race, asthma is the worst. The constant gasping for breath and the choking sensation of wishing to inhale fresh air and being unable to do so are horrible to experience or witness.

My mother choked and suffered with asthma for twenty years and I was powerless to help her.

Since my childhood, I had seen my mother suffer, without of course understanding the nature of her illness. As I grew older I began to take interest in the procedures pursued by the various physicians who were called in to give my mother some relief from her attacks, and I became aware of the different methods employed in trying to restore her breath to normal. For a few days she would feel pretty good, and then quite suddenly the attacks would recur; as soon as one doctor's medicine would cease to help her my father immediately consulted another. This procedure went on for years and years.

It was suggested that she go away, and for weeks and months at a time I would not see her. The country air helped for a spell, but eventually the attacks would return.

Then we heard of a very eminent physician who was reputed to specialize principally in asthma. He came to see her, and immediately proceeded to give her tests to discover to what she was allergic. My mother's body was black and blue, due to the needles that were injected into her. After about 150 jabs it was definitely established that feathers made her susceptible to attacks. However, one cannot sleep on the floor so not much encouragement was given. . . .

The doctor could offer nothing in the line of medicine except adrenalin, and since he realized that quick aid was necessary when the attack occurred he instructed my father in the art of injecting the adrenalin by the hypodermic needle.

At that time I was too young to be able to do it, but after several years I was given the job of injections. Nights to me were nightmares—two and three times a night I would awaken to give my mother the only relief which science could offer, injections.

Her condition grew worse, and still there was no permanent relief in sight. The climax came when mother suddenly developed a terrific pain at the base of her spine. Then her life became so unbearable that it seemed nothing short of death would ease her suffering.

It became my duty to stay away from the office to take care of mother, as the rest of the family could not be spared from business. I did the best I could, and fed her all the nourishing food suggested by the doctor in order "to give her strength." Her diet included chicken, soup, bread and coffee. All day I was alone with her, listening to her cries of agony. Finally, on one occasion, I called in one of our neighbors to help me do something as the doctor would not come until later in the morning and I was at my wit's end.

Emma's neighbor was acquainted with natural methods. What she told Emma sounded strange and incredible, and yet since Emma did not know what else to do, she decided to induce her mother to try these methods. She arranged for an appointment with the same doctor who had cared for her neighbor when she had had a stroke, and took her mother to him.

We'll let Emma continue her story:

The doctor felt confident that mother would get well if natural methods were used and the use of medicine was halted. His method was simply to cleanse the body of all toxic material and then rebuild it with a proper diet, good care, and the use of natural treatments. When mother heard that all the food she loved would have to be given up (coffee, fish, meat, eggs, butter, cake, and spices), she lost interest.

Needless to say, the other members of the family were also opposed to this unheard-of and highly irregular approach.

My father, brother, sister-in-law, aunts, uncles and what have you, said that I would kill mother if I dared put her on a "starvation" diet; imagine living on fruit juices for days at a time and then on a fruit and vegetable diet without such "nourishing" foods as bread, cereals, coffee, and eggs.

But, Emma insisted that the natural method be tried.

The weeks of cleansing and rebuilding were no pleasant tasks; it was difficult; but mother cooperated with me to the best of her ability, and gradually results became apparent. Her wheezing left her, injections were no longer part of our daily routine, and her breathing became easier. She began to walk upright, not stooped. All these improvements tended to change my mother from a lifeless individual to a personality of strength and belief. In spite of her disbelief in the entire procedure and regardless of what she or anybody thought about it, she recovered completely and fully. Today she is enjoying excellent health.

We wish to conclude by saying that Mrs. S., who was about 60 years old when she commenced these treatments, lived an additional twenty years, and never, during all of that time, did she have a recurrence of the ailment.

## A Program for Recovery

What are the measures that were of such great help in the case of Emma's mother, and in other asthma cases?

The first step is to place the patients on a protective

health and body-building diet. Excluded are all refined and processed foods, all concentrated fat foods, all concentrated sweets, and all stimulants and irritants such as spices and condiments, coffee, tea, tobacco, and alcohol. Milk and other dairy products are also excluded, until the attacks have been brought under complete control.

In the beginning, these patients do best when they dispense with solid food altogether for one to three or even several days. Hot vegetable broth, some of the hot herb teas such as chamomile, alfa mint, sassafras, and linden flower tea flavored with lemon and honey, the juices of fully ripened oranges or grapefruit, or other fruit juices such as apple, grape, papaya, pineapple, diluted or whole, may be used, but no solid food.

Following this, a diet composed primarily of raw and stewed fruits, small portions of lean proteins, and easily digestible vegetable carbohydrates is best.

These patients must make sure to eat only small amounts of food at a time, to chew their food well, and to eat only when hungry.

Furthermore, since they are usually in a greatly weakened condition, they must obtain a great deal of rest and sleep, and slow down in all their activities.

These patients are usually highly emotional, and a change of pace toward more leisureliness and a greater degree of tranquility is essential. They must learn to talk slowly, to think more slowly, to breathe deeply, and to get themselves under control when tense or worried. This will not only help them to obtain better control of their emotions and modify the spasms that play a part in bringing on an attack, but will also add to their enjoyment of life.

Hot baths to promote more thorough skin and kidney elimination, and enemas if necessary to maintain adequate and thorough bowel elimination, as well as a regulated program of moderate physical exercises, are of great help in these cases.

It should be evident that, to obtain gratifying results, this program cannot be applied haphazardly. Skillful and experienced guidance is necessary and this is why, whenever possible, these patients should be under the care of a doctor or practitioner who specializes in this type of care.

## Asthma in Children

That some children are born with a predisposition to asthma is undeniable. In these cases, asthma and eczema sometimes appear together, or show up separately at different times. However, even where the predisposition to these ailments exists, a well-regulated nutritional program and care along sound physiological principles will usually provide complete protection and, in many cases, will in time eradicate the existing sensitivity and weakness.

We have demonstrated this on repeated occasions and the following case history is merely an example of how this can be done:

*A Case History:* LARRY Z.

The following is a report of Larry's case history as written by his mother:

When he was eight months old, Larry broke out with eczema in all his joints and on his face. After taking him to a series of doctors and trying all kinds of medication we found one doctor who said he would have to be cured by diet. He cut out all dairy products and gave Larry soy bean milk, rice products, fruits and vegetables. Within six months, the eczema disappeared.

At four, Larry started a hacking cough, and as soon as he would go into the sun his eyes would itch and burn and get pussy. Medication would help the cough and the eyes, but they were too strong to give him for more than a week, and he would soon start the coughing and experience the itching eyes again. When he started school at five and a half years old, the school nurse came to tell me that while Larry coughed as much as he did he would not be allowed in school. It took notes from three doctors saying that he had allergic bronchitis, which was not contagious, before they would allow him back in school. In spite of this he still missed a lot of school because he would be up during the night coughing so much he was too tired to get up for school in the morning.

When he was about six and a half years old, he had his

first asthmatic attack. The doctors prescribed more medication. They advised removing his tonsils, and gave him 124 allergy tests. I asked whether a change of diet would help, and all said no, although Larry was about 20 pounds overweight.

Finally, we decided to take him to a doctor who used natural methods. After one day on this doctor's diet, Larry had his first full night's sleep in months. Within one month his cough had almost completely disappeared. In the first two and a half months we took him to that doctor he didn't miss a day of school. We had had to give him a pocket full of tissues because he would sneeze and cough up so much mucus that the teacher and children would turn away in disgust. Subsequently, I gave him one tissue at the beginning of the week and at the end of the week it was still unused.

Larry lost many pounds and became much more mentally alert. Neighbors told me that, not knowing he was on a diet, they offered him pretzels or candy or cookies and he told them he was on a diet and could not have any. He realized himself how much better he felt and wanted to stay on the diet.

When Larry had been on his diet for only a month he started coming home from school saying, "Mommy my brain is working so much better now."

By now, Larry's catarrhal condition had cleared up, and his patches of eczema had completely disappeared. His skin in the eczematous areas, formerly coarse, rough, and thickened, had become as soft and smooth as the skin of a healthy youngster should be.

His parents were truly happy and grateful, and it was interesting to hear the boy say that he planned to always take care of himself, since he did not want to be sick the way he was before. He would, he said, grow up to be a healthy man.

## 6

## ALLERGY AND THE RESPIRATORY DISEASES

Many of the diseases of the respiratory system such as colds, catarrh, asthma, and hay fever are blamed on allergy. The term allergy, however, does not really tell what is wrong with the patient. It suggests that a hypersensitivity to certain foods or substances such as pollen, drugs, or chemicals exists, but fails to explain how this oversensitivity has developed and what can be done for it.

Since drugs or chemicals are generally toxic, they may prove harmful even to the healthiest person, and should, therefore, be avoided. However, oversensitivity to a food that normally should not be irritating or toxic, or to changes of atmosphere or substances in the normal environment, indicates a special weakness or sensitivity that needs correction.

Interestingly, an allergic patient may be sensitive to a specific food or element on some days and not be sensitive to it on others. Too, the patient may be sensitive to a food when taking it in combination with other foods and not be sensitive to it when it is taken alone; as, for example, he may be sensitive to grapefruit with sugar, and not be sensitive to it by itself.

We remember the case of a young asthma patient who was subjected to all kinds of tests and finally was told that among other things he was sensitive to grapefruit and must not touch it. We took him off all *other* foods and placed him on nothing but grapefruit for three days. Returning to see us, he told us that those three days had been the best days he had in years; that where formerly the nights were a nightmare, he was able to sleep through the nights and was free of his attacks.

Needless to say, he followed faithfully the program we outlined for him, and ultimately made a fine recovery.

Allergy is often blamed for recurrent colds, for acute sinus or bronchial attacks, for the existence of asthma. This term, however, is also often applied to various skin disorders, such as hives, eczema, etc., and is also sometimes used to explain the existence of certain digestive disorders or other bodily pains or reactions.

Whenever starting the care of a patient suffering from some type of allergy, the offending elements should, of course, whenever possible be avoided. However, it is well to know that this is not the real answer to the problem, since the real task is to strengthen and rebuild the sensitive tissues so that the tendency to react unnaturally can be overcome.

Infants born with a tendency to catarrh or any other hypersensitive condition do best when they are breast-fed. Where this is not possible, a careful feeding program must be inaugurated from the very beginning. All grain foods, concentrated fats, and concentrated sugars should be avoided in the feeding of these infants. Since these children are usually also oversensitive to cow's milk, goat's milk, soybean milk, or almond milk is usually recommended. Raw and stewed fruits, raw and steamed vegetables, baked potatoes, brown rice, bananas, avocados, and other bland foods should gradually be added to the diet of these children, and should come to make up the bulk of their meals.

## Hay Fever

Hay fever is another link in the catarrhal chain that is often blamed on allergy. This ailment often shows up when earlier or acute colds and catarrhs have been suppressed, and, while it has proved intractable to conventional medical treatments, it can usually be overcome when the methods outlined here are employed.

It is imperative to realize, however, that a great deal of patience may be required. While the milder cases often show excellent results within a few months, the more difficult and severe cases may take more than one season before lasting benefits are attained.

In these cases the care should be started well in advance of the acute hay fever season and should be followed as a regular program of living until the disorder is brought under complete control.

These patients must also remember that, even after full

recovery, a return to the unhealthy habits of the past will be highly inadvisable since this is the surest way to bring about a return of the condition.

## Basic Causes of Respiratory Diseases

Fatigue is a great factor in causing colds, influenza, pneumonia and all the other catarrhal disorders. When the body is overtired its eliminative functions slow down and then the nasal passages, the sinuses and bronchial tubes, or some acute fever disease such as influenza, is called upon by the body defenses to take over the task of restoring the body to its normal condition.

When these conditions are treated in accordance with sound physiologic principles, health is restored and all that is required to maintain it, is to continue to follow a healthy way of living.

Where these conditions are suppressed, however, the acute respiratory disorders are bound to recur, while chronic diseases such as chronic bronchitis, asthma, hay fever, or some other chronic disorder is the ultimate outcome.

Overeating is another factor that ultimately leads to the development of these disorders. Overeating overloads the digestive system and causes the accumulation of an excessive amount of waste material which, in time, overtaxes the eliminative organs of the body. When these organs become overworked, other channels of elimination must take over the task of maintaining the inner cleanliness of the fluids and tissues of the body.

The excessive use of concentrated and fat foods such as cream, butter, eggs, the fat cheeses, the fat meats and fish, the gravies and sauces, also overload the digestive and eliminative organs and, in time, lead to the development of recurrent colds or other catarrhal disorders.

Refined and processed foods such as the white flour and white sugar products, the refined cereals, spaghetti, macaroni, white rice, puddings, cakes, pastries, pies, sweets of all kind, also play a part in unbalancing the internal chemistry of the body and lay the foundation for frequent colds and catarrhs.

Smoking, drinking, the use of coffee and tea, as well as

sharp and irritating spices and condiments, cause irritation to the delicate membranes and tissues of the internal organs and call forth the secretion of mucus in an attempt to expel these irritating substances.

All these influences, singly or in combination, contribute to the development of the various acute and chronic catarrhal disorders as well as influenza and other so-called acute infectious diseases and, furthermore, often lay the foundation for the various catarrhal or inflammatory conditions that affect the digestive system, such as catarrh of the stomach, spastic or ulcerative colitis, or catarrh of the gallbladder.

Undue exposure is also a factor that often plays a part in the onset of acute respiratory disorders. Chilling of the body checks or interferes with normal skin functioning and, furthermore, has a fatiguing effect on the other organs of elimination, and this reduces their ability to eliminate the waste materials from the system. The mucous membrane of the nasal passages and other respiratory organs must then take over.

## Lymphatic Glands in Respiratory Diseases

A point seldom realized is that the lymphatic system is an essential part of the defense mechanism of the body and plays a vital role in combating these diseases. One of the primary functions of these glands is to neutralize and carry off toxins that accumulate in the system and cannot be eliminated in another way. When they become overburdened with work they become swollen and ultimately break down.

This is why children who suffer from swollen or diseased tonsils and adenoids or from swollen neck glands, are often also subject to frequent colds and other catarrhal disorders.

The superficial view held in the past has been that tonsils and adenoids become infected from without, and this view gave rise to an orgy of surgery for tonsils and adenoids, under the mistaken idea that, by removing the swollen or infected glands, the channels through which infection sets in are being eliminated.

It is a sad commentary that so many fail to understand

that infection usually originates from within and not from without.

## A Summary of Facts Worth Remembering

The best way to take care of a cold or any other catarrhal disorder is to start by eliminating solid food for a day or two, or even several days. Juices, hot lemonade, and hot vegetable broth are permitted but no solid food should be taken. Abstention from food is essential when fever is present, but is also advisable, as a good start, in all chronic catarrhal disorders.

Following the fast, a diet of raw and steamed vegetables, raw and stewed fruits, with a moderate use of the easily digestible lean protein foods and the easily digestible vegetable carbohydrates, is usually recommended. This diet may vary in accordance with the individual case, and it is because of this that we stress that, where at all possible, these patients should be under competent professional care.

This program, adjusted to the individual case, will work wonders. However, for maximum and permanent results, consistency and patience are essential.

## Section Three:

# DIABETES: A METABOLIC DISORDER

# 1

## WHAT WE KNOW ABOUT DIABETES

Boyd writes: "The more we know about diabetes, the less we seem to understand it."[1]

While this does not sound too promising, the disease is not really as mysterious as it seems. It is well known that diabetes is a disorder of carbohydrate (starch and sugar) metabolism. However, it must not be overlooked that carbohydrate metabolism is only one phase of general metabolism and that, to obtain most desirable results in diabetes cases, not only must control of the carbohydrate disorder be restored, but the general metabolism must be rebuilt.

While diabetes has, in the past, been thought to be primarily the result of a disorder of some specialized cells of the pancreas (the islands of Langerhans), it is now well known that the liver, the nervous system, and the glands of the entire endocrine system, including the thyroid, the adrenals, and the pituitary gland are also usually involved. The portion of the brain known as the hypothalamus also plays an important role in this disease.

As a matter of fact, in some cases the disease may show up even when the pancreas is in an apparently normal condition. The pancreas may be able to secrete the insulin needed for normal carbohydrate metabolism, and yet some other factor may interfere with its complete or effective utilization. Boyd's statement that in the obese, middle-aged person, the liver may lose the power to store glycogen is particularly relevant in this respect. On the other hand, the pancreas may sometimes be found to be scarred and damaged, with calcified areas that have resulted from a previous inflammatory condition, and yet no diabetes may be present.

Under normal conditions, the starches and/or sugars (known as the carbohydrates) are first converted into glucose (grape sugar), and then carried by the bloodstream

[1] *Pathology for the Physician.*

to the liver, where they are stored in the form of glycogen for future use.

In diabetes, this function has become impaired, and as a result large amounts of sugar accumulate in the blood and spill over into the urine.

Some of the important symptoms associated with this disease are excessive thirst, a ravenous appetite, the passage of large quantities of urine, frequency of urination, loss of weight or obesity, depending upon the patient's age, the extent and duration of his illness, and his general physical condition.

Visual disturbances, as well as disorders of the circulation, the nervous system, and the skin are some of the later metabolic disorders that may show up in this disease. It is well known that sufferers from diabetes often suffer from a number of metabolic disorders, such as hardening of the arteries, cataracts, and hemorrhages in the eyes. Arthritis and gallbladder and kidney disorders also often accompany it. Sufferers from diabetes are also easily subject to infectious diseases and are, as a rule, prone to coronary disease.

Gangrene is one of the complications that often shows up in the more adavnced cases.

One of the points that must always be kept in mind in connection with diabetes is that an impairment in sugar metabolism leads to an impairment in fat metabolism, and this often creates a severe problem since it causes the formation of incomplete metabolic end products such as acetone and diacetic acid, which may accumulate in the blood. These metabolic end products often cause an acid intoxication and endanger the life of the patient.

Dr. B. A. Houssay, a leading authority on this disease, expressed this very ably when he stated that in diabetes "there is not only a disturbance of carbohydrate metabolism but of the whole metabolism, the metabolism of protein and the metabolism of fat." He reiterated this point by saying that "diabetes is not a disturbance of one metabolism; it is a disturbance of the whole metabolism and the whole balance of hormones."[2]

In connection with this, we cannot help recalling the

[2] *Symposium 1954*, "Newer Concepts of the Causes and Treatment of Diabetes Mellitus."

time when, to counteract loss of weight, sufferers from this disease were urged to eat a great many fat foods, such as butter, cream, and eggs. It is fortunate that doctors now realize that these highly concentrated foods can play havoc with sufferers from this disease and that, therefore, they should be excluded.

Many years ago we emphasized the fact that diabetes is the outgrowth of a disorder of the general over-all metabolism; all the facts that have come to light more recently only confirm this view.

## The Discovery of Insulin

Many of us still remember the hope and enthusiasm with which the discovery of insulin was greeted. When in 1922 Banting, Best, and Collip gave to the world their discovery of this remedy, both sufferers and doctors alike hoped that here at last was the solution to the diabetic problem.

Today, it is well known that this problem has been far from solved and that the most that insulin can do is to control the symptoms of the disease, while even this is often fraught with uncertainties and danger.

## The Findings of Dr. Somogyi

As a matter of fact, it is now becoming increasingly clear that the use of insulin often converts a simple or mild type of diabetes into a more severe and chronic condition.

The observations of Dr. Michael Somogyi[3] and his associates at the Jewish Hospital of St. Louis, Mo., are of interest at this point. In a report made public before the American Chemical Society, Dr. Somogyi pointed out that a study of 4,000 diabetic cases conducted by him and his associates over a period of fourteen years revealed that virtually all adult victims of diabetes can be restored to normal health without insulin injections, and that "Even the less than 1% of the adult diabetics who still require insulin can get along with 20 units a day or less instead of 50 to as high as 150 units daily now taken by a large

[3] *The New York Times,* September 19, 1949.

number of diabetic victims under present methods of treatment."

Dr. Somogyi then continued by asserting that when insulin is used in doses that lower the sugar below normal, it actually increased the severity of the disease, because it creates what he calls a state of "chronic insulin poisoning." This happens because:

Large doses of insulin lead to unbalancing of the delicately adjusted glandular system, particularly the pituitary gland at the base of the skull and the cortex of the adrenal gland above the kidneys.

These glands work in unison, along with the insulin-secreting pancreas, to maintain the blood-sugar level on an even keel. When too much insulin is given, it leads to a lowering of the blood sugar to a level below normal. This, in turn, activates the pituitary-adrenal system to elevate the blood sugar back to normal. . . .

The patient whose body is the scene of such a tug-of-war becomes a severe diabetic, a victim of a form of poisoning in which insulin, administered to reduce the blood-sugar level, indirectly but inevitably raises it.

## Insulin Shock

Insulin has not been without its accomplishments. By controlling excess sugar in the blood, it protects against diabetic coma. On the other hand, its use must be balanced by a carefully controlled carbohydrate intake to guard against insulin shock. Insulin shock develops when the sugar in the blood is reduced to an extremely low level. When this happens, a food that will provide sugar in a quickly absorbable form—plain sugar, orange juice, or some other sweet food—is taken to raise the sugar level in the blood.

Dealing with this point, Boyd states:

The diabetic under modern treatment is not likely to die of diabetic coma. He lives for many years and then dies from what are called complications, but are really late manifestations of the upset in metabolism which is the essence of the disease. . . .

Amongst the most important of these late results are

the renal (kidney) lesions, for the danger of death from diabetic coma has been replaced by the danger of death from renal (kidney) failure.[4]

## The Discovery of New Remedies

In the last few years several new remedies, to be taken by mouth, have been developed. Two of them, one known as tolbutamide (Orinase), and the other as chlorpropamide (Diabinese) are sulfa preparations. Another is a somewhat different chemical composition, and is known as DBI. These remedies, too, provide a certain measure of control, but have no effect as far as lasting results are concerned, and sometimes lead to serious complications.

## The Metabolic Functions Must Be Rebuilt

From all that we have stated above, it should be clear that if the sufferer from diabetes is to obtain real help, it is not enough that the symptoms of the disease be relieved; metabolic disorders that have led to the impairment of the sugar metabolism must be restored to as near normal as possible.

That this can be done in the great majority of cases has been repeatedly demonstrated.

*A Case History:* MRS. S. O.

To illustrate how this can be accomplished, we can do no better than present a few case histories. We shall begin with the case of Mrs. S. O.

By the time she was fifty-four, Mrs. S. O. had been ailing for many years. Then, when she was checked for an infected toe, doctors informed her that she was suffering from diabetes. To counteract the condition she was treated with Orinase, and while at first this helped to clear up the infection, it later recurred all over again.

She complained of severe pains in different parts of her body and of frequent abdominal pains and nausea, while

[4] *Pathology for the Physician.*

an extremely large goiter, pressing on the trachea, made her feel as if she were constantly choking.

Examination disclosed that Mrs. S. O. was a woman who weighted 206 pounds, had a blood pressure of 180 /64, and an extremely rapid heartbeat that galloped at the rate of 150-160 beats per minute (evidently this was due to a thyrotoxic condition, superimposed on the simple large goiter). To control the toxic goiter the patient was taking "thyroid pills" daily. What seemed to be of greatest concern to her, though, was that she was gradually losing all feeling in her legs. She was suffering from a sort of creeping paralysis from the hips down, which deprived her of stability, control, and the ability to walk.

With her son on one side and her brother-in-law on the other, she had had to be practically carried up the steps into our office. There, when we examined her for reflexes, none could be elicited from the right leg and hardly any from the left.

The following is the diet that this patient had been following while taking Orinase:

BREAKFAST    1.  Cornflakes or oatmeal with milk    2. One or two eggs    3.  Coffee    4.  Slice of buttered bread

LUNCH    1.  Meat or cheese sandwich    2.  Cooked vegetables    3.  Coffee

DINNER    1.  Raw vegetable salad    2.  Meat    3. Cooked vegetables    4.  Coffee or tea    5.  Jello or cake on occasions

She had also been taking coffee and cake between meals, but had recently switched to apples or bananas for her snacks.

## Program of Care

The first aim in the case of a patient suffering from this disease should be to awaken the body's own metabolic powers and promote its own functioning, or at least to help it to make a good start in this direction. To accomplish this, all extraneous influences, such as insulin or any of the other drugs commonly used in this condition should, whenever possible, be discontinued.

As a next step, a diet that provides all the necessary nutritional and protective elements to promote rebuilding is important.

In line with these precepts, Mrs. S. O. was taken off all medication and was placed on a carefully regulated dietary program. At first, she was advised to take half a grapefruit every two hours until evening, and then eat one solid meal, composed of about the following foods:

1. Large raw vegetable salad
2. Small portion of cottage cheese or farmer's cheese, or any lean meat, fish, or chicken
3. One or two of the following vegetables steamed, and eaten without salt or butter: string beans, squash, eggplant, artichoke, celery, broccoli, kale
4. Half grapefruit

This menu was carried out for several days and was then followed by a more complete diet that provided all the essential nutritional and protective elements needed for the maintenance of health and proper rebuilding. The following is an outline of the diet suggested:

BREAKFAST    Half grapefruit or raw apple, four or five ounces of cottage cheese, and one slice of whole wheat toast

NOON    1. Large raw vegetable salad    2. Two steamed vegetables or one baked potato and one steamed vegetable

EVENING    1. Large vegetable salad    2. Cottage cheese, pot cheese, farmer's cheese, or lean meat, chicken or fish    3. One or two steamed vegetables    4. Half grapefruit

Salt as well as all other condiments and all fats were eliminated from the diet, and neither coffee nor tea was permitted.

In addition to the diet, a program of general care to promote general rehabilitation was outlined. This program included the use of hot mineral baths every night before retiring; an abundance of rest and plenty of sleep; relaxation after each meal; and a long nap every day after lunch.

The patient was also urged to limit her activities, to get into the habit of doing everything slowly, to avoid tensions and excitements, and to prevent chilling of the body by keeping her feet warm.

To observe the results, blood tests were taken regularly and the patient was instructed to test her own urine daily for sugar and acetone and to keep a chart of her findings.

## Medical Report

Loss of weight was at first rather rapid, owing to the thyrotoxic influences and the withdrawal of the thyroid depressive pills. Because of this, we were rather concerned and insisted that she submit to a complete physical checkup at the hands of a well-known New York diagnostician. His report stated:

X-rays of the neck reveal marked deviation of the trachea from the midline to the right by the goiterous masses on the left side. There is also evidence of shifting of the mediastinum to the right due to the sub-sternal thyroid enlargement. An elongated calcified blood vessel on the right side of the neck is evidence of inflammatory processes.

The heart is mildly enlarged in all diameters. There is widespread osteoarthritis change throughout the cervical and thoracic vertebrae. The basal metabolism is markedly elevated and since the heart rate is rapid and the cholesterol level is below normal, it is evidence of a thyrotoxic process superimposed upon a colloid goiter. This frequently is a complication of such enlargements of the thyroid gland.

The fasting blood sugar was 250 mg. The tests for liver function as yet show no marked liver damage, although the presence of diabetes is presumptive evidence of liver dysfunction. This is confirmed by the rapid sedimentation rate.

This combination of thyroid and diabetic diseases requires not only expert dietetic regulation, but if excessive loss of weight continues, especially when signs of ketosis begin to appear, the introduction of insulin therapy is imperative to prevent irreversible changes in the central nervous system and the rest of the body, particularly since this patient has well established neuropathy due to the diabetes and muscular weaknesses due to the thyrotoxicosis.

Before long, the rapid loss of weight was checked. Her weight ultimately stabilized at around 165 pounds.

So far as Mrs. S. O.'s general health was concerned, we are happy to state that her diabetic condition improved almost from the very beginning, and came under complete control without requiring further use of insulin or any of the other remedies now being prescribed in these cases. Her blood pressure was reduced to about 150/76, her heartbeat came down to about 84-86 per minute, and what may seem almost unbelievable, her large and massive goiter shrunk considerably.

So far as her inability to walk is concerned, it is interesting to note that although there was at first a question whether this condition could be reversed, since the degree of deterioration could not be exactly determined, it is gratifying to report that as her general health improved, this condition too gradually improved as well. Today she is able to walk in the same way as any other normally healthy person, and it should not be necessary to state that she is highly elated about it.

When, during the early stages of the treatment, tests showed the presence of sugar in the urine, the patient was urged to omit solid food for a day or two. Thus, the condition was quickly normalized. As a precaution the patient continues the tests, but no recurrence of sugar in the urine has been noted. She eats liberally. She is now carrying on an active life and is able to work in the same way as she did before she became ill.

### Mrs. O's Report

The following is an excerpt from a letter in which the patient describes her experiences and the results she realized from following this program:

The first six weeks of natural treatment were the hardest because of the drastic change in diet and because of the elimination of medicine which was taken in large doses before. In the first week, I lost approximately 19 pounds which made me very weak and tired. However, as the loss of weight tapered off I regained my strength, my headaches disappeared and my health in general started to improve so much so that my attitude also changed.

I continued on the grapefruit, salad & steamed vegetable diet including fresh fruits and as I progressed additional foods were included.

When treatment started, I had no feelings in my legs and feet. After the first six weeks I noticed a remarkable change: I was able to move my toes. Gradually, my legs felt more relaxed and movement was made easier.

Two months after my first treatment, I was able to get out of a chair without assistance. About 4 months later, I noticed a great improvement because I was able to walk up the stairs at a normal stride. At this point, I realized how effective the treatments were, and at this writing I am more than satisfied because I can lead a more normal life without depending on the help of my family & others.

One day recently my daughter went to the drugstore, and the druggist asked her if her mother had died because we were not buying any more medicines, as before. He was a most surprised man and to this day can't believe that I, who was so sick with so many sicknesses, am able and well enough to do my own shopping and many household duties which I haven't been able to do before.

*A Case History:* GUS E.

Gus E.'s case also illustrates the benefits that can be derived from this type of care. This patient began to suffer from visual difficulties and went to an eye doctor for consultation. The examination revealed that he was developing cataracts and was also suffering from diabetes. Insulin was advised and he was instructed to return later for another examination for the eyes to find out when the cataract would be "ripe" for surgery.

The patient's wife, however, had had a certain amount of experience with the methods advocated here and therefore insisted that Gus try these methods before doing anything else.

This was about fifteen years ago. Gus was willing, and conscientiously followed the program that was outlined for him. When he started, he was in the early fifties. Today he is about sixty-seven. During all this time, he never had any need for insulin or any other diabetic remedy, and his cataracts have not only not matured to the point where they became ready for surgery, but his vision has actually improved. During all these years he continued to run his business, and he is still as active and alert as ever. The type of diet that Gus is following at present is described:

BREAKFAST    1.  Raw apple or peaches or blueberries in season    2.  One slice of whole wheat toast (without butter)    3.  One glass of raw skimmed milk

LUNCH    1.  Large raw vegetable salad    2.  Baked potato and one or two steamed vegetables

DINNER    1.  Large raw vegetable salad    2.  Four to six ounces of bland soft cheese, chicken, lean fish, lamb chop, or any other lean meat    3.  One or two steamed vegetables    4.  Half grapefruit, berries, or fresh peaches for dessert

Between meals, he is permitted to take grapefruit, blueberries, or peaches when they are in season. His wife says that Gus eats rather liberally, and never goes hungry.

On Sundays, when they go out for dinner, he can hardly wait until he gets his large steak, which is garnished with a plateful of raw vegetables. He tops off his meal with either a grapefruit or berries.

We do not mean to imply that at times Gus's sugar did not go up to above normal. Sometimes he would go on a binge and for days or weeks would eat much more than his body could handle. The periodic blood tests, however, would warn him that he had overstepped his bounds, and he would retrench, thus bringing his blood sugar down to within normal limits. He continues to be a vital and vigorous human being.

Thus, with countless other cases of diabetes that we have observed over a great many years, as with Gus E. and Mrs. O. S., a carefully regulated nutritional program and a hygienic way of living adopted to the requirements of the individual case have provided excellent results for many adults suffering from this disease. This has been true even in cases where the disease was of great intensity and even where insulin and other diabetic treatments had already been used for many years.

Occasionally, the disease may be of such a severe nature that insulin can be reduced only gradually, but these cases are rare. The plan in these cases should be to start with a well regulated diet and a sound program of living, and then reduce the insulin by degrees as the general health of the patient, and with it a more normal sugar metabolism, is re-established.

## A Difficult Case: ALICE B.

That some cases present difficulties is without question. This is especially true in the unstable or brittle type of the disease. It should be evident, that to obtain real results, these cases require much more than the use of a remedy that temporarily neutralizes the sugar in the blood.

We are thinking of the case of Alice B., who once showed a blood sugar of over 300 while taking large doses of DBI. She was extremely weak and debilitated, and so emaciated that she was actually wasting away. She had had rheumatic fever, which had resulted in damage to her heart. The diabetes was merely the last link in a chain of physical difficulties. Alice B. had received a complete diagnostic check-up at a hospital, and had been placed on DBI. She had shied away from the use of insulin when told that she would have to take 80 units a day.

She finally decided to visit the Florida Spa where the medicine was, at first, drastically reduced and within about a week completely eliminated. Because of her generally depleted condition, she was at first placed on a rather liberal diet. It included foods rich in protective elements, such as the leafy raw vegetables, but also included small amounts of the natural brown rice daily and, occasionally, baked potato. For protein, cottage cheese, fermented milk, or some other easily digestible protein food was used.

The patient showed improvement almost from the very beginning. She regained a great deal of her strength; she began to look much healthier, and in spite of the fact that she was allowed a rather liberal diet, with a fair amount of the natural carbohydrate foods. her blood sugar did not increase above the level it was when DBI was used.

To bring about a change in the blood picture, it was decided that the patient be placed temporarily on small quantities of insulin, with the idea in mind that the amount would be gradually reduced as her blood sugar levels permitted.

She was started on 12 units a day (instead of the 80 units that she was told she would need), which promptly lowered her blood sugar. The intake of food was kept at the same level and even increased at times, except that one day a week she was kept without food during the day, and permitted only one solid meal in the evening. The amount of insulin was soon brought down to nine units a day, and the sugar in her blood approached normal. Her diet remained liberal and ample, and she regained much of her strength and vitality. When Dr. Weinsier, the physician supervising the case of Alice B., told us that he felt confident that the amount of insulin given her might soon be reduced still further we knew that this patient, who had been foundering for many years, had finally come to realize that she was on the right road, and that from then on she would faithfully adhere to the program that had been outlined for her, since it was the only program that promised her lasting results.

After Alice B. had been at the Florida Spa for a number of weeks, Dr. Weinsier had this to report:

Mrs. B. is now taking brisk walks three times a day, and joining in the daily exercise class. The brisk walks are 11 times around the pool at present, although she started at a lower number. We plan to increase this number weekly until perhaps 15 laps or a mile is achieved.

Despite these walks, her pulse and heart sounds seem better, and there is no evidence of exhaustion or palpitation. She is unquestionably stronger, and perhaps we are helping to put together sufficient building blocks to the point where her liver and pancreas can rebuild and start functioning normally.

A later report by Dr. Weinsier stated the following:

Mrs. B.'s blood tests were completed. Cholesterol dropped

from 307 to 209. Cholesterol esters dropped from 185 to 115. The hemoglobin went from 82% when she first came, to 92% some weeks ago, and 97% now. She walks miles most vigorously and eats well. Blood sugar is now 211 (the latest report) on 7 units of insulin, and we plan to continue with this amount until a reduction in blood sugar justifies further reduction in insulin. She is maintaining her weight and energy, and looks wonderful.

We present the case of Alice B., not as one in which full or complete results may necessarily be attained, but as an example of how even very difficult or "brittle" cases of this disease should be managed, if favorable results are to be attained.

In the great majority of cases, diabetes is no problem. Control and actual correction of the disease can usually be established even in cases where insulin or any of the other antidiabetic remedies have already been used over an extended period of time.

The occasional unstable or difficult case may require special management. However, even in critical cases gratifying results can be obtained when careful adjustments are made in accordance with this plan of management, provided, of course, it is regulated to meet the needs of the individual case.

# 2

## DIABETES IN CHILDREN

In cases of children suffering from diabetes, we usually
have a more difficult problem. However, even in these
cases the curative forces of the body are at all times endeavoring to bring about a restoration of normal functioning, and we must remember that only when these forces
are given a chance to assert themselves can real results be
attained. Boyd very aptly compares the pancreas to the
liver, stating "that liver cells may be damaged ... either
by toxic factors or by lipotrope deficiency (deficiency in
fat metabolism), and that regeneration is concurrent with
destruction." He then quotes Warren and LeCompte to the
effect that:

The pathology of the pancreas in diabetes cannot be
considered as static. As seen at any one time, it represents
a balance struck between the factors tending to produce
degenerative changes of the islands and the regenerative
powers of the pancreas. . . . The pancreas in diabetes is
not simply the scarred field of the old battleground, but is
the actual field of conflict. It does not submit without a
struggle to injury, but endeavors to regenerate. . . .
*This leads to the hope that in young people, with more
resilient tissues, proper treatment may remove the cause
of injury and favor more or less restoration of the damaged islands.*

### Results in the Pre-insulin Era

A recently published medical book points out that insulin
has been a lifesaver to children suffering from this disease,
and to prove this point mentions that while in 1913 the
life expectancy of a ten-year-old child with diabetes was
1.3 years, the life expectancy of a diabetic child of the
same age today is 44 years.

Judging from this, insulin has surely been a blessing. This book, however, fails to point out that the reason these cases were so hopeless in those years was because so little was done for them. The major care consisted of restricting the intake of the carbohydrate foods, which at that time consisted primarily of refined, processed grain and cereal foods and white sugar products, and substituting in their place more of the protein and fat foods. We wonder what the statistical tables regarding the life expectancy of these cases would have revealed if, in place of these superficial dietary modifications, a sound plan of rehabilitation, similar to the one we are suggesting, would have been followed.

Thinking back to the early 20's when insulin was not yet in use or too well known, we remember some of the children's cases that came under our care and the great benefits that were attained when a program similar to the one outlined in this encyclopedia was followed. The nutrition of the children in those years was much worse than today, since the whole grain products were hardly known, while fruits and vegetables were considered luxuries, not basic foods. The diet of the children in those years in the average home was composed primarily of white flour and white sugar products, some protein foods, and a great deal of the concentrated fat foods, such as cream, butter, and eggs.

A change from this kind of diet to a physiologically correct nutritional program and other careful adjustments in the life of the child along sound hygienic rules proved of great help in those cases, and we see no reason why such a program could not provide similar results today.

## 3

# A PROGRAM FOR THE CARE OF DIABETES

Were we asked to outline a diet that would be suitable in all cases of diabetes we should reply that this cannot be done, since each case is an individual problem. Sufferers from this disease who are really interested in overcoming their ailment or who wish to bring it effectively under control in a natural way should, whenever possible, consult a doctor or nutritional authority who possesses a thorough grasp of the principles outlined here and knows how to apply them. Only such a program can provide maximum help. In the great majority of cases, such a program will bring about complete control of the disorder, and where complete control is not attainable, a much higher degree of sugar tolerance will be developed. This will enable the patient to handle many of the carbohydrate foods that could not otherwise be managed. A conscientious adherence to this plan of living and care, however, is essential if lasting benefits are to be derived.

However, while no specific program can be presented that can be applied to all cases, there is no reason why we cannot present, in general outline, the program that has been effective in many average or uncomplicated cases of diabetes.

At first, the patient must abstain from all solid food for one or two or even several days. Those who can do so are advised to stay on water only or, where this is not possible, either grapefruit juice or hot vegetable puree made of the green leafy vegetables, taken every couple of hours, may be permitted.

Following the period of food abstention or the modified food program, a simple natural diet, at first low in carbohydrates but rich in natural, protective body-building elements, is then advisable.

More of the natural carbohydrate foods are gradually added as the condition improves and the body can handle them without difficulty. However, at no time are the re-

fined and processed carbohydrate foods permitted, while
even the whole grain products should be used, when permissible, only in small quantities.

We often start with a breakfast of grapefruit, raw apple, blueberries, peaches, nectarines, mangoes, or papaya,
but where these fruits are still not advisable with raw vegetables such as lettuce, tomatoes, celery, and green pepper. Where a larger breakfast is indicated, the use of four
to five ounces of cottage cheese, pot cheese, or farmer's
cheese, which must be salt-free, or clabbered milk or
yoghurt, with the fruit or raw vegetables already mentioned is recommended.

For the noon meal, we advise a large raw vegetable
salad of green leafy vegetables such as escarole, chicory,
dandelion, romaine lettuce, parsley, cabbage, cauliflower,
Chinese cabbage, watercress, celery, and leek, or such
other green vegetables as cucumber, green pepper, zucchini, and kohlrabi. (Later in the treatment, some of the
root vegetables such as grated carrots and turnips may be
added.) To this we add one or two steamed vegetables of
the low carbohydrate family, such as string beans, squash,
okra, kale, artichokes, broccoli, and eggplant. Four to six
ounces of fermented milk or yoghurt or a half grapefruit,
strawberries, blueberries, peaches, or any of the other low
carbohydrate fruits, when they are in season, may be used
for dessert, if the patient is still hungry.

For dinner, a large raw vegetable salad and four to six
ounces of a protein food such as cottage cheese, pot
cheese, farmer's cheese, or ricotta cheese for the vegetarian, or chicken, lamb chops, or lean fish or any lean
meat for those who feel they cannot do without meat; one
or two steamed vegetables of those mentioned above; and
half a grapefruit or one of the berries or other low carbohydrate fruit may be allowed for dessert.

This diet should be carefully adjusted to the individual
case. A greater latitude may be allowed in the milder
cases, and less in the more severe ones.

Those who have seldom eaten or have used only small
amounts of green leafy vegetables are often under the impression that these vegetables do not provide much nourishment. But this is not true. The greens contain the finest
type of protein, although in small amounts; are rich in all
the protective vitamins, minerals, and enzymes; and supply

the essential trace elements without which complete health is impossible. Remember that the cow nurses her calf, supplies all our dairy needs, and provides the big beefsteaks that many think essential to life, and all this comes from greens, from the grass that she consumes.

In addition to the diet, cleansing warm water enemas are recommended when necessary to relieve constipation, and hot epsom salt baths are advised daily before retiring to promote kidney and skin elimination. When the bath is taken in the morning or during the day, it should be followed by a period of rest. The patient furthermore should make sure to obtain as much sleep and rest as possible.

The need for establishing a better circulation must not be overlooked, and this is why the feet must always be kept warm. A program of breathing and other simple physical exercises is recommended. All excitement and tensions must be avoided.

## A Complex Disease

As we were working on this chapter, an editorial appeared in the *Journal of the American Medical Association*, December 24, 1960, entitled "Diabetic Neuropathy" that made it clear that the appearance of sugar in the blood and urine is merely one of the many phases of the diabetic picture. It said: "The view is shared that diabetes is a generalized complex disease process, of which the carbohydrate metabolic disorder represents a single aspect." The editorial then goes on to say that "other aspects of this complex of diabetes are those seen in complications of pregnancy, in microangiopathy, such as retinopathy and nephropathy (diseases of the capillaries in the eyes and kidneys) and in arteriosclerotic involvement of the larger vessels."

Continuing further, the editorial states: "It is established that complications of pregnancy associated with diabetes may occur long before the eventual clinical manifestation of diabetes, and be identical with those occurring in the diabetic state," and then points out that phenomena that precede "the eventual clinical manifestations of diabetes ... include the overweight, oedematous baby, a marked increase in stillbirth and neonatal [newly born] fatalities, an increase in the number of congenital abnormalities, and hypertrophy of the islands of Langerhans in the offspring."

The editorial concludes that "inheritance apparently carries with it a specific vulnerability of the central nervous system and the vascular system."

As we were reading this statement, we couldn't help thinking of the time when many of the conventional disorders were said to have been caused by venereal diseases, and the term "damaged goods" was used to refer to the hereditary defects that showed up in connection with these diseases. It seems to us that the hereditary defects cited in this editorial are forms of "damaged goods" that could often be avoided if parents would prepare themselves for real parenthood.

What do we require for real parenthood? It should be evident that a well-planned nutritional program and a wholesome, healthy way of living are most essential. The prospective mother must realize that by keeping herself in good health she prepares herself for an easy and uncomplicated delivery and lays the foundation for healthy offspring. Furthermore, the fact that she understands the importance of taking care of her own health also conditions her to do the same for her children.

Parents whose children display the conditions mentioned in the editorial or who show any other signs of ill health should realize that the sooner they change their children's feeding and living habits to a more wholesome pattern, the sooner will they meet their real parental responsibilities and lessen the dangers for further breakdown.

Those who have to cope with a diabetic problem in one of their children should realize that only by turning to a physiologically correct program of living can they obtain the results they are seeking.

Where the illness is of a severe type and the use of insulin cannot be completely eliminated, the parents will still obtain the greatest amount of help if they will change the child's nutritional and other living habits so that only a minimum amount of insulin need be used. By working along these lines, the child's health may be rebuilt to the point where all medication may in time be discontinued.

Authorities realize that these cases must not be written off as hopeless. Boyd, writing about the crucial pancreas cells, the islands of Langerhans, whose malfunction results in diabetes, states: "There is no doubt that the islets are capable of regeneration."[1] This being so, our aim should

[1] *Pathology of Internal Diseases.*

be to plan a program of care that promotes rehabilitation. It should not be necessary to say that only a way of life based upon correct physiologic principles can accomplish this task.

The idea that diabetes is an incurable disease is all too commonly expressed, and yet is untrue in the great majority of cases. The realization that the body possesses vast regenerative powers should help doctors re-evaluate their approach to this disease, while patients who have resigned themselves to the thought that little can be done to overcome their ailment should realize that a sound program of care can lead to an entirely new and healthy life.

So, too, many sufferers from arthritis, one of man's most dread diseases, may find new hope in the application of natural methods.

In the next section, the nature of the bony structures and the diseases that afflict them are discussed in detail so that the sufferer from arthritis, a disease of the joints, will understand the basis for the program of care that we outline for him.

## Section Four:

# ARTHRITIS AND OTHER
# RHEUMATIC DISEASES

# INTRODUCTION

It is becoming increasingly apparent that we live in a period of unusually rapid changes in all fields of endeavor—economic, political, social, and scientific. The basic causes responsible for these changes have been operating for a long time, and have been accelerated by World War II.

All of us must become aware of the significance of these changes, and must be willing to accept the new truths they express, even though they clash with previous conceptions.

In the field of healing, Dr. Warmbrand's treatise on arthritis is indicative of these changes.

For years, some schools of healing contended that our approach to the treatment of disease in general and arthritis in particular was unsatisfactory. While we subdivided the patient into segments and treated the parts, they kept insisting on a constitutional or *organismic* approach, i.e., treating the individual as a whole rather than placing main emphasis on the local or specific disease or its symptoms.

While we directed our attack upon the symptoms, they maintained that the vitality of the individual as a whole must be restored in order to supply the energy needed by the tissues to correct the abnormal state.

The author is a leading exponent of this school of healing. His treatise presents a powerful argument in favor of this approach. Not only is his analysis of arthritis unusually rational, theoretically, but he has proved in scores of cases in actual practice the value of his method.

The amazing fact about his therapy is that it is apparently simple, as all great truths are. However, it is not so simple to get patients to discard all previous concepts of treatment and assiduously follow this regimen.

An essential part of his philosophy is that of *vitality*, which he considers so important, but which, however, has not received much attention in the past, probably because so little is known about it. Dr. Warmbrand maintains that the human organism is constantly being insulted by irritations of all kinds, physical, mental, and emotional. When the vitality is at is optimum, all the cells of the body are surcharged with this energy, either via the nerves or the blood vessels. The cells, in turn, are able to repair quickly any temporary damage done by these irritants.

When this vitality is lowered, the tissues are unable to neutralize the irritants or repair the damage completely. This is shown pathologically in congestion, inflammation, and ultimate tissue breakdown.

The total quantity of irritants in the tissues at any one time and their effect upon the body depend upon several factors: (1) The rate and quantity of irritants introduced into the body. (2) The rate and quantity of irritants created in the tissues, owing to impaired metabolism. (3) The rate at which the body neutralizes these irritants by means of its many protective and defensive functions, and is able to eliminate them via the excretory organs such as the skin, lungs, intestinal tract, and kidneys.

The author contends, rightly, that the less irritating toxic matter we introduce and permit to accumulate in the system, and the better the functioning of the organism as a whole, the less damage is done to our tissues. Unwholesome habits of living and other debilitating influences undermine vitality and contribute to the production and accumulation of these irritating toxins, which lead to disease.

While the claim made by the author may be contrary to accepted theories and practices, I believe that the more one studies this philosophy of healing the more logic one sees in it, and the actual results obtained through this method are convincing evidence of the intrinsic value of his approach.

The author is well known in the field of healing. He presents his subject from a strictly scientific point of view, employing at the same time, a style that makes for simplicity and understanding. He shows keen discernment in the presentation of his facts, and his analysis serves to clarify the subject.

We are greatly in need of more treatises by practitioners who, by sharing with us their special experiences, stimulate scientific reasoning and widen our horizons of knowledge.

To benefit from new concepts and new truths, tolerance and understanding are required. We must be prepared to lay aside convictions of a lifetime when new facts and new findings justify such a course.

HARRY SACKREN, M.D.

# A PLEA TO MEMBERS OF THE MEDICAL PROFESSION

The *Journal of the American Medical Association,* in an editorial[1] referring to the confusion that exists in medicine in regard to definition, causes, and methods of treatment in arthritis arrives at the following startling conclusion:

In the light of the evidence here discussed, the treatment of arthritis would seem to include such well established methods as *Physical Therapy and Orthopedic Treatment* prescribed as indicated by the nature of the individual case. The use of proper medication for the relief of pain is warranted. All other methods such as the use of vaccines, fever, sulfur, vitamins (including activated vaporized sterol) bee venom, histamine, penicillin and sulfonamide compounds, roentgen radiation and induced jaundice are still in an experimental and unestablished stage, and the weight of evidence points to the belief that most of them are useless. (Emphasis ours.)

What a significant admission and how vigorously and succinctly stated!

Thank you, gentlemen, for your forthright statement, for it substantiates our claims that while physical therapy has a place in the treatment of arthritis, most of the other methods employed in medicine for this disease are of questionable value.

It is true that in the summation the editors mention that the use of proper medication for the relief of pain is warranted. While this is a point with which we vigorously disagree, and for good reason as will be apparent from our discussion in this section, yet, even on this point, the qualifying statement that the use of medication is warranted for the relief of pain, and not as an aid to the correction of the disease, is significant.

[1] "The Treatment of Arthritis," *J.A.M.A.,* October 4, 1947.

Gold compounds, now in much use among specialists in arthritis, are properly evaluated in the editorial, and their failures noted.

The concluding statement of the editorial, quoted above, only verified many of the points that we have emphasized during our many years of active practice and are stressed in these pages.

We wish to congratulate the editors of the *Journal* for placing public interest above factional considerations. We are assuming that they were motivated in the presentation of these facts by the realization that a new orientation on the subject is imperative if the sufferers from this disease are to receive adequate help.

We have stated that the sufferers from arthritis are entitled to all the help they can get, and it is for this reason that we have applied ourselves to the uprooting of practices that are ineffectual or that interfere with recovery. The consensus among the lay public as well as among those engaged in the professions of healing is that the present-day approach to the disease is sadly lacking, and that a new and more fundamental approach is long overdue. The recognition that the old methods have proved a failure is the first step towards bringing about such a change.

In view of this, we are pleading with the medical profession, and all other professions devoted to the alleviation and correction of disease, to avail themselves of the information presented here, for only to the extent that the principles enunciated in this section are properly understood and conscientiously employed will the needs of the sufferers from arthritis be better served.

We are aware that those who are engaged in the profession of healing are motivated by a high standard of idealism and service, and we hope that they will permit nothing to stand in their way in the application of any constructive measure that can benefit their patients.

# FACTS ABOUT ARTHRITIS

Those interested in the question of health cannot help but feel a deep compassion for the many millions who are suffering from arthritis, and who, after having subjected themselves to countless forms of treatment, are at a loss to know what their next step should be.

## Millions Afflicted

It is estimated that about eleven million persons in this country are afflicted with arthritis. The fact that so many are afflicted, plus the intense pains and the crippling deformities that they suffer, creates a problem that must not be disregarded.

Not all arthritis sufferers are affected alike. In some cases the agonies may be unbearable, while in others mere discomfort or numbness indicates that the disease is yet in its earlier stages of development. In the majority of cases, the pains and the deformities develop gradually, and become more pronounced with time. Occasionally, however, the onset may be sudden, in the nature of an acute illness. In some cases the affliction may limit itself to one joint, while in others a number of joints or the whole body may be stricken.

Those who suffer from this disease in the earlier stages or who are affected by it only to a limited degree should bear in mind that they are potential victims of its more severe forms, and that the steps necessary to counteract the affliction and to remove the causes that have contributed to its development must be taken.

## Arthritis: A Rheumatic Affection

Arthritis is a disease of the joints. It belongs to the "rheumatic family," and differs from such other rheumatic disorders as lumbago, neuritis, and sciatica only in that while the latter involve the muscles or nerves, arthritis affects the joints.

## Early Symptoms

As a rule, the disease develops slowly, imperceptibly. It may take years before one becomes aware of its serious manifestations. Even where the onset is sudden, with high fever and severe pains, one must bear in mind that the factors that have given rise to it have been operating for a long period of time. The intense suffering and the extensive deformities that manifest themselves in the more severe forms of the disease and in its more advanced stages make it a dread and a menace, and cause much agony and despair.

A healthy body does not experience pain or discomfort. When the body is in sound health it is not handicapped by impediments or limitations in motion. Pains or discomforts in the joints, or limitations or impediments of motion should serve as signals warning that arthritis may be in the making, and that serious attention is required.

The disease in its earlier stages is often mild and, if immediately cared for, can be readily overcome. Unfortunately, first symptoms are often so fleeting and so superficial that only rarely are they recognized as the beginning of arthritis. A feeling of numbness or stiffness, creaking and cracking of the joints, occasional twinges, cold clammy hands and feet—these are some of the early symptoms of the disease. It is regrettable that in most cases these early manifestations are either completely disregarded or treated in a routine fashion, for such neglect or routine procedure contributes to the development of the more severe forms of the disease with their many difficulties.

It is essential that these early symptoms not be neglected. An aching or sore back may suddenly clear up and not recur for a long time; it is therefore easily forgotten. Yet such experiences, especially when recurrent, should serve as a warning that insidious influences are undermining the health of the patient. Numbness of the joints or stinging sensations are not always sufficiently annoying yet, if neglected, ultimately give rise to more serious conditions. A burning sensation of the feet or twinges are often early signs of the disease, but few recognize their serious import. A feeling as if ants were crawling under the skin should serve as a warning that something is wrong and that care is required. None of these earlier symptoms should be disregarded or overlooked if the more advanced forms of the disease with their marked deformities and intense suffering are to be avoided.

## The Changes in the Joints

In arthritis the joint is the seat of the damage. It will be easier for us to understand the nature of the disease if we obtain a clear picture of a healthy joint. The mechanical construction of our body has always been of fascinating interest, and if we are to gain a clear understanding of arthritis this knowledge becomes highly important. Fritz Kahn[1] describes the four different types of joints:

1. The ball-and-socket joint where the smooth round head of one bone fits into the socket of the other. This permits motion in all directions. The shoulder and hip joints are examples of this type of joint.
2. The saddle joint where the bones move in two directions. The vertebrae of the backbone, moving backward, forward, and sideways are an example.
3. The hinge joint, which moves only in one direction like the blade of a pen knife. The fingers and the knee joints are examples of this type of joint.
4. The rotary joint, which rotates about in its axis like a key. The elbow is an example of it.

Our skeletal framework gives shape and form to our body and serves as a means of movement and locomotion.

A more detailed study of a joint reveals several interesting points. The adjoining ends of the bones are covered by a semisoft elastic tissue called the cartilage, which cushions the joints and minimizes friction and strain. The inner surface of the joint cavity is lined with a membrane, known as the synovial membrane, which secretes a light, yellowish, semiliquid fluid that keeps the joint lubricated.

[1] *Man in Structure and Function.*

The ligaments and muscles hold the joint together and in place.

In health the bones are well-knit and firm, and the circulation of the blood and lymph,[2] which carries food and oxygen to the tissues and picks up waste materials for elimination, is unimpeded. The cartilages are pliable and serve to protect the joints against undue friction or strain. The synovial membrane secretes the fluid that is necessary to keep the joints lubricated. The muscles and ligaments possess the tonicity and springiness for firmness and balance.

In arthritis, many changes affecting the function and structure of these tissues take place. The joints become large and swollen, or shrivel up and waste away. The bones become either thickened or wasted and the adjoining surfaces often present irregular, rough, or jagged appearances. The circulation of the blood and of the lymph is impaired and this deprives the tissues of nutrition and oxygen, and interferes with the elimination of the waste materials. The cartilages lose their pliability and become brittle and dry. The function of the synovial membrane becomes damaged, causing either an excess or a lessening of the secretions. As the disease progresses the membrane often becomes completely worn out and the secretion dries up completely. The ligaments and muscles lose their tone and their flexibility, wasting away or becoming congested and thickened.

### Destructive Changes Develop Gradually

These destructive changes do not all develop at once. An impairment in circulation, with an inflammatory condition of the synovial membrane or the cartilages, is usually the change that manifests itself in the earlier stages of the disease. It is only as the disease progresses that the more advanced destructive changes develop and the more severe manifestations of the disease become apparent.

[2] The lymph is a clear yellowish or straw-colored fluid that carries away waste products from the tissues through the network known as the lymphatic system.

## How the Disease Develops

If we are to gain a complete understanding of the nature of the disease and how it can be corrected or controlled, the causes that give rise to it and that make it progress to its more advanced stages must receive serious consideration.

To begin with, it is well to realize that arthritis is not a purely local disease but a systemic disorder and the outgrowth of many systemic disturbances. These disturbances weaken the functions of the body, impair circulation, and create deficiencies. Starvation of the tissues, retention of toxins, chemical imbalance and stagnation, are the factors that affect the joint and give rise to destructive changes. Local injury or strain may weaken a joint and subject it to the disease, but when a body is in a healthy condition it possesses sufficient recuperative powers to counteract local strain or injury and to protect the tissues against permanent damage. It is only when the body is in a depleted condition or when its recuperative powers are weakened that it lacks the power to overcome local impairment, and only then does local strain or injury act as a contributory factor to the development of the disease.

## Associated Systemic Disorders

It is important to recognize the close relationship between arthritis and the many systematic disorders that either precede its development or are present in association with it. Constipation is present in the majority of cases and often exists for a long time before the disease begins to make its inroads. Digestive disorders often precede its development. Catarrhal conditions are frequently present. The existence of cold, clammy hands and feet, indicating a weakened nervous system and poor circulation, have already been mentioned. Fatigue, numbness, irritability, and backaches are some of the forerunners of the disease. These and many other disorders are generally present long before the actual arthritic symptoms begin to show up. It should be evident that all the disturbances that precede the onset of the disease or are associated with it must be either completely overcome or be brought under control before beneficial results can be attained.

Most people regard arthritis as a single, specific disease affecting only the joints, and fail to recognize the interrelationship of the different organs and functions and therefore fail to realize that only as these abnormal conditions are overcome can the body be restored to health.

When this close relationship between the general constitutional disorders and the arthritic manifestation is fully recognized, it becomes obvious that any approach that fails to eliminate or overcome the underlying causes of the disease is bound to fail in providing permanent results.

## Why the Disease Persists

A short analysis of the evolution of the disease from its early prearthritic symptoms to its more pronounced stages will make this even more clear. When the early prearthritic symptoms become annoying, remedies are usually prescribed to provide relief. Bicarbonate of soda to neutralize acidity, codeine to relieve pain, the barbiturates or bromides to check nervous symptoms—these are some of the typical remedies used. These drugs may help to relieve distressing symptoms or lessen discomfort, but since they accomplish this by means of sedation or stimulation and since they do not eliminate causative factors, they have no corrective value and fail to overcome existing systemic disturbances. It is deplorable that most sufferers fail to recognize the futility of these conventional remedies, so far as permanent correction is concerned. Very seldom are they aware of the temporary nature of these remedies, and seldom do they recognize the need for more fundamental changes.

Cathartics induce bowel action, but do not overcome intestinal sluggishness; in fact they only increase the intestinal weakness. So-called alkalizers may relieve digestive upsets, but as long as the causes of the "acid condition" remain, the symptoms will recur, with even greater damage as the ultimate result. Barbiturates or bromides may quiet nervous symptoms, but in time cause greater impairment to the nervous system, and are responsible for many breakdowns. A stimulating drug or physiotherapy may temporarily improve the circulation and provide relief, but unless fundamental corrective measures are employed, the underlying disturbances are not overcome and the diseased condition continues to grow worse. These or similar remedies may mask or modify symptoms, but they fail to promote the needed correction and ultimately cause more disease.

## A Summary of Principles

For clarity it is well that a few of the basic principles relating to the disease and its correction be summarized.

1. The disease is of a constitutional nature, and is the outgrowth of many systemic disturbances.

2. These systemic disturbances occur as a result of abuses to which the body has been subjected, and can be completely overcome only when these abuses are eliminated.

3. In our endeavor to correct the disease or bring it under control, our primary objective must be to eradicate or overcome all abnormal conditions that have contributed to its development. This can only be accomplished when the abuses that have given rise to the perversions are eliminated and measures that promote general rebuilding are employed.

4. While the conventional remedies may relieve pain or modify symptoms, they neither eliminate the harmful influences nor do they in any way succeed in overcoming the underlying disturbances. What is more, being suppressive or stimulative in nature, they actually interfere with the adjustment processes of the body and cause more damage.

## The Reason for Failure

Those who have no knowledge of these basic principles wonder why they have failed to obtain results and are at a loss to know what to do next. The recurrent pains, growing more severe with time, and the accompanying deformities only increase the confusion and anxiety, and prove conclusively the fallacy of trying to overcome the affliction through the use of measures that merely suppress symptoms but fail to correct the underlying causes of the disease.

Most persons are under the impression that these remedies possess specific curative properties. They do not realize that the power of cure is a prerogative of the organism, and only to the extent that its basic physiological needs are satisfied and all influences that impair function are eliminated can the body be maintained at its optimum degree of health.

### The Different Forms of Arthritis

Arthritis occurs in many forms. The following are the most common:

1. The *hypertrophic* type of arthritis, also known as arthritis deformans. This form usually begins with a softening and erosion of the cartilage and later becomes marked by a thickening or enlargement of the affected joints. It occurs most often in the middle-aged or older individual, and the process is usually regarded as a sign of the aging of the tissues.

2. The *atrophic* or wasting type of arthritis, also known as rheumatoid arthritis. This type starts with an inflammation of the synovial membrane, and ultimately leads to extensive wasting or degeneration of the tissues. It usually affects younger people and occurs more often in the long and lanky type of individual. It is the more serious type of the disease, and the degenerative changes may become extensive unless proper corrective measures are instituted in time.

3. So-called *infectious arthritis* such as "tubercular," "gonorrheal," and "streptococcus" arthritis are really forms of atrophic arthritis. While a specific germ is supposed to give rise to these forms of the disease, they are really of the atrophic or wasting variety and can be corrected only as the debility of the body is overcome and the accumulated toxins that favored their development are eliminated.

4. *Still's disease,* a form of atrophic arthritis affecting children, and spondylitis deformans, known as the Marie Struempel type of arthritis or Van Bechterow's disease,

the former a disease in which the spine becomes ankylosed or stiffened. I shall discuss them more fully later in this section.

Arthritis may affect any joint in the body. No joint is immune. It may be observed in its early stages where destructive changes have not yet had a chance to develop, or in the more advanced stages with extensive deformities. Where deformities exist, it is known as arthritis deformans. When many joints are affected, it is known as polyarthritis.

## Related Conditions

When the irritating toxins that give rise to this disease affect specific parts of the body, the local disturbance is often classified in accordance with the part that is affected. An inflammation of the shoulder caused by these toxins is known as bursitis; of the lower part of the back, as lumbago; of the muscles, as myalgia or myositis; of the nerves, as neuritis or neuralgia; of the sciatic nerve as sciatica or sciatic rheumatism.

These inflammatory conditions, except where caused by injury or pressure, are the direct result of the same irritating poisons, and are basically of a rheumatic nature. If neglected or improperly treated, they may ultimately lead to the development of arthritis with its severe pains and its extensive distortions.

Early diffused pains recurring at different times are often an indication of a generalized rheumatic or arthritis condition, and if not corrected often lead to the more advanced stages of the disease.

As mentioned earlier, neuritis, sciatica, or back pains are not always of rheumatic origin. Local factors such as injury or pressure may give rise to them. However, in the majority of cases it is the irritating toxins of body metabolism that are responsible for their development, and even where local strain or injury or pressure has given rise to them it is still imperative that general care be made part of the corrective program. If this is not done, the local damage may serve as a focal point for the accumulation of toxins with consequent destructive changes.

## Intense Suffering Experienced

It is needless to stress the severe suffering or the intense crippling that is frequently associated with this disease. It is well known that to many of the afflicted every day is a nightmare, every hour a torment. The feeling of hopelessness that becomes more evident with each failure to obtain help and the many deformities that grow more pronounced as time goes on only intensify the despair that already exists.

I have already pointed out the futility of resorting to measures that merely modify or suppress symptoms. If we are to succeed in our endeavor to overcome or counteract the disease, we must do more than provide mere relief. We must eliminate the harmful influences that have contributed to its development, and institute measures that promote general rebuilding.

## 2

## FALLACIOUS CONCEPTS

### Change of Life

Change of life, or the menopause, is often associated with arthritis and often considered a causative factor. Women frequently begin to suffer from this disease during the menopause, and because of this some investigators assume that a definite causal relationship exists between them. Close observation, however, will reveal that this is placing the cart before the horse. While it is true that many women begin to feel arthritis pains at this stage of life, the inception of the disease can often be traced back to a long time before. It is merely that the abnormal condition, existing either in a quiescent state or in a mildly active form, becomes active or accentuated during this period.

The normally healthy woman suffers no pain or discomfort during the menopause. The changes that occur during this period are of a perfectly normal nature and proceed gradually and without pain.

It is only in those cases where disturbances already exist, either in an inactive form or in their early stages, or where the body is greatly depleted, that pain or discomfort manifests itself or becomes accentuated during this period. The woman who develops an active arthritic condition during the menopause, will, upon checking back, recollect many discomforts, and probably some of a definite prearthritic or mildly arthritic nature, long before the menopause began to manifest itself. The stress and strain placed upon the organism during this time merely hastens or intensifies the development of a condition that is already in the making.


### Exposure

Chilling of the body or overexposure is often mentioned as

a major causative factor; it has been pointed out that the rigors of the battlefields and the dampness of the fox holes have contributed materially to the number of arthritis sufferers.

Undue exposure unquestionably contributes to the development of the disease. However, here too the reasoning is fallacious, and the major underlying factors are either overlooked or disregarded. There is no doubt that the stress and strain of the battlefields and the dampness of the fox holes had an unwholesome effect upon our soldiers, for such influences are not conducive to good health. But, since the soldiers were also subjected to a highly concentrated and unbalanced diet and to many other extremely debilitating influences, why place emphasis on only one factor and disregard the others? It should be obvious that arthritis is not the result of one single factor, but the outgrowth of many undermining influences, and that when the body is in a strong and healthy condition it can readily cope with unfavorable climatic changes.

It is only when our resistance is undermined and our vitality is depleted or when the initial stages of the disease already exist that climatic influences or abrupt changes in temperature activate the disease or intensify its manifestations.

### Injuries as a Cause of Arthritis

Injuries are often mentioned as a cause of arthritis. There is no question that they do contribute to the development of the disease. Falls, blows, and sprains all injure the joint and make it a point of least resistance to the inflow and deposit of toxins. However, when one possesses good health and a clean healthy bloodstream, injuries can be easily overcome and leave no deleterious aftereffects. Only in cases where the body is depleted or where an overload of toxins has been permitted to accumulate does the impaired joint become a focal point for the disease.

An arthritic condition that had its beginning in an injury must still be cared for in accordance with the plan outlined in this volume, for only as the health of the body as a whole is rebuilt, can the injured parts be benefited and health restored.

## 3

## FUNDAMENTAL CHANGES NECESSARY

If our efforts to restore the health of the patient are to prove successful, it is important that we understand how the disease originates, for only then can we gain a full understanding of the factors that have contributed to its development and what we have to do to bring about its correction. The measures that are employed must not merely provide relief but must eradicate all systemic disturbances that acted as contributory influences or that are found associated with it. Constipation must be corrected, digestive disorders must be overcome, the nervous system strengthened, circulation rebuilt, anemia counteracted. Excessive weight must be eliminated. The functions of the kidneys, the skin, and the liver, where impaired or weakened, must be restored to normal.

### Our Method Easy and Simple

The measures that promote such readjustments are within the reach of all, and are not difficult to apply. As a matter of fact, it is their very simplicity that is often responsible for the skepticism with which they are received. Most persons are in search of complex and mysterious remedies and are often unable to grasp the fundamental values of our simple approach.

If lasting results are to be attained, a well-integrated plan based upon a sound and well-balanced mode of living and the employment of constructive health-restorative measures are essential. Such a plan must be based upon a change to a wholesome, well-balanced diet, which supplies the body with all its nutritional requirements. It must provide an abundance of rest and sleep and, whenever indicated, must include a well-regulated program of exercise and outdoor activities. Fresh air and sunshine are important. It must also embody a proper adjustment to the problems of life, so that poise and proper emotional control may be developed. Moreover, all influences that have a debilitating or devitalizing effect, such as late hours, sexual excesses, overeating, and the use of tobacco and alcohol, coffee and tea must be curbed or eliminated.

In addition to these readjustments, measures that strengthen the weakened organs and rebuild their functions must be employed. The application of heat, massage, actinotherapy or the ultraviolet rays, and other forms of physiotherapy, applied in accordance with the need of the individual case and properly correlated to all the other fundamental needs of the body, will be of great aid in bringing about lasting results.

## Nutrition

The food eaten by the average individual leaves much to be desired. The diet of most persons is generally deficient in the essential nutritional elements. White bread, processed cereals, puddings, white sugar, coffee, tea, spiced foods or foods prepared with condiments, and chemically treated, denatured, or devitalized foods overtax the digestive organs and deprive the body of many elements that are essential to good health. Such foods are not only of no benefit to the arthritic patient; they are actually detrimental. It is such foods that have contributed to the development of the disease, and if no change is made will only add to the damage.

Most persons are under the impression that, to rebuild health, the eating of large quantities of food is necessary. This is a mistaken belief. Those who think this way overlook the fact that it is *not the food we eat, but the food we digest and assimilate that nourishes the body*. Eating beyond digestive capacity or partaking of food that is not easily digestible overtaxes the digestive organs, increases fatigue, and adds to the toxins in the body. This only aggravates the disease.

It is well to emphasize some of the rules of nutrition that should be kept in mind in connection with arthritis. It is becoming increasingly more evident that concentrated starches and sugars are not well utilized by sufferers from this disease and only aggravate it. The liberal use of concentrated protein foods overloads the system with purine bodies, and ultimately causes much harm. Fat and other "rich" foods overtax the digestive organs and increase the damage. Meat soups and beef broths, at one time regarded as highly nutritious because of their so-called sustaining qualities, contain primarily the extractives of the meat, and only add to the accumulation of toxins.

## Fundamentals of Proper Diet

A diet composed of natural, easily digestible foods providing all the essential nutritional elements must be substituted. A diet composed of raw and properly steamed vegetables, raw and stewed fruits, fruit and vegetable juices, the luscious berries, the easily digestible starches such as baked potatoes and, to a lesser degree, well-ripened bananas, and a restricted intake of such carefully selected protein foods as fresh, unfermented cheeses, green soy beans and avocados will serve the purpose. These wholesome foods, properly combined and used in their natural state or prepared to make certain that none of their valuable vitamins and minerals are destroyed or wasted, provide the essential nutritional needs of the body and aid the arthritic in his efforts to regain his health.

## Emotional Factors

Emotional readjustments play an important role in the rebuilding of the health of the arthritic. Nervous strain, worry, excitement, irritations, fear, fretting, unhappiness, deplete the energies of the body and contribute to the development of functional and organic disorders. Since emotional or nervous disturbances are often the result of hardships or problems incidental to life, some of which are beyond our control, most persons assume that they are unavoidable. While it is true that hardships add greatly to emotional stress and cause many of the nervous reactions from which the individual suffers, it is a mistake to assume that our emotional faculties cannot be rebuilt or controlled. We are aware that many of the conditions leading to emotional upsets cannot always be avoided, yet experience has demonstrated that a well-regulated mode of living plus a clear understanding of our problems will provide us with the physical and mental balance that is necessary for emotional stability. Just as we can promote health by providing the body with its proper physical care, so can we acquire poise, calmness, and balance by strengthening and rebuilding the nervous system and by a rational approach to our problems.

### Rest and Exercise

Appropriate exercises and an abundance of rest aid greatly in the restoration of health and are of great value in counteracting the arthritic condition. The need for sufficient rest in these cases is frequently disregarded. How often do we find the arthritic forcing himself to do strenuous exercises and taking long walks under the mistaken notion that he must keep active in order to keep his joints in a flexible condition, when in reality his need is for more rest! Overactivity or forced activity, when rest is indicated, leads only to more fatigue with more inflammation and consequently more damage to the afflicted joints.

Dr. Logan Clendenning, author of *The Human Body*, states, "Body rest needs more emphasis. People are constantly bragging about how they are a little better because they can walk around or perhaps perform some motions. Thus they get worse again. The walking around simply brings back the disease."

However, let no one believe for a moment that rest alone, without regard to diet or emotional poise and other indicated bodily requirements, will be sufficient to restore health. Rest must be regarded as merely one of the many basic needs of the body, and must be properly coordinated with all other needs, if real benefits are to be attained.

Regarding exercise, it is important that a distinction be made between exercises that are performed haphazardly and irregularly and those that are performed in accordance with the need of the individual case and followed systematically. The former often lead only to greater exhaustion and cause even more damage, while the latter aid in the promotion of a better circulation and provide better cellular nutrition and drainage.

Rest, too, can easily be overdone, and an excess may lead to further atrophy of the tissues, and cause more extensive crippling.

Ralph K. Ghormley in discussing this question points out that, in cases where activity has not been arrested, when "one opens a thigh to remove fascia for surgical procedure, one will be struck by the smooth surfaces of contact between the fascia and the underlying muscle" and that "these surfaces fairly glisten and are not adherent" while "on the other hand, when one opens a thigh that has been at rest, either in a cast or in a splint, or as a result of rest in bed, one finds that the fascial surface, as well as the surface of the underlying muscle, is dull and does not glide; often times many small adhesions have formed between the muscle and fascia."[1]

"If it is to be used properly, rest must be neither too much nor too little, but adequate," is an apt statement, and it is important that the needs of the patient be properly understood in order that rest and exercise be properly coordinated.

## The Role of Physiotherapy

In discussing the benefits that can be derived from the application of physiotherapy, it is well to repeat that although heat, massage, the ultraviolet radiations, and other similar measures are of definite value in these cases, these treatments must be employed as part of a completely integrated program of health-building if permanent benefits are to be derived.

These treatments, when properly administered and applied in accordance with the indications of the individual case, and when employed in conjunction with the other physiological requirements, are of great help in promoting recovery. They contribute materially to the rebuilding of circulation, relax the nervous system, promote better elimination, and aid reabsorption and drainage.

[1] Ralph K. Ghormley, "The Abuse of Rest in Bed in Orthopedic Surgery," *J.A.M.A.*, August 19, 1944.

## Therapeutic Fasting: A Physiological Rest

It may surprise many to learn that limited feeding programs, and often even total abstinence from food for certain periods of time, are of tremendous benefit in these cases.

I have already stressed the importance of rest as one of the prime needs, if rebuilding is to take place. This point, however, is often sadly misunderstood. The impression generally prevails that when we talk of rest we refer primarily to physical or bodily rest, and that staying in bed or obtaining sufficient sleep takes ample care of this need.

This is not really the case. Unquestionably, physical or bodily rest is helpful and often a necessity, but it takes care of only part of the need. We often overlook the fact that energy is wasted in many ways, and that all these leaks or dissipations of energy must be checked if health is to be rebuilt. One way in which energy is dissipated is when the organs of digestion and elimination are overtaxed. It is well to remember that when the organs of digestion become overworked *they are unable to digest food properly,* and the result is an increase in the creation of poisonous by-products. By the same token, when the kidneys, and the other organs of elimination are exhausted, *they cannot adequately eliminate the waste products* and the result is that much more toxin accumulates in the system.

When at this stage we continue with our habitual ways of eating, we overtax the organs of digestion and elimination only further, and their functions become increasingly impaired. This increases the production and accumulation of toxins. A short fast or a restricted intake of food at this point provides a much needed rest to the overworked organs and assists in their rebuilding, and this in turn enables them to do their work more effectively.

That the rebuilding of energy requires more than mere physical or body rest should be apparent. We waste a great deal of energy when the nervous system is overtaxed or abused, and this often occurs even when the patient is kept in bed. How often does a person find that he is extremely fatigued and tired even after a full night's sleep!

This is because even after ample rest or sleep his nerves are still in tension, and this interferes with the rebuilding of the depleted energies. Sleep or rest alone, if one does not counteract all the other energy-dissipating influences, falls far short of providing the necessary results.

There are many who resort to fasting or a restricted food intake with skepticism, and then are amazed at the benefits that follow its application. However, it is well to warn the reader that one must not embark upon these procedures without expert guidance, and that all precautions for their proper application must be carefully observed.

We dissipate energy when we are under tension, when we are unable to maintain a calm or composed demeanor, or when we are easily swept off balance by fear or panic. Hatred, greed, jealousy, and unhappiness also add to the dissipation of energy. All these debilitating influences waste energy, and mere sleep or physical rest is not enough to counteract it. All these energy-dissipating influences must be eliminated or overcome if vitality is to be rebuilt.

## Chronic Fatigue and Arthritis

Those afflicted with arthritis usually suffer from chronic fatigue. The functions of the different organs have slowed down, and sluggish circulation with a retention of poisonous waste products accompanies the condition. Fasting or a restricted intake of food provides rest for the tired organs, aids in the elimination of the accumulated poisons, and helps in the rebuilding of vitality.

In some cases, abstinence from food is clearly indicated and yet for various reasons cannot be put into practice. In such cases a fruit juice diet, properly applied, is the next most advisable step. The citrus fruits, oranges, grapefruit and limes, are valuable sources of needed minerals and vitamins and are easily utilized by the system. But here, too, individual needs must be considered, for while the citrus fruits may be of great value in the majority of cases, they are in some instances definitely not indicated because of individual predisposition.

The question of vitality and body fatigue needs further

elucidation. We know that our body possesses stored-up energy much in excess of the energy required for our ordinary activities or regular body functioning. These stored-up reserves, however, must not be used recklessly. As a matter of fact, we should carefully husband these energies, making certain that no more be expended than can readily be replenished. This is why rest is necessary when our activities are carried to the point of fatigue. This is why it is imperative that we eat sparingly or at times abstain from food altogether; for overeating or partaking of food when our digestive organs are unable to digest food properly only adds to fatigue and to the toxic state. This is the reason we urge the use of easily digestible foods and foods that do not produce an excess of toxic materials: the first, to lighten the burden of the digestive organs; the second, to safeguard the eliminative organs from undue strain. Again, this is the reason why dissipations or excesses and indulgences in habits of injurious nature such as tobacco, alcohol, late hours, should be curbed. And this is why we emphasize the need for emotional calm and poise.

These reserve powers are to serve us when unforeseen emergencies arise. If they are continually drawn upon by a reckless or improper mode of living, a deficit to life is the inevitable result. This deficit does not, as a rule, become apparent immediately, for excesses draw upon these reserves only gradually, but their cumulative damage to life and health ultimately manifests itself in full force. When, at a comparatively early age, signs of degeneration affecting the vital organs are noted and a slowing up of the physical and mental capacities occurs, they are but the cumulative results of these depletions.

## Life's Problems Deplete Energy

The problems of daily life, the hustle and bustle of our present-day existence, coupled with careless or harmful habits of living, add to the wasting of valuable reserves. It is the height of folly to permit these depleting influences to operate unchecked, for it is this neglect that inevitably leads to chronic fatigue and toxemia, with their premature bodily deterioration and disease.

Scientists, referring to the inherent capacities within our bodies, often point out that we have yet to learn how to make full use of all our powers. It is true that our capacities for life and accomplishment have barely been fathomed, and that once we acquire an understanding of how to check needless dissipations of energy, the gain to life and well-being will be enormous. This, however, will be accomplished not by stimulation that needlessly and recklessly squanders our reserves but by a program of living that carefully preserves and properly directs the energies that we possess.

## The Spiritual Needs of Man

Man's yearning for spiritual expression is well known. The powerful influence that religion plays in the lives of the many and its persistence through the ages provide proof of the need it fills. The spiritual uplifting that faith and prayer provide and the calm and hope that they engender make them powerful influences for good. My plea to those who have turned to spiritual or religious guidance in their search for an explanation of the problems of life and their solution is that they realize that complete spiritual fulfillment is attained only as we follow a clean and wholesome way of living.

To maintain the human body, "the temple of our soul," in a state of purity and health (physical as well as spiritual) should be the *first law* of all who subscribe to spiritual or religious teachings.

Adherents of some faiths abstain from the use of flesh foods because of their spiritual abhorrence of the destruction of life; but use with equanimity such denatured and harmful products as white sugar and white flour foods, spices, coffee, tobacco, liquor, and otherwise injure themselves by indulging in practices that have a deleterious effect upon the body.

Indulgence in unwholesome food and drink and other harmful habits debilitates the body. It is incomprehensible that persons who believe in the sacredness and purity of life do not also recognize the importance of *not defiling* their own bodies by a careless as well as a physically and spiritually harmful mode of eating and living.

Rules embodying the principles of clean and wholesome living are found in the teachings of many of these spiritual and religious movements, and "it passeth understanding" why so many of their followers fail to put them into practice. A leader of the Theosophy movement once mentioned to me that Buddha taught that *Man can find salvation only through his own physical body,* while a search of the writings of the Bahai movement, the Unity Groups, and groups of similar teachings discloses emphasis upon a simple and clean way of living and the avoidance of such health-destroying practices as smoking and gourmandizing.

Persons devoted to these spiritual ideals should possess the willingness and strength of character to overcome habits or practices that contribute to the premature deterioration of health and life.

"The basis of all religion is truth" is an oft-quoted Hindu proverb. This is merely another way of saying "know the truth and the truth shall make ye free." Both consider the knowledge and practice of the basic truths of all phases of life, and certainly rational living, or living in conformity with the hygienic needs of the human organism, is one of the basic truths that should never be disregarded. As the Romans said, "A sound body brings a sound mind."

## Poise Essential

Contentment, cheerfulness, serenity, are attributes that enrich our lives and maintain our well-being. They are attributes that help greatly in the rebuilding of health. It is not difficult to change a disturbed, maladjusted, or depressed nature into a more serene and contented one, provided we are conscious of our objective and know how to strive for its attainment.

Discontent or tendencies to morbidity are not solely the result of environmental influences or difficulties inherent in life. While these factors contribute to the shaping of our emotions, the state of our health plays an important role. The secretions of the glands, the functions of the organs, the chemistry of the tissues and the body fluids are all interrelated and influence the nervous system, affecting our emotional reactions and our conduct.

Intelligent living, added to adequate physical care, promotes better health and strengthens the nervous system.

Sound thinking, plus the use of will power, can train our mind and our nerves to react more objectively to the problems that confront us, and enable us to handle them more adequately. By coordinating these two factors, intelligent living and sound thinking, we gradually succeed in developing a more constructive outlook and counteract the tendencies to morbidity.

## A Well-Rounded Program Essential

A program embodying all these principles, conscientiously planned and systematically applied, offers the only sound approach toward the control or eradication of arthritis. In the earlier stages of the disease, such approach would be an act of utmost wisdom and would save untold suffering. In the more advanced stages it is still the only sound approach to better health. Those who in their persistent search for help have found naught but discouragement and failure will find this the only program that can promote recovery.

## 4

## THE EFFECTS OF DRUGS

A comparison of the results that follow the different forms of treatment should help us determine which of the methods will really benefit the sufferer from arthritis. I have already mentioned that mere relief is insufficient, and that only by removing underlying causative factors and promoting physiological readjustment can we attain permanent results. The old conventional remedies may provide relief, but the experiences of the sufferers from this disease have amply proved their ineffectiveness so far as permanent benefit is concerned. I have already mentioned that these preparations are not only ineffective from the standpoint of permanent correction, but actually add to the damage. This will be evident when the physiological effects of these remedies are fully understood.

### *Aspirin*

Aspirin, known technically as acetylsalicylic acid, is a coal-tar derivative and belongs to the salicylate group of drugs. It is regarded as a remedy *par excellence,* and is so extensively employed in treatment of arthritis that it often becomes a habit and a routine. There is no question but that aspirin may provide relief, but at what a price! The following statement by Dr. Paul Dudley White, internationally known authority on heart disease, is significant. In discussing the effects of aspirin in cases of rheumatism, Dr. White recognized the harm that can result from its use when he stated:

The possibility that long continued salicylate therapy may depress the production rate of immune bodies in the organism makes one hesitate to recommend such chronic treatment unreservedly. It is of considerable importance to recognize that evidence of the persistent activity of the rheumatic infection *may be masked by the long continuous use of salicylates, which abolishes temporary symptoms and signs including fever and leucocytosis.*[1] (Emphasis ours.)

Translated into simple language this means that aspirin, used over a long period of time, may undermine the body's powers of immunity and mask the acute symptoms of the disease, converting an active rheumatic condition into a chronic state. Does a patient benefit when his ailment is converted from its acute state to a chronic one? What a promising remedy!

Pursuing the matter further, the following statements from the *U.S. Dispensatory* on the effect of the aspirin are of interest:

In the first place, Christone and Lapresa have found that it requires forty minutes for the decomposition of acetylsalicylic acid by the gastric juice and that its toxicity is three times as great as that of sodium salicylate. Moreover, there have been reported a very *considerable number of cases of acetylsalicylic acid poisoning in human beings* with symptoms very different from those caused by the salicylate, and in many of these cases of poisoning the dosage has been so small as to practically exclude salicylic acid poisoning. . . .

In a case reported by Graham (*J.A.M.A.*, 1911) after two doses of five grains each there occurred marked cardiac weakness with pulse rate of 136, and edematous swelling of the face and mucous membranes, with eversion of the lids and lips from the swelling. . . . [The normal dose of acetylsalicylic acid is from five to fifteen grains.]

Frequently, however, even in quantities not excessive, it produces a very different type of intoxication. Among the most common symptoms are profuse sweating, cold extremities, either with or without a fall in body temperature, rapid or irregular pulse, and occasionally albuminuria (albumin in the urine).

Need we say more to prove the toxic effect of aspirin?

[1] Paul Dudley White, *Heart Disease.*

## Cinchophen

Cinchophen is another remedy that is sometimes employed in arthritis. Cinchophen is prescribed to promote the excretion of uric acid from the system. Nevertheless, it is an extremely dangerous drug and can cause great harm. In fact, it is regarded as so dangerous that many physicians are loath to prescribe it. Dr. Irving S. Cutter, Dean of the Medical School, Northwestern University, Chicago, Illinois, in one of his syndicated articles wrote the following about this preparation:

A word of warning should be sounded relative to the use of cinchophen and its modification; while some persons are able to resort to this compound with impunity, others may be poisoned. Some fatalities and much invalidism have been reported following its use. . . . Why is it dangerous? Apparently it disturbs the epidermis (the skin), the digestive tract, the heart, the kidneys, and the liver. . . . All cases do not terminate favorably. Sometimes the degeneration of the large digestive organ (the liver) occurs so extensively that repair cannot be effected. There is every reason, therefore, to look upon cinchophen as potentially harmful.

If the chemical is considered necessary in any one case, its behavior should be watched with the greatest care. *Unfortunately, the toxic effects may come on suddenly with so much injury to vital structures that nothing can be done to save life.* (Emphasis ours.)

Dr. Ernest P. Boas, Associate Physician, Mount Sinai Hospital, New York City, and Clinical Professor of Medicine, Columbia University, in his discussion of drugs that will augment the excretion of uric acid through the kidneys, states:

Cinchophen is the most effective of these, but in view of the fact that it may cause acute hepatitis and jaundice, it should not be used unless all other measures fail. . . .

If cinchophen must be used . . . the patient should be instructed to report promptly the development of itching skin and nausea, or other gastrointestinal symptoms. If any such symptoms arise, the drug must be stopped immediately. *Fatal liver degeneration may result in persons who are sensitive to cinchophen.* (Emphasis ours.)

Comroe states, "This drug is not advised because liver damage (with more than 200 deaths) has followed its use, and because as yet no safe method of administration has been presented."

A well-known physician once remarked to me that because of its "peculiar effect upon the liver" and because it is known to have caused death, many leading hospitals have discontinued the use of this drug.

### Codeine

Codeine is obtained from opium or prepared from morphine, and contains many of the toxic properties of these drugs. The *U.S. Dispensatory* mentions that it is used in many conditions "for which opium is usually administered" and "although less efficient than morphine it has the advantage of *being less constipating and less liable to habit formation. Symptoms of poisoning by it have been vascular excitement, exhilaration, then depression with great anxiety, nausea and vomiting; pale, cool, clammy skin, slight contraction of pupil and sleeplessness with slight delirium.*"

Codeine is often prescribed to relieve the excruciating pains of this disease. It is, however, regarded as having no therapeutic value and its use only leads to more enervation with an increase of toxemia and damage.

### Vaccines

Vaccines were once quite the rage in the treatment of so-called "infectious" types of arthritis. The vaccines that were used were either freshly prepared from the patient's own secretions or were stock vaccines put up ready for use. The principle behind this form of treatment was that the vaccines would stimulate the production of antibodies to combat or destroy invading bacteria.

The majority of sufferers are only too well aware of the failure of this form of treatment. That its application was often followed by dangerous consequences has now been admitted, even by many of its most ardent advocates.

Comroe mentions that the editorial committee of the American Rheumatic Association considers the cautious use of vaccine therapy justifiable in certain cases of progressive atrophic arthritis, "provided that both physician and patient are aware of the difficulties and that every care is taken to prevent harmful reactions." Summarizing the views generally prevailing on the subject, Comroe states that "Some individuals have obtained remarkable benefit with them, others slight or no benefit, and still others feel that vaccines may do harm."

Where improvement follows its use, let us bear in mind that this may be the result of suppression or may be merely a psychological reaction. In either case, it is not lasting.

Vaccines are supposed to aid in building up the immunity of the body, yet advocates of this practice concede that they do not know how they work and can never be certain of obtaining results. While the aim is to increase immunity, it is admitted that the effect may frequently be the very opposite. It is recognized that relief of pain following the use of vaccines often results from the fact that the reactive powers of the body have become impaired or suppressed. This certainly does not mean increased immunity! When the suppressive effect wears off, greater sensitivity with increased suffering often follows. Comroe quotes Holman, who summarized this by saying: "When we think we are immunising, we may be desensitizing, and when immunity peters out, we may then have an unexpected sensitization." In other words, when we think we are building immunity we may actually be suppressing the reactive powers of the body, and when this desensitization wears off it may be followed by greater sensitivity and more pain.

So far as the psychological effect of vaccine therapy is concerned, it is interesting to note one of the experiments described by Comroe in which the injection of a plain salt solution and small doses of aspirin for patients suffering from osteoarthritis resulted in improvement in 86 per cent of the cases. It is known that any form of treatment that raises the hopes of the patient has a profound psychological effect and makes the patient feel better. This, however, is not a lasting value.

## New Miracle Drugs

First the sulfa compounds, then penicillin, then streptomycin,[2] and more recently other antibiotics such as Aureomycin and Chloromycetin were introduced as remedies against what is commonly identified as "infection."

The theory explaining the action of the sulfa compounds is that they counteract or destroy infection by choking off the supply of oxygen to the bacteria. *It should not require much reasoning to realize that these remedies cannot overcome the existing bodily perversions or eradicate the many causes that have contributed to the development of the disease. Germs may be destroyed and symptoms may be suppressed or modified by the use of these preparations, but unless the causes of the disease are eliminated and the depleted or broken-down condition is overcome the disease will never be corrected or be brought under control.*

That the sulfa drugs cause great damage is already well known. Diseases of the blood, injury to the kidneys and liver, nervous disorders, impairment to the heart, and skin diseases are only a few of the many aftereffects that often follow its use. These remedies often inactivate the acute processes of the so-called "infection" or suppress some of the symptoms of disease, but they neither overcome the lowered resistance nor eliminate the toxic condition that exists.

The sulfa drugs and the antibiotics[3] such as penicillin, streptomycin, Aureomycin, and Chloromycetin have been proved to be powerful bacterial poisons. As such they may be effective in checking or modifying certain disease symptoms or their manifestations. However, since disease does not originate in germs but in bodily perversions or metabolic disturbances, the mere modification or suppression

[2] The New York *World-Telegram* in its July 1, 1947 issue reported authoritative medical opinion to the effect that streptomycin has proved itself wanting as a remedy in tuberculosis and stated that "in many cases it is poisonous to the patient and causes severe reactions, including deafness and sometimes mental disorders." This view has since become well known in the medical profession.

[3] Anti-biotic, anti-life; opposed to life.

of the symptoms of disease or their manifestations, without the eradication of the underlying abnormal bodily conditions, will fail to bring about basic systemic correction.

It should also be apparent that, irrespective of how these products operate, they cannot adversely influence bacterial growth without, at the same time, affecting the cellular structures of the body.

## Gold Therapy

The gold salts are often recommended as being of value in the treatment of arthritis. The use of gold salts is not new. Comroe points out that as early as the eighth century the use of gold was advocated as a panacea for all ills. In 1500 Paracelsus recommended its use in combination with mercury as an elixir of life.

With the beginning of this century, the use of the gold salts received renewed impetus. At first applied in cases of pulmonary tuberculosis, it later came to be regarded as a helpful remedy in arthritis.

Nobody knows exactly how the body reacts to the gold injections. Comroe says that the gold probably acts as a stimulant, and induces a mild, prolonged form of shock therapy.

That this remedy is highly toxic is agreed to by all. Many untoward complications follow its use. Various skin diseases, stomach and intestinal ills, kidney and liver disorders, catarrhal conditions, headache, dizziness, severe neuritis, eye impairments, deafness, secondary or pernicious forms of anemia, hemorrhages under the skin, ulcerations of the mouth and gums, soreness and numbness of the tongue, and general debility are among the complications that have been observed.

As many as one third of the cases treated with gold salts develop a generalized itching of the body, and a mortality of about 1 per cent has been reported following its use. The dangers of this remedy are so well recognized that it is generally recommended only in cases where other forms of treatment have failed, and *physicians generally require that a waiver be signed, relieving them of any responsibility, should serious complications or death follow its use.*

Dr. William B. Rawls,[4] an advocate of gold therapy, states in the August 5, 1947, issue of *New York Medicine* that "although chrysotherapy (gold therapy) has been used in rheumatoid arthritis for 18 years, there is still a difference of opinion of its real value." Aware of the dangers of this remedy, Dr. Rawls advocates the use of small doses rather than larger ones but admits that even from small doses "toxic reaction may result." He warns, "Liver damage may occur and may cause death. Loss of weight and sudden anorexia (loss of appetite) should be considered symptoms of toxicity and possible liver damage even though jaundice may not have developed."

While stating that involvement of the central nervous system does not occur frequently, Rawls admits that "deaths from gold encephalitis (inflammation of the brain) have been reported."

His statement that "at present there is no method for detecting oncoming toxemia and no proved method of treatment" is of grim interest.

Gold therapy is usually prescribed only in cases of rheumatoid arthritis, and the benefits claimed for it occur most frequently when it has been applied in the earlier stages of the attack.

We do not question that modification of the disease or relief of its symptoms may follow the application of the gold salts, just as they follow other forms of therapy. However, we must not forget that neither causative factors nor underlying bodily perversions are thereby removed. *The nature of the disease may be merely altered from an active or acute state to a less active or chronic state.* Does such modification justify the risk involved in the use of this remedy?

Gold therapy has received a great deal of publicity as one of the more promising weapons in the treatment of arthritis. In view of the intense suffering and the extensive crippling that often accompany this ailment, what a tragedy it is that this is the best that is being offered to its victims, and what a shame it is that the natural approach, with its great potentiality for results, is so little understood.

[4] William B. Rawls, "An Evaluation of Present-Day Therapy in Rheumatoid Arthritis."

## Spas, Bathing Resorts, and Change of Climate

Sufferers from arthritis frequently visit spas or bathing resorts or travel to distant places such as Arizona or Colorado in the hope that mineral baths or a change of climate will, in some miraculous manner, promote their recovery.

We do not object to a visit to the spas or change of climate. Any change that takes the patient away from the monotony or strain of his daily existence is of benefit. However, it is essential that we realize that such a change is not sufficient to restore health. The mineral baths and the relaxing effects that result from a change of climate are undoubtedly helpful, but the benefits are only of a temporary nature, unless the sufferer also recognizes the necessity of a complete reformation in his mode of living.

This brings to mind the case of Mrs. C., whose experience with Arizona proved rather tragic. Mrs. C. went to Arizona hoping that a change of climate would help get rid of her arthritis. However, instead of getting better she became much worse. She was able to walk when she left for Arizona, but had to be brought back, seven months later, on a stretcher. When Mrs. C. finally recovered it was as a result of having followed the methods outlined in this encyclopedia.

Many similar experiences can be mentioned, which prove the fallacy of hoping to overcome this disease solely by a change of climate or a visit to the baths. We remember a trip through Europe in 1929 on which we visited many of the spas and health resorts. On these visits we were particularly impressed by the fact that many persons who visited these resorts had to make yearly pilgrimages to them in order to gain a measure of comfort. Most of them told of temporary benefits that they derived, but they always had to return yearly for relief from recurring pains.

Among the places visited were the famous spas in Czechoslovakia, Karlsbad, Marienbad, and Franzenbad. In Karlsbad we met one of the residents, who was hobbling about on crutches, crippled from arthritis. One might have asked why the baths, which were supposed to be the most famous in the world, had failed to help him!

## 5

# CORTISONE: THE FAILURE OF ANOTHER DREAM

It is when gold salts and aspirin fail or have to be discontinued because of their toxic reactions that various cortisone preparations are tried. However, Rudd, Freyburg, Hartung, and Lowman make it clear that these remedies can be very dangerous: "Patients with active peptic ulcers, severe hypertension, cardiacs, diabetics, and psychotics should not be given systemic corticosteroids. All these conditions may rapidly worsen and even prove fatal."

The authors state that *treatment of patients with these remedies may lead to the development of these disorders*, and add that "Another common complication which develops chiefly in the middle-aged group is progressive osteoporosis (softening of the bone)."

Another point of profound significance made by the authors is that when these remedies are stopped, "all the disease symptoms and the signs return ... that this happens because corticosteroid hormones suppress the disease manifestations but do not cure rheumatoid arthritis."[1]

When, in 1949, Hench and his associates demonstrated that spectacular relief could be attained with cortisone, the whole world was electrified. Here at last was a remedy that would solve the problem of the millions of arthritic sufferers, most doctors and patients thought.

Since then, a variety of related drugs have been offered to the public. Soon afterward came ACTH, and more recently prednisone and prednisolene. But almost from the very start there were scientists who were skeptical. They realized that natural law cannot be circumvented, and knew that unless the underlying causes of the disease were eliminated, no true correction could take place.

Waldemar D. Kaempffert, now deceased, one of the most highly regarded lay science editors of his time, was

[1] Lowman *et al., Arthritis—General Principles, Physical Medicine and Rehabilitation.*

among those who placed a big question mark on the value of these remedies soon after they were introduced. Mr. Kaempffert wrote in the Science Section of *The New York Times:* "Whenever a new drug is discovered with astonishing properties, cautious and skeptical physicians wonder whether the benefits that follow its administration may not be accompanied by evils worse than the affliction itself."

He reiterated his doubts a few months later by stating: "Though both cortisone and ACTH are still more precious than radium and, therefore, not in general use, it is this department's prediction that both are on their way out so far as arthritis is concerned.... Some of the leading pharmaceutical houses are of the same opinion."

How sound Kaempffert's prediction was has now been fully recognized. The *Journal of the American Medical Association*, summing up editorially what is now well known of the dangerous side effects of these drugs states:

During the 11 years in which naturally occurring and synthetic corticosteroids have been employed in clinical medicine, *a gradually increasing list of untoward side-effects has accumulated.* Most reactions were recognized and reported in the first two years of clinical experience with these drugs. *It was then known that the major or serious effects consisted of peptic ulceration, osteoporosis with spontaneous fractures, mental disturbances including psychoses, and activation or extension of infections. A few years later necrotizing arteritis, associated in some cases with neuropathy, was added to the list.*[2]

There is not much to be happy about when the remedies that are supposed to help the victims from these diseases can cause ulcers, softening of bones with resulting fractures, mental and psychic disturbances, severe infections, destruction of arteries, and deterioration of nerves!

While the above quotation does not mention it, diabetes and the reactivation of tuberculosis are other serious byproducts, often resulting from the use of these drugs.

The editorial continues: "*Still another adverse effect now comes to our attention, namely, the formation of circumscribed posterior subcapsular cataracts (PSC)....*

[2] *J.A.M.A.,* September 10, 1960.

*Seventeen (39%) of 44 corticosteroid-treated patients with rheumatoid arthritis were observed to have PSC, whereas none of 19 nonsteroid-treated patients with rheumatoid arthritis exhibited this lenticular lesion."*[8]

Dr. William S. Middleton of the Department of Medicine and Surgery, Veterans Administration, lists *manifestations of moonface, acne, hirsutism (excessive hair growth) hypertension, diabetes mellitus, peptic ulcer and pathological fractures (especially compression fractures of the vertebrae) from demineralization,* as among the serious complications that may follow the use of these preparations.

Dr. Middleton concludes by saying "hence these potent new agents are in truth double-edged weapons."[4]

A very serious complication developing in rheumatoid arthritis is the condition known as neuropathy (degeneration of nerves). Reports recently published on this condition are highly significant.

In one of them, Drs. F. D. Hart and J. R. Golding discuss their observation in a series of 42 cases of rheumatoid arthritis that developed peripheral neuropathy. They point out that "the patients in whom the condition was most severe, and 4 of the 5 who died, were treated with steroid, as were most of the patients reported on in the world literature."[5]

Dr. V. L. Steinberg, discussing a series of 18 cases of rheumatoid arthritis with neuropathy observed at the London and Chase Farm Hospitals, reports that 15 of these cases received cortisone or cortisonelike drugs and that "five patients died within one year of the onset of the neuropathy, and all were receiving steroids or corticotropin (ACTH)."[6]

Another report appearing in an earlier issue of the *Journal* describes four patients, three with rheumatoid arthritis and one with pemphigus vulgaris, who were treated with the various cortisone preparations for periods of three months to two and a half years.

"In each patient the destruction of the femoral head,

8 *Ibid.*
4 "A New Drug Is Born," *J.A.M.A.,* September 24, 1960.
5 *J.A.M.A.,* September 17, 1960.
6 *Ibid.*

with consequent disorganization of the hip joint, was observed," the report says, and then states: "It is suggested that the corticosteroids have a damaging effect upon joints."[7]

Since these drugs can cause extremely serious disorders, the sensible doctor tries to avoid them, and when they are already in use, discontinues them as rapidly as possible. Their discontinuance, however, is often accompanied with a great deal of suffering.

Commenting on her experiences with metacorton and the difficulties she encountered when trying to give up the use of this remedy, one patient told us that when she started using it, she felt like sixteen; she could run and swim; she seemed newborn. It was only when she tried to stop using it that she became aware how bad it really was. Not only did her pains return; she actually felt much worse than before. However, what frightened her most was that each time she tried to stop the medicine she felt "paralyzed." Three times she tried to stop using it, but each time she tried, she felt so bad that she had to go back to it.

She finally discontinued the remedy when reports in the press made her realize that its use was accompanied by grave risks. Seeking a new approach to her problem, she finally found her way to the natural methods stressed in this book.

When starting this care she was in a wheel chair, but after about six to eight months she improved to such a degree that she could walk and dance like any normal person.

When we listened to this patient's story, we could not help but think of another patient, a woman who was treated with cortisone in the early years of its discovery, and then turned to natural methods when rumblings of its dangerous side effects began to be heard. In her case, the most significant effect she suffered when discontinuing the remedy was that she lost all power to walk and stand on her feet, although she was really not paralyzed. It took a long time before this patient rebuilt her strength and vitality, and before she regained the confidence to get on her feet again.

[7] *J.A.M.A.*, August 27, 1960.

We have seen any number of cases where serious complications followed the use of these remedies, and in view of all this we cannot stress too strongly the fact that the sooner the sufferer from arthritis dispenses with the use of these drugs, and the sooner he turns to a natural, well-regulated program of rehabilitation, the sooner will he rebuild his health.

## GOUT AND WHAT WE KNOW ABOUT IT

Gout is really a form of arthritis. Its distinguishing characteristics are that it usually affects only certain joints, and that the deposits that accumulate are composed of uric acid crystals.

Uric acid is an end product of protein metabolism or, in other words, a toxic by-product of protein digestion. It is normally eliminated through the kidneys. In gout, we find an increase of uric acid in the blood and an accumulation of these crystals in the joints. The quantity in the blood may be increased to as much as two or three times above normal.

Because of the increase of uric acid in the system it was at first assumed that the disease originated from a diet rich in uric acid, and that a reduction in the intake of foods rich in this element would bring it under control. Further observations, however, exploded this assumption and it is now generally recognized that it is not the mere intake of these foods but a disturbance in metabolism that is responsible for gout. This disturbance impairs the proper utilization of these foods and interferes with the functions of elimination.

This is clearly evident from the fact that such other disturbances as constipation, indigestion, headache, neuralgia, depression, irritability, eczema, hives, kidney and liver ailments, a weakened lymphatic and blood circulation, and even heart symptoms are often found associated with the disease or precede its onset, proving that gout, too, is not a mere local disorder but part of a general derangement of the body.

Gout frequently begins with an affection of the big toe. It does not, however, limit itself to this joint. Other joints that may be affected are those of the feet, the ankles, the wrists, and hands. It seldom affects the spine, the hips, or the shoulders. In its acute stage it manifests itself by periodic flare-ups. The affected joint becomes red and angry-looking; the attack is accompanied by intense and agonizing pains. These attacks are precipitated by an increase of uric acid in the blood, which sets up an inflammation in the joint.

In the chronic stage, the uric acid crystals deposited in the joint have caused damage to the tissues. In the more advanced stages, extensive crippling sets in. In the severe cases, the damage may proceed to the point where the skin breaks and discharges "chalky" uric acid crystals.

I can never forget the impression one of these cases made upon me. I was called to see a young man who exhibited frightful deformities of the joints of both hands and fingers and knees. Many of his deformed joints showed gaping openings, from which "chalky" crystals were eliminated.

One of the interesting developments in gout is the appearance of nodules or bumps on the cartilage (soft bone) of the ears. These nodules, known as tophi, may attain the size of a pea. They develop from the deposits of urate crystals. They may disappear, but others will form.

### Gout and Its Relationship to Other Diseases

Gout offers a vivid illustration of the close relationship that exists among many diseases. Scientists recognize a close relationship between kidney stones or gallstones and gout. It is the accumulation of gravel or concretions in the joints that produces gout. Similarly, it is the accumulation of gravel or concretions in the kidneys or the gallbladder that produces kidney stones or gallstones. Lichtwitz mentions this interesting relationship and quotes Garrod who wrote, "in later years gout develops when in early life gravel and calculi (stones) are formed." Lichtwitz also points out the close relationship between gout and such diseases as migraine, asthma, urticaria, and polycythemia (a blood disease—with a pathological increase of the red cells).

It should be evident that gout and hardening of the arteries bear a close relationship to each other. In gout, we have the accumulation of concretions in the joints, while in hardening of the arteries the infiltration of this hardening material is found in the walls of the blood vessels.

Such afflictions as iritis, glaucoma, and cataract (diseases of the eyes involving congestion and hardening), and diseases of the ears involving calcification or hardening with consequent impairment of hearing or bodily incoordination all bear a close relationship to gout and to each other. Since basically all diseases (barring those resulting from injury) involve a disturbance in metabolism and are accompanied by a retention of toxins in the body, this close relationship between the different diseases should not be surprising.

In some cases we find the presence of both gouty and arthritic manifestations. In these cases, the patient is said to suffer from gouty arthritis. This is only of academic interest, inasmuch as treatment and care of both conditions is basically the same.

At one time gout was regarded as a "rich man's disease." Overindulgence, eating excessively of rich foods, heavy meat eating, and the use of alcohol were considered its causative factors. However, the disease is found with equal frequency among the poor classes. Osler says that "in England, the combination of poor food, defective hygiene, and an excessive consumption of malt liquors make the 'poor man's gout' a common affliction." Evidently, the rich man does not possess a monopoly on this disease.

### The Use of Colchicum

In gout, the drug most favored is colchicum. It is believed that this drug promotes the excretion of uric acid from the system. In this connection, however, it is interesting to note that Jackson and Blackfan[1] believe that while an increased output of uric acid follows the use of this remedy, this is due rather "to an increased formation than a more active elimination."

Lichtwitz, too, rejects the idea that this remedy promotes the excretion of uric acid. He claims that colchicum "does not influence ... the excretion of urates," but that "it acts on the capillaries, bringing on dilatation and paralysis" which provides relief by "alleviating the blockade (obstruction-congestion) in the congested veins."

Colchicum is a rather dangerous remedy. The U.S. Dis-

[1] "U.S. Dispensatory," *J.A.M.A.*, 1906.

pensatory emphasizes that "full doses of colchicum administered during the acute attack (of gout) will often abort it," but also points out that "the treatment . . . is not without serious danger and most clinicians urge caution in the use of colchicum during the attack."

A little further, it states:

"When taken internally in therapeutic doses, colchicum usually produces . . . intestinal pains and looseness of the bowels. . . . When larger amounts are exhibited, the purging is more pronounced, and there may also be vomiting. . . . In an overdose, it may produce dangerous and even fatal effects and those that it kills, succumb as the result of a gastroenteritis (an inflammation of the stomach and intestines)."

We accept the statement by Osler that "in gout there is probably defective oxidation of the food stuffs combined with imperfect elimination of the waste products of the body." We also agree with Garrod, who holds that it is the lessened alkalinity of the bloodstream that is responsible for the deposition of the urate crystals. If these are the factors that are responsible for the development of gout, why not bend our efforts toward their correction, rather than accept a remedy that at best merely aborts an attack?

It is well that we ponder this carefully, for it is the suppressive approach that is responsible for the development of the more chronic stages of the disease, with their severe pains and tragic deformities.

There is no question but that relief from the agonizing pains is greatly to be desired. However, relief obtained by means of stimulative or suppressive measures is certainly not desirable, and usually results in damage to health and life. Such relief is, as a rule, not lasting, and often leads only to greater suffering. *We should seek permanent relief which is attainable only* by the re-establishment of a normal metabolic pattern.

# 7

## THE TRANSITION PERIOD

While stressing the fact that a complete change in the mode of living and the application of rational measures are essential, it is nevertheless important to bear in mind that because of the nature and severity of arthritis, results in many cases may not follow as rapidly as we would desire. A great deal of time and patience may be required, and many disturbing reactions may occur before results are finally attained. Where the inroads of the disease are not pronounced and where few or no suppressive remedies have been employed, improvement follows more rapidly, and the reactions or crises that are to be expected during the corrective phase may be only of a mild nature. Where extensive damage and extreme debility exists, or where intensive suppression has been employed, much time and patience may be required, and painful reactions may occur before the condition is finally brought under control.

### The Reason for Reactions

The reason for reactions or crises during the transitory period must be clearly understood. The transformation from the diseased condition to health involves many bodily readjustments. The inflammation must be dispelled. The depleting effects of the suppressive or stimulative remedies must be eradicated. The toxins (the end products of body metabolism) and the drugs that have been used in the past and that often accumulate in the system must be eliminated. Existing deficiencies must be corrected. The organs that have become weakened or damaged must be strengthened or rebuilt. These are some of the changes that have to be brought about before the arthritic can regain his health, and the acute reactions or crises that manifest themselves during the corrective periods are merely signs of the increased activity in the system that is necessary for the changes that take place.

## Reactions Vary

The reactions will vary with the individual case. Recurring pains, swelling of the joints, shifting of pains from one joint to another; sometimes fever, skin eruptions, boils, and other disorders such as cramps, diarrhea, dizziness, nausea, headaches, and restlessness are some of the reactions that occur at one time or another during the curative period. These reactions merely indicate that the body's eliminative functions and reparative processes are actively engaged in the process of eliminating the toxins and promoting repair, and should therefore not be feared. It is imperative, however, that proper care be provided if these constructive processes are to be carried to a successful conclusion.

We cannot stress too strongly that these acute reactions are curative processes and that while in advanced cases they may be accompanied by severe pains or other disturbing symptoms, they are nevertheless of a constructive nature. On no account should suppressive measures be employed, if real and lasting results are to be attained.

Pain and fever are two of the reactions that require special consideration. There are many measures that will relieve or control pain but we have already pointed out that the remedies used for this purpose are either suppressive in nature and as a result tend to undermine the vital powers of the body, or have a stimulative effect forcing a temporary increase in certain functions but ultimately lead to greater exhaustion and damage. When relief follows the use of these measures, the sufferer often assumes that actual recovery is taking place, only to find himself sadly deluded; in reality, these measures promote merely a temporary change with greater impairment as the ultimate result.

In connection with these delusions, it is important that we emphasize that cortisone preparations provide spectacular relief, not because they induce healing and repair, but because of their powerful effect on the body's mechanism, and in time only create more damage and greater debility.

## The Modus Operandi of Natural Methods

When treatment with natural methods is begun, suppressive or stimulative measures are immediately discontinued. The tissues of the body that have been weakened or whose powers to react to the toxic disturbances have been numbed or suppressed begin to reawaken and regain their powers to react to the accumulated poisons. The reactive functions that have been kept in check by these unnatural, abnormal remedies are freed from their artificial restraints, and again begin to react freely and unhampered. As vitality is restored and the reactive powers increase, the elimination of toxins is accelerated.

Acute pains, recurring at various intervals during the curative stages, are to be expected, and are to be accepted as indications that the corrective or curative processes have been freed from the artificial influences that hampered them in their work. These pains could again be artificially and forcibly suppressed; the constructive way, however, is to rid the system of its accumulated poisons and to overcome the inflammatory condition so that real health is restored. The suppressive or stimulative approach is the old approach, and its serious and crippling results are only too well known. The natural approach is the corrective approach and ultimately leads to better health.

## Fever: A Constructive Process

Fever is another reaction that occasionally develops when the suppressive or stimulative measures are eliminated and the retarding influences are removed. When fever sets in, it may manifest itself as a generalized fever affecting the whole body, or it may occur as a local reaction affecting an individual joint or only part of the body. Most persons fear fever. They regard it as a danger signal, and in their anxiety accept any remedy that holds out a promise to check it. While there are many remedies that tend to suppress fever, it should be evident that this does not eradicate the cause of the fever and only interferes with recovery.

*Fever is a symptom of increased metabolism.* As such, it is not a dangerous process; merely an intensification of the bodily functions reacting to a definite need. It is constructive in nature and must not be suppressed. When fever is checked or suppressed, this constructive function of the body is interfered with and this ultimately leads to more disease. When fever develops, its curative value should be readily recognized and only those measures that promote the free elimination of poisons through the kidneys, skin, intestines, and other organs of elimination and that help in the process of readjustment should be employed.

Many authorities have recognized that fever is a constructive process and if not artificially interfered with, will lead to improved health. Medical literature reports many alleged "spontaneous" recoveries from so-called "incurable" diseases following a febrile condition. Asthma, arthritis, and even cancer have been observed to disappear following the occurrence of erysipelas, measles, or other acute diseases.

W. G. MacCallum of Johns Hopkins University very aptly stated:

Only in the last decade has it become vaguely appreciated that there is real evidence that fever, on the contrary, is a reaction elaborated, to a considerable degree of perfection, which aids in the defense of the body against the advance of an injurious agent by facilitating the production of the substances which are formed in the body to neutralize poisons or kill bacteria.

From this point of view it would seem, to say the least, shortsighted to give a patient in fever an antipyretic drug which will cut short the febrile reaction.[1]

If only the dangers inherent in the use of fever-suppressing drugs were universally recognized, much needless suffering and tragedy would be avoided.

### Natural Fever vs. Fever Therapy

Fever therapy was at one time considered of great value in the treatment of arthritis. The temperature of the body

[1] W. G. MacCallum, *A Textbook of Pathology.*

was artificially raised by drugs, vaccines, or the electric current, to as high a degree as 106 or 107, and maintained at this level for many hours.

Those who stressed the value of fever as a constructive process watched with keen satisfaction the development of this type of therapy, for its application was a recognition of the beneficent role of fever in the body economy. This, however, does not mean that we can recommend this form of treatment. We would be remiss in our duty if we did not stress the essential difference between fever that arises naturally as a result of the body's own curative reactions and fever that is artificially induced. While the first is an active process of the body responding to an acute need, and arises spontaneously as one of a number of concomitant or associated physiological phenomena that are part of the body's defense mechanism, the latter is a forced rise in body temperature, brought about regardless of whether or not the body is prepared to cope with the task and carry it through to its logical end. If in the first instance no suppressive measures are employed, the results are bound to be beneficial; in the second instance, while improvement may be noted, this is attained at a great expenditure of energy, and its permanent results are questionable.

Lately, this type of therapy has been largely discontinued.

## The Powers of Your Body

Most persons are aware, in a vague sort of way, that the body is a wonderful mechanism. Both in its construction and in its ability to maintain the processes of life, the body presents marvels that no human ingenuity could ever devise. The precision with which it functions, its equilibrium, its powers of adjustment, have all been viewed with deep wonder by the scientists of all ages. These powers, if not interfered with, are always asserting themselves for the preservation and protection of life.

The organism is at all times exposed to changing conditions, and constantly demonstrates its ability to adjust itself to these changes. When difficulties or obstacles arise, this ability on the part of the body becomes easily apparent.

We have seen that pain is a warning. Pressure or inflammation interfere with circulation, and the body cries out for relief. This is one of the body's reactions to interferences. We have discussed how fever acts as a curative process. This again is illustrative of the body's adaptive mechanisms to meet a changed condition.

*All disease symptoms are specific reactions to definite conditions or needs.* When diarrhea sets in, isn't it simply an attempt by the body to expel an irritant by way of the intestines? Aren't boils and eruptions but forms of elimination carried on by means of the skin?

Many doctors are aware that a cough is an eliminative process and part of the protective mechanism of the body. Note how Cabot[2] describes it: "A cough in itself is usually a good thing, because it helps to take out of the lungs what ought to come out," and in admonishing us not to use medicines to check a cough, he says: "We can all help to train people out of the idea that every cough needs medicine. In the first place very few coughs can be stopped by medicine and in the second place, the drugs would probably do harm if they could check the cough."

These marvelous powers of the body can be observed in innumerable ways. Could there be anything more wondrous than the growth of healing tissue to repair a wound? Is there anything more inspiring than the mobilization of the body's healing forces during an acute process?

The rate of our heartbeat and our breathing fluctuate continuously to conform to the demands on the body. We are calm or tense, hot or chilled, nervous or at ease, all in response to certain definite influences.

These are but a few of the many wondrous reactive powers of the body, which in health serve to maintain equilibrium and in disease to promote restoration.

We are dwelling at length on these points for it is essential that we realize that disease symptoms are also expressions of the adaptative powers of the organism, and are not to be feared. Fear often influences us to submit to treatments that suppress the symptoms and lead only to more damage. A proper understanding of the meaning of these symptoms, however, disperses fear and aids us in finding the correct approach.

[2] Richard C. Cabot, *A Layman's Handbook of Medicine.*

## 8

# NUTRITION IN THE TREATMENT OF ARTHRITIS

A more detailed discussion of foods and their effects is in place. Foods supply the body with the building materials as well as its fuel, and if our body is to be well nourished, this subject must be clearly understood.

A well-balanced diet should contain the following elements:

Proteins
Carbohydrates (starches and sugars)
Fats
Minerals and vitamins

## The Proteins and Arthritis

Protein foods provide the building materials of the body and are essential for adequate nutrition. However, the types of protein used by the sufferer from this disease are of extreme importance. The heavy, concentrated proteins create a great deal of uric acid and other poisonous by-products, which are harmful in this disease. The arthritic must make certain that he obtains his proteins from foods that are easily digestible and produce a minimum of toxic by-products.

A great deal of confusion exists with regard to the protein foods. Many are under the impression that meat, fish, and eggs are the only foods that supply the right kind of protein. This is a grave mistake. It is known that millions of people in different parts of the world live on very little meat or no meat at all; and yet, how vigorous and sturdy most of them are compared to us! They obtain their protein from dairy products, the lowly potato, nuts, grains, and the green leafy vegetables and fruits.

Do not raise your eyes in wonder when you hear it said that green leafy vegetables and fruits contain valuable protein. These foods provide a rich, complete protein in easily digestible form, although in much smaller quantities than the more concentrated protein foods.

All foods contain protein; there are none without it! The question is merely which of them provide the more valuable protein. For the sufferer from arthritis it is without question that the more easily digestible and less concentrated protein obtainable from vegetables, fruits, the potato, and soft, nonfermented cheeses are the ones to be recommended.

## Why We Object to Eggs

Eggs are considered a valuable source of protein, and yet we object to their inclusion in the diet of the arthritic. We regard them as particularly harmful in these cases. Eggs are not easily digested, owing to their rich fat content. In addition they contain a relatively large amount of a waxlike substance known as cholesterol, which when not properly disposed of contributes to the formation of gravel and stones, and leads to hardening of the blood vessels. Since our need is to dissolve deposits and soften hardened tissues, and since the metabolic functions in this disease are definitely impaired and may therefore be unable to adequately utilize and/or dispose of cholesterol, the use of eggs is inadvisable!

## Milk and Milk Products

Milk is a good source of complete protein, and for that reason we favor the use of such mild, soft cheeses as cottage cheese, pot cheese, farmer's cheese, or the Italian bland cheese known as ricotta. However, since all concentrated protein foods are sources of uric acid, only moderate quantities of these cheeses should be used, and in the early stages of treatment it may be advisable to restrict their use or omit them altogether.

Milk, too, should be used sparingly, or even be eliminated in the early stages of the treatment. Allergists are aware of the fact that in cases of allergy milk is not always a suitable food. Since allergy is regarded as a factor in many cases of arthritis, why use a food that may prove to be detrimental?

## The Complete Protein

In connection with the question of protein, great stress must be laid on what is known as the *complete protein*. A complete protein contains all the "building stones" that are needed for the growth of tissue, while an incomplete protein lacks one or more of these elements.

It has been mistakenly assumed that meat is the only source of protein in complete form, but this is incorrect. Dairy products, green leafy vegetables, the lowly potato, soy beans, nuts, and many of the fruits are wonderful sources of complete protein, and will adequately supply all that is needed for the body.

Another point worth remembering in connection with this fact is that only 10 per cent to 15 per cent of the total protein requirement need be supplied from complete protein sources; the balance can be obtained from incomplete protein foods, which will collectively provide adequate nutrition. Sherman pointed out that 4 ounces of milk or a proportionate quantity of apple protein will supply all the complete protein needs of the body, while Ragnar Berg waxed enthusiastic about the fine quality of the protein contained in spinach.[1] Anyone who depends upon a diet which includes liberal quantities of the green leafy vegetables, potatoes and other root vegetables, an abundance of fruits, and some dairy products or soy beans, need never fear that he will fail to obtain all the protein his body requires.

## The Danger of the Concentrated Sugars

Concentrated sugars are not easily tolerated by the arthritic. There are sound reasons for this. One reason is that

[1] We do not recommend the use of spinach, particularly if it is to be cooked, because of its high oxalic acid content, which interferes with the assimilation of calcium.

concentrated sugars supply fuel in concentrated form and cause intensive stimulation. This leads to dissipation of energy and consequent fatigue. The fact that concentrated sugars create a great deal of lactic acid, which is destructive to bone tissue, is another reason for it.

Carbohydrates are essential to our diet. However, they should be obtained from fruits and vegetables. The sugars and the starches in fruits and vegetables are easily digested, do not cause overstimulation with resultant added wear and tear, and do not produce an excess of lactic acid in the system.

All foods that contain sugar in concentrated form are harmful to the arthritic and for this reason we recommend that such concentrated natural carbohydrate foods as figs, dates, raisins, and honey be used only sparingly. Sugar from no matter what source leads to excessive fermentation and overstimulation, with detrimental aftereffects.

Sweets are fuel. As such, if used in small quantities and taken from nonconcentrated natural sources, they "keep the fires burning" just right and do not deplete the vitality of the body. If used in excessive amounts or in concentrated form, the intensity of the fire is increased and the vitality of the body becomes burned out. Apples, pears, grapes, berries, and the root vegetables are good sources of sugar and may be used in liberal amounts by the arthritic. They supply our needs in just the right amount, while the objectionable vitamin-and-mineral-depleted sweets such as candy, chocolate, pastries, and ice cream, which contain sugar in concetrated form, must be avoided.

It is said that the Arab sustains himself on his long trips through the desert with a few dates and a sip of water. Many persons use these sweet fruits in excessive amounts. Dates, figs, and other dried sweet fruits can be eaten as a condiment or in place of a less desirable sweet dessert, but they must be used sparingly. For children these sweet fruits may be used in place of candy. The arthritic should during the curative period, omit all concentrated sweet fruits, but may use the natural sweet fruits occasionally, and in small amounts after the condition has been brought under control.

## What We Know About Grains

The grains have come to be regarded as essential foods. Bread is supposed to be the "staff of life." However, after we study the effects of the grain foods on the human body, we cannot remain too enthusiastic about them. They are concentrated starch foods, and highly acid-forming. Thus they are difficult to digest and cause an excessive amount of lactic acid fermentation—a detriment to health. If used at all they should be used but sparingly, and then only in the whole, unrefined form. White flour products should be completely omitted.

Since those who suffer from arthritis need food that is easily digestible, they should obtain their starches from such easily digestible carbohydrate foods as potatoes, carrots, beets, and parsnips. These foods are not only easily digestible, but also alkaline in reaction and therefore doubly beneficial.

The whole grains are highly recommended for their rich mineral and vitamin content. However, there is no need to depend upon these foods for our minerals and vitamins, for these valuable elements are available in great abundance in raw vegetables and fruits, which lack the detrimental effects of the grains.

## Confirmation from Dental Sources

A great section of the dental profession has become aware that the injudicious use of sugars and grains can cause much harm. In their search to discover the causes of caries or tooth decay, many dental researchers have observed the harmful effects of concentrated sugars and grains, and have pointed an accusing finger at them. Says one writer:

There is probably general agreement that caries (decay) is initiated by the fermentation of carbohydrate food stagnating between the cusps of the molar teeth, between the teeth themselves and round their necks. . . . Inefficient mastication leaving stagnating mucus on and around the teeth encourages the development of tartar. On the other hand, the consumption of soft, *sticky carbohydrate food leads to the production of acid* and this *attacks the enamel.* Thus starchy or sugary foods favor decay, while the more fibrous foods, such as fruits or raw vegetables and fish and meats, tend to cleanse the teeth. . . .

The less vitamin and the more cereal present in the diet, the worse was the structure of the teeth. It seems possible that the influence of carbohydrates upon dental caries *is not only due to their fermentation in the mouth, but also to their effect, in association with the fat soluble vitamin, and after their digestion and absorption, upon the structure of the teeth.*[2]

The New York *Herald Tribune,* October 23, 1938, carried a report by John J. O'Neill, commenting on the findings of Drs. L. J. and P. H. Belding. According to this report, grains "are responsible for the diseases of civilization, including appendicitis, arthritis, coronary occlusion, dental caries, kidney-stones, peptic ulcer, pernicious anemia, rheumatism, and cancer."

*The New York Times*[3] in its story on the same report stated that according to the report of these two doctors, "caries are entirely absent among people who subsist on a meat diet and rare among those whose carbohydrate is derived from the simple agricultural products such as tubers."

The Research Department of the Queens Hospital in Honolulu, Hawaii,[4] conducted an extensive investigation into the effects of the grains of the Hawaiian people and came to the conclusion that the introduction of grain foods among their people *has been responsible for a tremendous increase in respiratory and blood vessel diseases and has had a ravaging effect upon their teeth,* and that changing back from the grain foods to taro and sweet potatoes produced a remarkable improvement in the health and the teeth of the natives.

For the arthritic, these observations by the dental pro-

[2] *Literary Digest,* October 6, 1928.
[3] *The New York Times,* October 18, 1938.
[4] Martha R. Jones *et al.,* "Taro and Sweet Potatoes vs. Grain Foods in Relation to Health and Dental Decay in Hawaii," in *Dental Cosmos,* April, 1934.

fession are of special significance, since it should be evident that foods destructive to the teeth are also destructive to other bony structures of the body.

Incidentally, how many are aware that under favorable circumstances sugars and starches generate alcohol? There are many persons whose intestinal tract is a veritable "still." And certainly for the arthritic, alcohol in any form is injurious! A craving for sugars and bread in many cases is really a craving for alcohol.

## Fats

Fats, too, are fuel foods. They are digested at a much slower rate than the carbohydrate foods and are difficult to digest. Since arthritics must confine themselves to easily digestible foods, the use of fats must be restricted. A moderate use of cold-pressed, unsaturated oil in raw salads, yes, but none or very little should be used in cooking or baking. And, of course, no fried foods!

The question may be brought up whether fatty foods may not be essential to the maintenance of health. Yes, undoubtedly, a certain amount of fat is needed in our diet, but this must come to us in its natural form, as part of the whole food and not in a concentrated form.

Many of the concentrated fat foods that are used are the result of man's ingenuity. We extract the fat from milk and make butter, and from other foods and obtain oil. In Nature, the fat in a food is only one of its many elements, and by eating the whole food we obtain the fat that the body may require in proper combination and in small quantities.

This is how we should obtain our fat. When taken in concentrated form, separated from its other food elements, it is much more difficult to digest, and the fatty acids that develop as a result of its improper or incomplete digestion are extremely harmful to the body. Concentrated fats are also a rich source of cholesterol, and I have already discussed the injurious effect of an excess of this element in arthritis and its other related conditions.

The fat foods that supply large quantities of cholesterol are egg yolk, butter, cream, milk, and animal fat. An excess of this element may result in a disturbance in metabolism. Since an excess of cholesterol contributes to the development of disease, it is important not only that the cholesterol-rich foods be omitted, but also that the perversion in metabolism that favors the accumulation of this element in the system be corrected.

## Fruits and Vegetables

We have been told a great deal about the value of fruits and vegetables, and it should not be necessary to emphasize their importance. Yet, how few really use these foods liberally!

People are served small helpings of some vegetable as relish, and most of them barely touch them! How many are there who include a large raw vegetable salad in their daily diet? Only too few! A salad composed of the crisp raw vegetables, served fresh with a wholesome, natural dressing or even no dressing, is a gift of the gods. Most persons unfortunately spurn these gifts; and so they live on the foods that pollute the bloodstream, deposit mineral residue in the joints, accumulate morbid matter in the tissues, and eventually build arthritis and other diseases!

The fruits and vegetables, either raw or steamed so that only a minimum of the essential minerals and vitamins are lost or destroyed, should be the most essential foods of our daily diet. We need an abundant supply of their vitamins and minerals, for in arthritis these elements help in dissolving the accumulated deposits and in purifying the tissues and the blood stream.

## Vitamins and Minerals

In arthritis, many deficiencies exist. These deficiencies result not only from incorrect diet but also from many other debilitating influences that impair the metabolism of the body.

We are mistaken when we think of wrong diet as the sole cause of deficiencies. Any influence that undermines health contributes to their development. Poor circulation, digestive disturbances, chronic fatigue, nervous tension, and glandular disorders, all are contributory factors. Deficiencies help create some of these disturbances but, in turn, these disturbances increase the deficiencies.

A mere change of diet, therefore, is not sufficient to overcome them. All other adverse influences must be corrected.

The use of vitamins and minerals in concentrated form is often recommended in an attempt to overcome deficiencies, but fails usually to provide permanent results. Improvement is sometimes observed following their use but in most cases this is only of a temproary nature. Often the results are of a purely psychological nature, though occasionally they supply an actual need and therefore actual improvement is noted. However, we must never overlook the fact that unless we change to a wholesome natural regimen and correct all the disorders that brought the existing deficiencies the results will not be long-lasting.

Those who do not realize this fail to see the picture in its entirety. They stress the lack of a particular vitamin or mineral but fail to realize that where the body is deficient in one element, other elements are usually lacking as well, even though this is not always apparent. Deficiencies usually occur in manifold forms. Supplying the body with one element, where many elements are lacking or where actual rebuilding is necessary, will fail to correct the damage.

Your body lacks iron? Your body needs calcium? Your body is short of vitamin A? By all means, let us supply these needs! Not merely iron or calcium but also sulphur, phosphorus, magnesium, copper, and all other mineral elements. Not merely vitamin A, but also all the other vitamins with which we are acquainted; and in addition, all the vitamins that haven't yet been discovered but that may be important to our bodily economy, as well as the many enzymes that are essential to the maintenance of good health, and about which little is said. This we can do with a diet of wholesome, natural foods. At the same time, let us also do all that is necessary to restore normal bodily functioning, for only then can we be certain of correcting all existing deficiencies.

## The Danger of Vitamin D Preparations

Vitamin D preparations in massive doses had gained great popularity as a form of treatment in arthritis, but the bad aftereffects that began to manifest themselves following its use considerably cooled the ardor with which it was originally advocated.

The New York *Post,* June 12, 1947, in a report from the annual convention of the American Medical Association, stated that Drs. C. H. Slocumb of the Mayo Clinic and Smith Freeman of Northwestern University reported that too much vitamin D. hardens numerous body tissues until they are much like stone, and already had caused seven known deaths.

Too much vitamin D? How much is too much, or too little? This ambiguity is meaningless in the light of the statement that "No popularly used preparation of Vitamin D is safe from producing kidney damage, calcium deposits, and other toxic symptoms even in doses of 50,000 to 100,000 units daily, unless given carefully."

Doses of vitamin D may run up to nearly a million units daily.

In the June 21, 1947, issue of the *Journal of the American Medical Association,* Drs. Paul Kaufman, Donald Beck, and Richard D. Wiseman reported the case of a woman who, following the use of vitamin D over a period of 14 months in doses of between 150,000 to 200,000 units daily, developed extensive calcifications in her joints as well as in her tissues, her lymph glands and her arteries, and finally died from vitamin D intoxication. Microscopic examination revealed extensive deposits of calcium in her heart, lungs, pancreas, kidneys, bronchial tubes, and parathyroid glands.

Does this mean that vitamin D is harmful? By no means, if it is obtained from natural sources and not in the form of concentrates. We should obtain our vitamin D from fruits, berries, and green leafy vegetables and by exposing our bodies to the sun or, where this is impossible, by judicious use of ultraviolet radiation.

It is surprising *how seldom* the green leafy vegetables and the luscious fruits and berries, bathed in the sun's rays during their ripening process, are thought of as a source of vitamin D. We recall when much was made of irradiated foods: irradiated milk, irradiated yeast, irradiated cereals, and so forth. But where are these foods that are irradiated to a greater extent than the foods that grow and mature under the direct rays of the sun?

Why is vitamin D in concentrated form dangerous? Because it causes extensive calcification. In arthritis, our need is not to promote mere increased or decreased calcification but to bring about an improvement in general metabolism with the restoration of a more normal calcium metabolism. When this is brought about, correction will take place and the calcification or decalcification that may be indicated will take place, to the extent that it is possible, as a matter of course.

Vitamin D? By all means! In addition to all other vitamins and minerals and enzymes, *and from natural sources* if we are to do a good job and avoid stalking a blind alley.

## 9

## BUILDING A CLEAN BODY

Cleaning house—cleaning the poisons out of the body—is important in arthritis. Not merely "dusting off" the surfaces, but cleaning out the nooks and crevices is necessary. The poisons from the deepest recesses must be "cleaned out."

The body cleans house in many ways. Many persons are under the impression that when we mention elimination, we refer primarily to the bowels. This is not the case. We use this term to describe the work done by all the organs of elimination: not only the intestines, but also the lungs, the kidneys, and the skin. Since the retention of toxins contributes to breakdown, increased elimination is imperative if stagnation is to be overcome and correction brought about.

### How Can We Promote Better Elimination?

Each organ of elimination must do its work effectively if health is to be restored. The lungs breathe in oxygen and expel carbon dioxide, which is a poison. The kidneys eliminate many of the poisonous by-products of metabolism. The skin is another very important eliminative organ. Through its vast network of sweat glands, poisonous wastes and gases are constantly being eliminated. The intestinal tract is another organ that serves to rid the body of poisonous waste material. All these organs must function at their best if results are to be obtained.

When these organs have become impaired, we have at our disposal many measures that can help in restoring them to health.

## Regular Bowel Function Important

Intestinal sluggishness contributes to breakdown and disease. It causes fermentation and putrefaction in the intestines and leads to flatulence, stagnation, poor circulation, sagging of the organs, and fatigue.

If you think that laxatives and cathartics can help you here, you are mistaken. Run from them as you would run from the plague for they cause only more damage. The same is true of mineral oil. You can strengthen your intestines and promote better functioning only through a change to better food and better eating habits, plus measures that strengthen and rebuild the tissues.

## The Enema in Constipation

As a temporary aid, the enema may be used to advantage. Many think that the enema is habit-forming but they are mistaken. Only stimulants or sedatives are habit-forming. We have met many persons who shrank from the use of the enema because they thought that it was habit-forming, and yet resorted to the use of laxatives or cathartics regularly. Laxatives and cathartics are habit-forming and weaken the intestinal tract, while the plain water enema merely washes away the accumulated residue, and therefore has a place in our program.

This does not mean, however, that the enema is to be accepted as a permanent procedure. It is to be used merely as a temporary expedient until the necessary corrective measures have restored normal intestinal functioning.

## The Hot Bath

The hot bath helps to rid the body of toxins through the skin and promotes better kidney function. It also has a wonderfully relaxing and soothing effect. We advise the addition of two or three glasses of epsom salt or sea salt to the water. The bath should be as hot as can be borne with comfort for a duration of about ten to thirty minutes, the length of time depending upon the individual's condition.

Following the hot bath, the patient should, without drying, slip into a robe and retire, with a hot water bottle at his feet. If perspiration set in, it is to be welcomed, for perspiration is one of Nature's ways of eliminating toxins from the system.

## The Importance of Circulation

That a healthy circulation is essential for the maintenance of good health is obvious, for it is the blood stream that carries food and oxygen to the tissues and carries off their waste materials. Poor circulation usually precedes the development of arthritis and if the disease is to be overcome or be brought under control, the rebuilding of a healthy circulation becomes imperative.

There are many ways that help rebuild circulation. Such treatments as baking, massage, hot baths, and exercises are helpful. It is important, however, that we realize that these treatments improve circulation only temporarily and that for permanent restoration the influences that have weakened or undermined the circulation must be eliminated or overcome.

There are many factors that impair circulation. Among these, chronic weariness or fatigue is one of the most important. The retention of waste matter that clogs the tiny blood vessels and the drainage system is another. Deficiencies that result from wrong food or depleted functions constitute another factor. Lack of sunshine and fresh air, and insufficient rest and sleep deprive the body of beneficial influences and weaken the circulation.

Excessive weight is a burden on the body and interferes with circulation. Fallen arches that result from strain and bad shoes also cause poor circulation. Tight clothes obstruct the free flow of the blood stream. Anything that impairs or weakens circulation must be eliminated if the arthritic is to be helped.

## Metabolism

The term metabolism is often mentioned in connection with health, and we refer to it in our discussion. You may wonder what we mean by it. This term refers to the all-embracing integrated functioning of the body. When we stress the necessity for normal metabolism we mean to convey the need for an all-embracing integrated normal functioning of all the organs if health is to be maintained.

Life and health depend upon normal metabolism. Healing and repair are at their best only when metabolism is restored to normal. The elimination of poisons, and repair and growth, are dependent upon it.

Many factors impair metabolism and thereby interfere with the elimination of toxins and impede the healing processes of the body. Overeating, the eating of denatured or heavy, concentrated foods, improper combinations, unwholesome habits, a weakened digestive system, and general fatigue, are some of these factors.

Fortunately, correction is possible. Healthful living in place of unwholesome habits, plus various forms of physiotherapy treatment where indicated, will rebuild the functions of the body and enable the recuperative process to bring about repair and healing.

## 10

## THE BASIC PROGRAM OF TREATMENT

From all that we have said in these pages, it should be evident that if the arthritic is to regain his health he must discard many of his old habits and adopt an entirely new program of living. How exactly should he go about it?

If the sufferer has within his reach a doctor or practitioner who follows this line of practice, the safest policy is to place himself under his care. Experience is a great teacher. There are no two cases alike; each patient presents his own individual problem and must be managed in accordance with his own particular needs. The practitioner who has made this practice his specialty is fully equipped to handle such cases. He is qualified to administer the necessary physiotherapy treatments, he can advise on the proper selection and preparation of foods, teach how to relax, supervise one's way of living, and guide one through the many adjustments that have to be made. His experience has also prepared him to know how to help the patient during the difficult periods that occur during the curative stages.

Let us make sure that we possess a clear understanding of the role of the doctor. The real meaning of the word "doctor" is "teacher." The doctor does not cure; Nature cures. Our own recuperative powers do the job of curing. The real doctor, however, can help by making use of corrective aids, and by teaching us how to reorganize our way of living so that the recuperative powers of the body are helped to do an effective job.

We must be willing and determined pupils, but at the same time we must make certain that the doctor who is to help us is aware of *how* the disease develops, knows how it can be corrected and is willing to give unstintedly of his time and effort to realize our aim.

Assuming, however, that there is no one to whom one can turn for help and guidance, what is to be done? Must the sufferer resign himself to his present unfortunate condition and give himself up as being incurable?

Not at all! He can still benefit from the information embodied in this encyclopedia, and to the extent that he follows its principles, to that degree will he benefit.

While each case is a problem of its own and therefore no one approach can fit all cases alike, a general outline is nevertheless possible, and if followed faithfully is bound to give results.

A complete change of diet is imperative. The arthritic must discard all denatured, concentrated foods and subsist on a diet of natural, easily digestable foods. His diet should include a raw vegetable salad at least once a day, and plenty of fresh fruits and berries in their raw, natural state should be used. Bread, cereals, eggs, sugars, coffee, tea, canned or preserved foods, the concentrated cheeses, pastries, cakes, puddings should be omitted. Salt, pepper, mustard, vinegar, and other condiments are harmful and must be excluded.

The following is an example of a suitable diet:

MORNING  1. Fresh fruit or berries  2. Glass of skimmed milk or buttermilk

OR

1. Fresh fruit or berries  2. Shredded wheat, unsweetened whole wheat crackers or whole rye crackers  3. One glass of skimmed milk or buttermilk

OR

1. Fresh fruit or berries  2. Wheat germ or ripe banana

NOON  1. Raw vegetable salad  2. One or two steamed vegetables (no salt or butter)  3. Raw or stewed fruit or berries (unsweetened)

OR

1. Large fruit salad (composed of fresh fruits) or berries  2. Small portion of cottage cheese, pot cheese, or farmer's cheese, or avocado (in season) or young green soybeans

OR

1. Raw vegetable salad  2. One or two steamed vegetables (no salt or butter)  3. Half grapefruit, fruit cup or berries (in season)

OR

1.   Freshly prepared raw vegetable salad     2.   Cottage cheese or pot cheese or farmer's cheese, or avocado or soybeans     3.   One or two steamed vegetables     4. Raw fruit or berries

OR

1.   Raw vegetable salad     2.   One or two steamed vegetables     3.   Whole wheat or whole rye crackers     4. Baked apple, raw shredded apple, or unsweetened stewed fruit

OR

1.   Raw vegetable salad     2.   Half avocado     3. One or two steamed vegetables     4.   Baked apple, or raw shredded apple, or unsweetened stewed fruit.

OR

1.   Raw vegetable salad     2.   Cottage or pot cheese or farmer's cheese     3.   Berries in season.

DINNER     1.   Large fresh fruit salad     2.   Cottage or pot cheese or farmer's cheese (when not used at lunch)     3.   Baked apple or pear or unsweetened stewed fruit

OR

1.   Raw vegetable salad     2.   Corn on the cob     3. One or two steamed vegetables     4.   Baked apple

OR

1.   Raw vegetable salad     2.   Green lima beans     3. One or two steamed vegetables     4.   Berries (in season)

OR

1.   Raw vegetable salad     2.   Vegetable soup     3. Two or three whole wheat or whole rye crackers     .4. Baked apple or stewed fruit or unsweetened berries.

OR

1.   Raw vegetable salad     2.   Potatoes baked or steamed in jacket     3.   One or two steamed vegetables (no salt or butter)     4.   Berries in season or unsweetened stewed fruit

These meals illustrate the kind of diet that is suitable for the arthritic. They can be varied to suit individual taste, provided wholesome, natural foods are used.

If one has been a hearty eater, these meals may not seem sufficient. In reality, however, they provide more real nourishment than the so-called conventional meals. While we omit many foods that are included in the average diet, these meals supply all the needed protein, carbohydrates, minerals, and vitamins, and are easily digestible. All food eaten in excess of this type of diet will only tax the digestion and overburden the organism.

After a certain amount of progress has been made or when health has been regained a greater latitude is permitted, though it is not essential. An increase in some of the whole grain products, some of the milk products, unsulphured dried fruits, and soybean products is permissible.

One may complain of the monotony or the tastelessness of the diet. When one has become accustomed to food prepared with salt, pepper, mustard, vinegar, and other taste-stimulating condiments and spices, this way of eating may at first seem uninviting. The meals may seem limited or appear to lack flavor.

The taste buds, once perverted, are no criterion of the quality or value of the food eaten. However, as health improves and the craving for the appetite-arousing foods or condiments is overcome, a true appreciation of the delicate flavors that are inherent in the natural foods is acquired, and the craving for unwholesome foods disappears. Then, one learns the true joys of eating!

While the natural foods possess fine delicate flavors of their own, which we learn to appreciate as our taste buds regain their normal functioning, we can well understand that a change from the conventional foods to this simple way of eating might be difficult for some. Where this is the case, the use of various natural flavorings to enhance the palatability of the food is permissible.

## On the Question of Meat

We are often asked what we think of meat as a food for the arthritic. Meat supplies a biologically complete protein, but since it is a rich source of the acid by-products of metabolism, the arthritic would do well to obtain his protein from nonmeat sources.

All concentrated protein foods must be used sparingly, and the soft bland cheeses, soybeans, and the green vegetables are valuable sources of protein and of superior value to meat for the sufferers from this disease.

We do not really regard meat as a necessary or valuable food. While we recognize that it provides a complete protein, we are also aware that it is highly putrefactive, that it contains the toxic end products of the animal's body metabolism, and that its minerals and vitamin contents are of inferior quality.

The exception mentioned above is made only because we recognize that an intense craving for meat may in some cases generate the fear of inadequate nourishment and become a psychological hazard. The worry and uncertainty associated with this fear would then interfere with recovery. The arthritic in his desire to get well should discard all preconceived notions and boldly make the changes that are most desirable in his condition, and to the extent that he is able to do this, to that extent will he benefit.

## Eating Habits

In addition to a correct diet, our eating habits are important. Most people eat too much, eat too fast, do not chew their food thoroughly, and often eat when not hungry.

The following rules of eating must be carefully observed:

1. We must not overeat. Any excess of food creates toxins and overburdens the digestion.

2. We must learn to eat slowly and masticate our food thoroughly. Bolting food without chewing it well interferes with digestion and causes excessive fermentation.

3. We should eat only when hungry. Eating when not hungry leads to overeating with its bad aftereffects.

4. We should not eat when emotionally upset or disturbed or when in severe pain. Food eaten under such circumstances turns to poison and causes damage.

## Emotions

The emotions can play havoc with our efforts to regain health. Many arthritics are tense, irritable, impatient, and fail to realize how important it is to develop poise and self-control.

Slow down! Take it easy! Relax! Bitterness, resentment, anger, hate, are damaging to health. One who wishes to get well must erase these harmful emotions and replace them with kindness, patience, and understanding.

It is not always easy to make these changes, but nonetheless we must fight it through if we are to succeed. Reading, relaxation, interesting hobbies, meeting people, developing a constructive philosophy, all help. No matter how difficult it may seem at first, it can be done! Instead of brooding or being resentful, we must change to a congenial outlook and the results will surprise us!

## Sunbaths

Regular sunbaths, whenever possible, are very helpful. Sunbaths should be taken with discretion. The best time to take them is in the morning or late afternoon. It is best to start with a few minutes' exposure on each side, and then gradually increase the duration until a full hour's sunbath is taken. The mid-day period should be avoided, for the hot rays of the sun are weakening.

## Injurious Habits

All habits that are injurious to health must be eliminated. Tobacco, alcohol, late hours, excesses of one sort or another are injurious to health and interfere with recovery.

Some may find it difficult or be unwilling to give up some of these habits. It is important to bear in mind, though, that unless all these adjustments are made, one will fail to attain complete results. Certainly the regaining of health is much more important than the somewhat doubtful pleasures gained from drinking, smoking, or any of the other dissipations that may have become part of one's existence.

## Medication

Medication, whether taken by mouth or in the form of injections, must be discarded. The patient is often afraid to discontinue his medication, for medicines provide a temporary lift. They enable the patient to get out of bed or relieve pains for the moment. The patient is afraid to give up this crutch. However, if health is to be regained the crutch must be discarded even if this means more pain or suffering in the interim. Continuing with the crutch only keeps one chained to the disease without any hope of salvation.

## Piecemeal Job Insufficient

Minor variations may have to be made in this program because of circumstances or the need of the individual. Essentially, however, this program should be followed as closely as possible and in its entirety. Doing only some of the things and neglecting the others or doing it piecemeal will defeat our purpose.

## Curative Process Requires Time

One who is really desirous of rebuilding his health must embark upon this program with determination, and must not permit extraneous influences to deter or sway him from his course. He should endeavor to gain a full understanding of the principles involved, realize what is to be done, and be determined to follow through faithfully and willingly.

"A journey of a thousand miles begins with but one step" is a favorite Chinese proverb. Impatience or the expectation of quick results will lead only to disappointment. Being overenthusiastic at the first signs of improvement and becoming discouraged when reactions occur will not help. Considering the nature of the disease and the degree of damage that often exists, the sufferer must realize that, in many cases, the task may be difficult, and must be prepared to accept the reactive processes calmly, permitting neither overenthusiasm nor discouragement to lead him astray.

Some find it difficult to persevere. Those who have not suffered too much or too long frequently fail to realize that profound systemic derangements may exist that have to be overcome before correction is possible. In their search for help they are willing to accept any remedy that provides relief, and are not aware that relief promiscuously obtained is not only of no value, but may actually lead to more damage.

Those who have suffered much and have submitted to different forms of treatment with but indifferent or disappointing results often do not possess the necessary stamina or patience to embark upon a new or radical course. We must always bear in mind, however, that only to the extent that we apply ourselves diligently to this new task are we able to obtain results.

Do you remember our discussion on the reactions that we may have to contend with while the curative processes re-awaken and the body is attempting to rid itself of its toxins? Bear in mind that the greater the suppression has been, the more intense the reactions are likely to be.

In most cases these reactions are not too severe and do not last long. In some, however, the reactions may occur in intense form or extend over a long period of time. A skillful practitioner, standing by during these difficult periods, would be of tremendous help. However, if such help is unavailable what should one do during these periods of crises?

At first we must keep remembering that these crises are curative processes and the steppingstones towards better health. On no account must we permit ourselves to succumb to the temptation to reach for the symptom-relieving, pain-suppressing drugs that convert a simple disease into its more advanced, chronic state. Resorting to these drugs again would only lead to more damage.

Then we must employ all the constructive health-building measures enumerated in this book to hasten the elimination of toxins, rebuild circulation, and restore the functions of the body, for only to the extent that we are able to accomplish this do we help to bring the reactions to a rapid and successful end.

The following are some of the measures that are helpful in bringing these reactions to a more rapid conclusion:

1. A regular, thorough cleaning out of the bowels by means of the enema once or even twice a day.

2. The hot epsom salt or sea salt baths applied as outlined in another part of this book once or twice a day.

Where the full tub bath cannot be used, hot foot baths with the addition of 1-2 tablespoons of dry mustard to the water can take its place.

3. Prolonged baking or steaming of the painful joints is helpful. An electric pad or a hot water bottle or a baking lamp can be employed to good advantage.

Where pains persist and remain intense, prolonged steaming of the painful joints is especially beneficial. Steaming is done by placing a towel dipped in hot water over the painful area and applying a baking lamp over it.

This should be done for at least 30 minutes at a time and repeated frequently.

During periods of intense pain a short fast or a carefully restricted diet is definitely indicated. Complete abstention from food for a few days often reduces the severity of the pains or even overcomes them completely. Where complete omission of food is impossible or impractical a fruit juice for two to three days is often a good beginning. A glassful of unsweetened, freshly squeezed orange or grapefruit juice, every two hours, sipped slowly without any other food, serves to promote better elimination, aids in purifying the blood stream, and relieves pressure and congestion. Following the fruit juice diet, a diet composed of fresh fruits, raw vegetable salads, and baked potatoes is suitable. It is well to take one kind of fruit every two hours, and a raw vegetable salad with one or two baked potatoes for the evening meal. Where this seems insufficient, another raw vegetable salad, with baked potatoes, is permissible at noon.

This diet is advisable at the beginning and should be continued for the first few weeks, to be followed by the menus outlined in this section.

In those cases where, because of "allergies" or digestive difficulties or nervous disorders, the fruit juices, the raw fruits, or the raw vegetables cannot be tolerated, stewed fruits and steamed vegetables are the next most advisable foods, provided no sugar is added to the fruits and no butter, salt, or other unnatural condiments to the vegetables.

## Complete Rest Essential

At the start or when the pains are of an acute nature, rest, not exercise, is of first importance. After the acute inflammation has subsided, exercises are then in place. We should begin with moderate exercises, done slowly, then gradually increase them in accordance with the strength of the patient. We must be careful not to overdo, and never to exercise beyond the point of fatigue. In acute bursitis (one of the many forms of localized arthritis), placing the arm in a sling for rest and support and having the joint well covered to provide warmth helps to overcome the acute condition. In an acute attack of the knee joint, an "ace" bandage provides warmth and support and is of great help. Flannels, bandages, hot compresses, or any other form of application that provides heat is helpful in these cases.

A routine of this kind brings about many profound changes. We are endeavoring to promote elimination, increase circulation, and correct the existing deficiencies. However, these objectives cannot be attained at once, nor without certain changes manifesting themselves in the interim. Two of the changes that often occur at the beginning are a loss of weight and a feeling of weakness.

## The Question of Weight

Those who are overweight need not be concerned when there is a loss in weight. They should actually be pleased by it, for almost everybody realizes nowadays that obesity is a detriment to health. Those who are below normal weight do not lose as much or as rapidly as the overweight, but they, too, have to expect that there will be, at first, a loss in weight.

Certain deep-seated ailments cause loss in weight. In these cases the problem is not one of forcing an increase in weight but of overcoming the existing affliction. If this can be accomplished, the weight will take care of itself. Assuming, however, that the patient is not suffering from one of these ailments, and his loss of weight is merely the result of the changes that are necessary in order that beneficial results be attained, then there is no cause for worry; as soon as the digestive and assimilative processes are restored to normal, he will regain weight.

Gain in weight is not dependent upon the amount of food we eat, but on how well the body can digest and assimilate it. Those who are overweight continue to maintain their loss, even when a greater latitude in diet is allowed. Our way of living promotes neither excess weight nor frailty but tends to establish a normal weight.

Now, on the question of weakness: Arthritics as a rule are anemic and, in many cases, greatly depleted. The changes suggested here involve limiting the intake of food, the elimination of many of the heavy concentrated foods, and avoiding all foods and habits of a stimulating nature. A person may be greatly weakened or depleted and yet not be aware of it since heavy concentrated foods and stimulants *mask* the depleted condition. Only when these foods and stimulants are eliminated is the exact weakness of the body fully disclosed. This weakened condition *is not created, it is merely revealed,* by the changes that are being made.

Another factor that adds to the feeling of weakness is the fact that the intensive eliminative measures place an added burden on many of the bodily functions, and this involves an increased expediture of energy. When the functions of the body are increased, energy is used up.

To compensate for the energy that the body is lacking, rest, sleep, relaxation, fresh air, sunshine, and easily digestible foods are called for. More rest and sleep and peace of mind, the benefits of the outdoors and the nourishment attained from wholesome, natural foods replenish the energies and promote healing and repair.

When the digestion is improved and the energies are regained, some of the heavier or more concentrated foods can again be handled with ease. However, until these improvements have been established only foods that require minimal expenditure of energy for digestion and provide optimum nutritional value are indicated.

The changes recommended in this volume involve a

profound change in outlook and practice. To obtain the greatest benefits from their application requires patience, perseverance, and courage.

Fear, confusion, uncertainty and lack of confidence retard progress and make for failure. We must understand what we are aiming for, grasp the logic of these applications and put them into practice. Then, results will not fail us.

## 11

## ONLY NATURE CURES

The desire to get well without effort leads many persons astray. The attempt to get "something for nothing" often boomerangs. Many wish to get well but not all are willing to make the necessary effort. They seek "a vicarious sort of atonement," expecting to reap benefits without giving up their "sinful" or harmful habits.

Anyone who is truly desirous of regaining health will find that a change to a sound way of living offers the only approach with a genuine promise for beneficial results. There may be suffering in the interim, but the results will in the majority of cases be beyond his fondest expectations.

It is of interest that many a patient, when warned of the reactions that may occur and the pains that may manifest themselves before permanent results are finally attained, often remarks that, since he is suffering anyhow, this does not frighten him. Friends and relatives can be of real help during these difficult periods. They should abstain from rendering thoughtless suggestions or opinions, but should instead offer well-chosen words of encouragement. The intelligent counsel and comforting words of a wise and patient friend or relative can lend strength and courage. What a blessing this is to the patient in distress!

When sufferers from this disease, accustomed to seek relief in conventional remedies, are told that the power of cure is an inherent quality of their own bodies, and can operate freely and fully only when the harmful or retarding influences are discarded and a more rational mode of living is instituted, many are either unwilling to accept this concept or are unable to grasp its significance. It is only after repeated failures that some begin to question the soundness of the old approach and become interested in investigating this new way. It is only then that they begin to comprehend what we mean when we say that results are attainable, provided they possess the willingness and the determination to follow our rational plan.

They come to understand that a program based on the principles of rational living, including wholesome, natural foods, emotional balance, and the use of the outdoors with its restorative and invigorating effects, plenty of rest and sleep, and the scientific application of various forms of physiotherapy provides the only method that can benefit the arthritic and promote his recovery.

## 12

## STORIES THAT TELL THE STORY

Case histories have their place in a book of this kind for
they illustrate from actual experience what can be accomplished. Two or three case histories do not, as a rule, have
much significance. However, when they are illustrations of
the experiences of thousands of similar cases, then they
serve as actual proof of what can be accomplished. The
following three case histories are typical examples. We
shall let the patients speak for themselves.

A *Case History*: MRS. J.F.

This is the story of Mrs. F.:

For three years, I suffered with arthritis, lumbago, sciatica, neuritis, and neuralgia.

It started as sciatica. One morning on attempting to get
out of bed (after a week spent in bed with grippe, accompanied by fever), I discovered that I could move the
lower part of my back and legs only with great difficulty.
After that, if I stooped to pick up something, I couldn't
straighten up, because of the pain that would grip that
part of my body. This condition would disappear for a
short interval, only to return suddenly.

I tried not to pay too much attention to this, but soon
became conscious of a pain shooting down my left leg,
which though at first was not persistent, after a while became more obstinate, and settled down to a constant, nagging feeling like a dull toothache.

I was forced to sit without permitting any pressure on
that side because of the severe pain this would bring on.
My doctor prescribed salicylates and codeine, which I
took regularly, but to no avail, for I noticed no improvement. At times the pain and stiffness in my knee was so
bad, I was forced to drag my leg when walking.

Several months passed and I began to notice that my

arm also ached. At first, very slightly, but as time went on, my wrist, elbow, and fingers developed that maddening toothachy feeling.

When weeks passed and the continual pain in my leg and arm had so frayed my nerves that I was frequently in tears, my doctor suggested that we try a different type of treatment. Injections of a milk-like fluid were shot into my upper arm and sometimes the buttocks. Immediately after this, there was a swelling where the fluid was injected, which was accompanied by redness and soreness. However, the next day, although the arm remained quite sore, the regular pain seemed much less severe.

We continued these injections in the hope that some day the pains wouldn't return. This went on for months. I still was full of hope, in spite of jokingly referring to the arm as beginning to look like a pincushion and a sieve.

Gradually I was beginning to become more and more aware of a similar pain in my jaw. I became frantic. I was ashamed to mention this new involvement to my doctor, but when weeks passed and this new pain just wouldn't go away, I visited my dentist and pleaded that he pull several teeth in that region of the jaw where the pain had grown so intense I just couldn't stand it any longer. He took x-rays, tried to calm me, and promised to extract the teeth if necessary. I was back in his office within a few days—in tears, because the constant, nagging pain in my arms, legs, and jaw was more than any mortal could be expected to stand. In spite of the codeine, I spent pain-racked, sleepless nights which seemed endless. (Codeine helped when I first started taking it, but after a period of time, it began to lose its effect.)

After consulting my physician, the dentist extracted two beautiful, perfectly normal-looking teeth. Here, I wishfully thought, was the focus of infection—the cause, the doctor said we had to look for and get rid of—and I was very happy that at last I'd get rid of my misery. However, as weeks passed, I sadly realized that although the teeth were gone, the pain was still with me.

For three long years I suffered and grew progressively worse. I, who always loved life and laughter, had become a confirmed invalid—refusing to see friends because for weeks at a time I was bedridden and couldn't move, ashamed of the frequent uncontrollable crying spells brought on by the growing fear that perhaps I should never get well again.

While my doctor continued to see me, he freely admitted there was nothing further he could do, and I felt doomed. At the age of thirty-six, I saw stretched ahead of me a pretty bleak future, without the least hope of improvement—an invalid, to be waited on hand and foot. I no longer could play the piano, which would have helped me to forget. In fact, there was *nothing* to which I could look forward.

This was the state I was in when a friend told me of a new method of treatment. I didn't believe anyone could help me, but it was a straw to grasp, and when you are desperate you do just that. To be frank, I accepted this new treatment with such an antagonistic attitude that it fairly shouted "I know it can't help me, but here I am anyway." I honestly didn't believe it possible anything could be done for me with this treatment where so many doctors had failed.

I was placed on a fruit juice and vegetable diet, told to take daily hot epsom salt baths—and most important— throw away all the medicines I had been taking. I was also instructed how to control my emotions, to develop a calm outlook, and how to relax and rest. In addition, I received physiotherapy treatments regularly.

My family and friends, unfamiliar with this approach, ridiculed the idea of making such a drastic change in my eating habits. We were accustomed to eating conventional, overcooked, devitalized foods, and habit is difficult to overcome at first. They predicted dire consequences. "But I am so very ill already—how can I get worse?" I asked them.

They just couldn't understand how a method that sounded so simple could produce good results, especially where the varied medical prescriptions had failed for so many years.

*Too simple*—therefore they couldn't comprehend!

But I was helped! The improvement wasn't sudden. In fact, it was so imperceptible at the start that I wasn't too much encouraged. However, as time passed, little by little, I noticed a gradual lessening of pain; I was able to sleep and my nerves became less temperamental. After several months—I awoke one morning, without the accompanying ache in my arms and legs! Was it possible? Not even one little ache! I couldn't believe it was actually true, but true it was—and even today, as I walk along briskly, I think how wonderful it is to be able to move one's arms and legs without pain.

Of course, this didn't "just happen." It took time, patience and perseverance; for many a day I was very discouraged at what seemed to be the slowness of the cure. But the important thing is, I *did* get well again—something I hadn't believed to be possible.

A *Case History*: MRS. PAUL A.

Mrs. A., in telling of her experiences, writes:

I was a sufferer from arthritis for over thirty years. It started with neuritis in my shoulder, and progressed steadily into bursitis, gout, and arthritis. In search of relief and cure, I sought the advice and treatment of many doctors, and spent some time in the Neurological Institute in New York.

Prescriptions were changed as often as doctors were changed, and as frequently as doctors' prescriptions failed to give relief. A grand array of drugs and injections was administered. Drugs deadened my pains temporarily, but my condition continued to get worse. Injections of colloidal sulphur were taken for a long time without effect.

Colloidal gold injections were recommended as my last hope. The latter treatment I refused to take since my doctor very wisely explained the bad effects of the gold treatment on some individuals. I quickly decided that the gold cure was worse than the disease itself.

I have submitted to all of the electrical and heat treatments such as short wave localized and body applications of diathermy, baking in electric lamp ovens, tonic baths and massages. After the last dependable physician assured me that medical science had no cure for arthritis, in desperation I decided to place myself under the care of a practitioner who had been treating arthritis successfully without drugs.

I started, discouraged and quite skeptical but determined to follow instructions and submit to physiotherapy treatments.

The instructions were simple, but to me it meant a profound adjustment in all my ways: I had to change my food, my habits, my whole way of living. And I stopped all my medicines.

After a few weeks, slight relief and hopefulness appeared. After a year, notwithstanding painful reactions, which I endured with patience, the painful attacks became less frequent and of shorter duration. At the end of two and a half years, I no longer had pain in any of my joints or elsewhere in my body. Moreover, I now have a healthier body, clearer mental capacity, loads of energy and eagerness to meet each day's work and problems as they appear.

These methods are so simple, I marvel at the ease with which my body responded and my arthritis was conquered.

*A Case History:* MR. ED K.

This is the story told by Mr. K.:

It was in the month of October in the year 1940 that my feet began to hurt. One month later they were very painful and swollen. Walking became extremely difficult. Doctors thought that I was suffering from fallen arches and suggested the baths. Alternating hot and cold baths were prescribed, but my condition showed no improvement.

During that winter, I purchased twelve different pairs of shoes, hoping that they would afford me some relief; this, too, seemed to be of no avail.

About a year later, doctors came to the conclusion that my swellings and the deep pains were the result of arthritis, and suggested a series of injections which I received weekly for several months. They also prescribed six aspirins daily, which I took faithfully.

The injections and the aspirins did not help me and by the following spring my whole body was affected by the disease. I suffered severe pains all over my body; every time I opened my mouth the pains in my jaw were excruciating.

No doctor seemed to help me, and, disgusted with their failure, I finally decided to give up all doctoring. I started to read on the subject of arthritis. As a result of what I learned from reading about the disease, I started to take care of myself by applying different forms of hot baths and applications, and modified my diet by excluding all spices and many of the rich foods, but continued with the six aspirins a day.

I followed this for five years. On and off there were some periods of relief, but on the whole my condition continued to grow worse. My feet became completely crippled and I developed a severe case of sciatica.

About a month before the pains in my feet started, a skin disease developed, later was diagnosed as psoriasis,[1] which has been with me for years.

Then, a friend advised me to try physiotherapy treatments. I readily accepted his suggestion. The treatments were given to me in conjunction with a carefully regulated diet. Aspirin was completely prohibited.

The results were eye-opening. Within a short period of time the pains began to disappear, the swellings diminished, and I began to feel like a new man. About eight months of these treatments and healthful way of living completely overcame my arthritis.

## The Limitations We Encounter

*While stressing* the fact that the hope for the arthritic lies in this approach, we may be confronted with certain limitations and it is well that these limitations be recognized so that we may know to what extent improvement is possible. In cases of long standing, complete fusion or ankylosis of the joint may exist. Where this condition has developed, the bones are completely grown together and motion is completely lost.

When a condition like this exists it can not be overcome. In a case of true ankylosis, no motion can ever be restored again. However, we must be careful to distinguish between a case of true ankylosis and one in which the stiffness or fixation is the result of inflammation, infiltration, or adhesions. While in cases of true ankylosis the

[1] An obstinate skin disease occasionally found associated with arthritis.

bones are completely knit together and nothing can be done to restore motion again, in those cases where the fixation is caused by inflammation, infiltration, or adhesions *the bones are not grown together and partial or even complete restoration of motion may be brought about as reabsorption and correction take place.*

We have already referred to the type of arthritis known as spondylitis deformans, or the Marie Struempel type of arthritis, in which either the whole spine or parts of it become ankylosed. Where this condition is fully developed, the joints that are affected remain forever locked, and no known treatment can ever free them again.

The Marie Struempel type of arthritis usually begins with an involvement of the sacroiliac joint, and then gradually extends until the whole spine becomes affected. Where the sacroiliac joint or any other part of the spine is involved, health-building measures should immediately be instituted, lest neglect or haphazard care lead to the development of this irremediable condition. Where ankylosis of some joints already exists, it should serve as a warning that continued neglect or lack of proper care will lead to further damage and possible ankylosis of joints not yet fully affected.

Where destructive changes in the joint have advanced to an extensive degree and much damage has taken place, it should be evident that only partial restoration is possible; but even in such cases a great deal can be accomplished provided the sufferer is determined to do all that is necessary and continues to persist.

While not all cases of stiff joints can loosen up, there are many cases in which flexibility can be restored either completely or partly, depending upon the extent of the damage.

We will never forget the first case of arthritis that came under our care. It was our first experience with a difficult case of an ailment regarded as incurable and, while we believed that our methods would yield results, it required a supreme effort to inspire the patient to persist.

The interesting fact in this case was that not only was the arthritic condition completely overcome, but that both elbow joints and one of the knees, which had been extensively crippled, were restored to complete freedom of movement after about two years of care.

The presence of stiffness with calcium deposits need not be accepted as an indication that true ankylosis exists, and proper measures, persistently employed, will often help restore motion in joints that were previously regarded as incurable.

## A Case History: MOLLIE B.

The above case is only one of many in which calcium deposits were completely dissolved and motion restored. Here is another:

Mollie B. suffered from severe pains and stiffness of the left shoulder for many years. A diagnosis of bursitis with extensive calcium deposits was made.

In a case of simple bursitis, with mere swelling or inflammation and no calcium deposits, the problem is comparatively simple. Intensive elimination of toxins by means of hot baths and enemas, a wholesome diet, and the application of heat directly to the joint, along with rest; and then mild, regulated exercises, will yield quick results.

Where calcification has set in, however, the problem is much more difficult. Mollie, an outpatient in one of the leading New York hospitals, was advised to submit to an operation for the purpose of scraping away the calcium deposits. She refused, and in search for help found her way to natural methods.

In such cases, results do not come quickly. Calcium deposits do not dissolve easily. You do not just "wash away" the deposits. All functions that have been impaired must first be rebuilt and the body strengthened before the deposits can be dissolved. Mollie was pale, anemic, and extremely weak. Besides the pains in her shoulder she also complained of pains and aches in other parts of the body. Low blood pressure, dizziness, and digestive upsets were among her other disturbances.

Mollie was "a willing pupil" and before long began to show signs of progress. Better digestion, improved circulation, increased vitality, and a lessening of her dizzy spells were the first indications of improvement. Gradually, her shoulder pains began to diminish. However, it took about a year and a half of intensive care before she was free from all her pains, and before complete motion was restored to the affected shoulder.

At about that time, she met Dr. H., who was chief physician of the clinic where she had been told that an operation would be necessary. He was surprised to see how well she looked. She had grown thinner, but she was radiant, cheerful, happy, and free from pain.

"What have you done?" was the first question he shot at her. Mollie, at first reluctant to tell, finally explained that by changing her diet, and using daily hot baths with plenty of rest and sunshine, she had succeeded in conquering her disease.

Skeptical of everything she said, Dr. H. persuaded her to return to the clinic for a check-up. There he subjected her to a searching examination. To his amazement, every test proved only the extent of her recovery. She had no pain, motion of the shoulder was unimpeded, and the new x-rays, checked against those taken previously, showed that all calcium deposits had completely disappeared.

At Dr. H.'s request, Mollie returned for another check-up six months later. This time it was performed in the presence of six other physicians. This check-up confirmed his previous findings, and Dr. H. reluctantly had to admit that there was no doubt. Mollie had fully recovered. "Evidently diet had something to do with it," was his remark to the other physicians.

As a sidelight, it is interesting to note that after the second examination, Dr. H. suggested that Mollie abandon her new way of living and resume her old habits for six months, and then return to the hospital for another check-up. Needless to say Mollie refused to accommodate.

## Do All Cases Respond Alike?

Not all cases respond alike. In cases where destructive changes have not as yet occurred, further progress of the disease is checked and improvement is brought about in a relatively short period of time. Where extensive destructive changes have already developed, our approach is still the only one that protects the patient against further damage and promotes correction to the extent that this is possible.

The results that manifest themselves even in the advanced cases of the disease are often amazing, but one must not become discouraged should his case be a difficult one and require patience and perseverance.

We have pointed out that even though progress is made in the correction of the disease, the pains are often bound to recur. Recurrence of pain and other symptoms, it must be remembered, are to be expected during the curative stage and are to be accepted as an unavoidable part of it. On no account should anything be done to tamper with or suppress these symptoms, if a thorough job is to be done.

In some cases, after a certain degree of improvement there is an apparent standstill with no further progress. This does not mean that the ultimate in improvement has necessarily been reached. It is often merely a lull during which gain is consolidated and further strength is accumulated for the next step.

## 13

## THE THEORY OF INFECTION

The theory of infection has played an important role in the endeavor to explain the origin of arthritis. . . . According to this theory, the disease develops when disease-producing germs invade the organism by way of the teeth, tonsils, sinuses, or other so-called "foci of infection" or portals of entry.

While at one time this theory received enthusiastic acceptance, grave doubts have arisen as to its soundness, and today many noted authorities question its validity. Yet in spite of this the treatments that have grown out of this theory are still being followed extensively.

Logic and observation easily disprove the validity of the theory. Even those who subscribe to it admit that "predisposing factors" such as weakness, strain, deficiencies, chills, must undermine the resistance of the body before germs can gain a foothold. If this is the case, isn't it an acknowledgment that the body must first be weakened or depleted before an infection can set in and the disease develop?

### Germs Not Self-Contained Evil

It is well known among scientists that the nature and the characteristics of germs are modified or even completely changed with a change of environment. It is also known that the same germs may be benign or virulent, depending upon the environment and the influences that surround them. These facts are frequently overlooked or disregarded, and yet when properly considered they place the blame squarely where it belongs, namely, upon the condition of the body which makes up the environment in which the germs grow and multiply. It is well known that only where the body is depleted or weakened can the germs gain a foothold, and only an environment that is favorable to their growth and development enables them to thrive and become active.

*Once this is clearly understood, it becomes evident that the condition of the body, not the presence of germs, is primarily responsible for the development of the disease. It also becomes evident that when the tonsils, the teeth, the intestines, the gallbladder, or other so-called "foci of infection" have become affected, here too unhealthy body influences have been responsible for the impairment.* When these organs are impaired, the need is not for surgery or the administration of remedies that destroy bacteria but for the application of measures that rebuild the organism and restore normal functioning.

The indiscriminate removal of organs or tissues in the hope that this will correct the condition has proved a costly delusion.


## The Tonsils and Their Importance


A brief discussion of the function of the tonsils and their importance to body metabolism will clarify this point still further. The tonsils are lymphatic glands and serve to neutralize and eliminate toxins from the system. They become inflamed or congested when the lymphatic system becomes overburdened with work. Now, these valuable glands can be removed by surgery, but this certainly will not result in better lymphatic drainage. The important thing is to restore lymphatic drainage to normal. This will relieve the tonsils of their excessive burden and restore them to a normal condition. This is readily accomplished with a more wholesome and hygienic program to promote the elimination of toxins by way of the kidneys, the skin, the lungs, and the intestines, and re-establishes normal body chemistry.

Dr. Richard C. Cabot, outstanding diagnostic authority, recognized this fact when he stated:

The so-called "Quincy throat" or peri-tonsillar abscess has its origin very deep in the tissue; far from their faucial surface. *How do we know that the infection does not come from within rather than from without?* Such a question has often occurred to me when I observed in a child, first endocarditis or arthritis, and later tonsillitis. Such a sequence suggests that an *infection widely generalized within the body has been carried first to the heart or the joints and later to the tonsillar tissues. Have we any good reason to believe that the tonsils are not often infected in this way from within rather than from without?*[1] (Emphasis ours.)

## Harmful Effects of Surgery

Many sufferers have become aware that surgical practices are usually of no help and may cause much harm. How often do we hear patients regret the fact that they have submitted to these useless operations? Sooner or later, many begin to realize that the indiscriminate extraction of teeth, the removal of tonsils, the extirpation of the appendix, gallbladder, uterus, or ovaries, and the repeated drainings of the sinuses, not only offer no solution to arthritis, but lead to needless mutilation and damage. Where relief occurs, it is generally only temporary.

## Opinions of Recognized Authorities

Dr. Ernst R. Boas recognized the harm that results from these practices when he stated: "For many years it was believed that foci of infection in the teeth, tonsils, prostate gland, or gall-bladder, were the cause. This view has been relinquished even by former most ardent advocates, after hundreds of patients have been operated on and mutilated without benefit."[2]

Dr. Bernard I. Comroe points out that "although focal infection has been incriminated for more than twenty-five years as a cause of rheumatoid arthritis, definite experimental evidence on this point is difficult to obtain"[3] ... and on the subject of atrophic arthritis he points out that "the statements of most observers who claim that focal infection is an important cause of this form of arthritis *are*

[1] Richard C. Cabot, *Differential Diagnosis.*
[2] Ernst R. Boas, *Treatment of Patients Past Fifty.*
[3] Bernard I. Comroe, *Arthritis and Allied Conditions.*

*often based upon impression rather than carefully controlled observation. At the present the pendulum is swinging away from complete acceptance of the theory of infection in atrophic arthritis."*

Dr. Richard H. Freyberg, Associate Professor, Clinical Medicine, Cornell University, mentioned that the infectious nature of rheumatoid arthritis *is only a theory,* and stated that he had *"yet to see a patient who had rheumatoid arthritis for more than a year in whom there has been any evidence of benefit to the articular diseases from the removal of foci of infection from the oral cavity, pharynx, abdomen, or pelvis."*[4]

Dr. Victor G. Heiser,[5] in a lecture delivered before the American Association for the Advancement of Science, reported certain findings that bear significantly on this question. Dr. Heiser was describing in detail the observations of research workers of the Rockefeller Foundation who, by feeding the diets followed by various sections of India's millions of people to large colonies of animals, were able at will to reproduce in the animals the same state of health and well-being and the same types of disease that were observed among the human population following the diets.

The highly significant conclusion arrived at by the investigators was that *"A host of other diseases generally never associated with faulty diet were also definitely connected with the type of food eaten by the individual man or animal."*

What were those "other diseases never associated with faulty diet" that they were able to reproduce, at will, by changing the diet of man or animal? "Among the parts of the body which developed various types of diseases in the animals fed the faulty diet were: chest, ear, nose, upper respiratory passages, the eye, gastro-intestinal and urinary tracts, the skin, blood, lymph glands, nerves, heart and teeth."

Sinusitis, adenoids, infections of the middle ear, pneumonia, and bronchiectasis were some of the afflictions that the experimenters were able to reproduce in the animals,

[4] Richard H. Freyberg, "Focal Infection in Relation to Rheumatic Diseases: A Critical Appraisal," *Journal American Dental Association,* September 1, 1946.
[5] *The New York Times,* June 21, 1940.

"at will," by feeding them the diet that produced these diseases in man. Since these afflictions are usually regarded as infectious in nature, is this not but another proof that lowered resistance and impairments resulting from nutritional deficiencies rather than invading micro-organisms are the primary causative factors?

That specific germs are present in specific diseases is not questioned. Each specific microorganism thrives best in the environment best suited to its needs. In other words, each specific environment promotes the growth of its own particular type of microorganism. But is it logical to conclude from this that the germs create the environment? Isn't it rather that a diseased or abnormal environment provides a favorable soil for the growth of a particular type of bacteria?

These experiments conducted by the Rockefeller Foundation have conclusively proved that, when humans or animals are fed faulty diets, many so-called infectious diseases develop, and when they are fed a wholesome diet, freedom from infection is maintained. We do not know whether Dr. Heiser and his co-workers realized the full significance of this observation, and whether they recognized its implications in relation to the theory of infection, but the facts nevertheless speak for themselves.

## Osler's Explanation of Germs

In the writings of Osler and other noted authorities, we find ample support for our concept. In his discussion of tuberculosis, Osler points out that "fortunately, the human body is not a very good culture medium of the tubercle bacillus. The adult human individual in normal health seems to be practically immune to natural infection." He states further that "the ultimate result in a given case depends upon the capabilities of the body to restrict and limit the growth of the bacilli."

Osler describes three kinds of tissue soil:

1. Tissue soil in which the bacilli "find lodgement, but nothing comes of it; they wither away 'because they have no root.'"

2. Tissue soil "in which the seed finds the soil suitable and grows, but the conditions are not favorable, as the . . .

protecting force of the body gets the better in the struggle."

3. Tissue soil in which the seed "fell on good ground and sprang up and bore fruit a hundred fold."

In expressing these views, Osler expounded a truth that pertains not only to tuberculosis but to all other so-called infectious diseases.

## Care of Local Infections

A reorientation in the recognition of the fundamental causes of arthritis does not mean that local impairments should be neglected or disregarded. The teeth may require attention, fallen arches may need help of a local nature, other local weaknesses may require special care. However, the care provided must not only correct or improve the local condition but must also eradicate the factors that contributed to its development. While local care of a special nature may be necessary and should therefore be provided, it is always well to bear in mind that only when the underlying causes are corrected is the source of the trouble really overcome and real improvement possible.

## 14

## OUR THEORY CONFIRMED

The International League for the Control of Rheumatism stresses the systemic nature of the disease and emphasizes the benfits obtained from a carefully regulated diet. Referring to the systemic nature of the disease, it says: "Our observations tend to confirm once more the correctness of all opinions holding that we have to consider the organism as a whole, and that the action of the whole organism has a decided effect on the course, symptoms, and cure of the disease." In another part of its thesis it states, "On the basis of the available findings of Biochemistry and Biophysics, we must admit that in any kind of disturbance of separate organ functions or of systems, or of the whole organism, we have a change in the metabolism and nutrition of the cellules and tissues: in other words, that any kind of disease affects the normal range of change in the metabolism."

In stressing the benefits of nutrition in this disease, the League has the following to say: "Of whatever nature the Polyarthritic may be, whether it appears as a superstructure of rheumatism proper with typical cyclicity and acute cardiac lesion; whether it is of an infectious nature or whether its development with disturbance of metabolism; in all cases, as our observations have convinced us, the nature of nutrition is a self-sufficing therapeutic factor."

Many other noted authorities recognize the need for a new approach in the treatment of disease. Dr. Ray Lyman Wilbur, Dean Emeritus, Stanford University, has the following to say on the subject: "Medicine based on pills and potions is becoming obsolete. . . . Biologic thinking is replacing empiricism. . . . Those treatments involving the use of heat, cold, water, electricity, movement and massage, having striking biologic responses, including effects on psychic reactions, are more potent than many of the drugs

gathered through many centuries by trial and error."[1]
What an admission, and how important that the sufferer
from arthritis heed this advice!

The drift from the conventional medical treatments to
natural methods of healing has been apparent for some
time. The phenomenal growth of physiotherapy, gaining
special impetus during the world war in response to a particularly acute need, and the acceptance of the different
unorthodox methods of healing such as osteopathy, chiro-
practic, and naturopathy by the various state legislatures,
are only some of the signs of this change. One could cite
the sensational successes of the Sister Kenny treatment,
which is but the application of hydrotherapy and manipu-
lative treatments plus psychotherapy in the handling of in-
fantile paralysis. There are the significant findings of the
official Bernard M. Baruch Committee, of which Dr. Ray
Lyman Wilbur was chairman, which were instrumental in
obtaining further grants from Bernard M. Baruch for research in the field of nutrition, physiotherapy, and other
forms of drugless healing. Finally, the positions of prominence gained in the health field by such individuals as
Trall, Jennings, Graham, among the old-timers, and Til-
den, Jackson, Kellogg, Macfadden, Hay, among the more
recent ones, is another sign of this trend from "empiricism" and a practice based upon trial and error to a more
fundamental approach.

However, while this drift is accelerating, humanity still
has a long way to travel before a sound system of healing
based upon these fundamental principles attains complete
recognition.

A system powerfully entrenched, cloaked with the
mantle of authority, possessing the vigor and strength that
position and custom impart to it, is not easily uprooted.
Orthodox medical practice is no exception. However, the
pace at which our ideas are taking hold approaches that
of an avalanche, and its ultimate success can no longer be
questioned.

Anyone in the throes of arthritis who has followed the
uncertain and confusing practices of the past and is dissat-
isfied or who is yet in the earlier stages of the disease and
wishes to save himself costly mistakes should be grateful

[1] "Medical Education Today," *J.A.M.A.*, March 20, 1944.

that this era makes these new methods available to him. He should greedily reach out for them for only in that way will he be able to undo the harm and protect himself against further damage.

We must never overlook the fact that *Nature is the great healer,* and that all correction and repair is achieved through the curative forces of the body. We contribute to this correction only to the extent that we intelligently provide all the body's physiological needs and remove the obstacles that interfere with the body's corrective processes.

Dr. Walter Estell Lee takes his profession to task for overlooking this important point when he stated, "The trouble with our profession is that it persists in too much meddlesome therapy—using the term in its broadest sense—to the detriment of Nature. We are losing sight of 'the patient himself,' and many of us are substituting machine-made diagnosis for clinical acumen, ready to use advertised remedies for intelligent cooperation with nature, fads for facts."[2]

Dr. Theodore R. Van Dellen in a syndicated article, September 3, 1947, admits that "Rheumatoid arthritis is still a puzzle to the medical profession" and "it may be that the term is a misnomer and *the joint symptoms are merely manifestations of a generalized disturbance. . . .* In the future it is highly possible that the *physician will concentrate more of his attention on the general condition of the victim of rheumatoid arthritis and less on the joints.*"[3]

### Arthritics in the Making

We pointed out earlier that there are over 11,000,000 people in this country suffering from arthritis. From years of observation we are convinced that the actual number of sufferers from this disease is greatly in excess of this number. There are millions who are treated for various stomach and intestinal disorders, nervous conditions, heart diseases, asthma, prolapsed organs, gallbladder conditions,

[2] Walter Estell Lee, "Surgery of the Extremities," *Progressive Medicine,* December, 1922.
[3] Theodore R. Van Dellen, "Diet and Rest Help Sufferers from Rheumatoid Arthritis."

and many other diseases, who also suffer from aches and pains in different parts of the body without realizing that these pains and aches are of a rheumatic or arthritic nature. The rheumatic or arthritic condition may be merely in the process of formation or may already have reached a definite stage of development, but since the patient's concern is with his primary ailment, the rheumatic pains and aches receive, at best, only secondary consideration, and often are completely disregarded.

"My back is just breaking," "The pains in my shoulder are unbearable," "I cannot stand those shooting pains in my legs," "My back feels so weary and achy, I cannot find a place for myself," are some of the remarks one hears from these patients, but they seldom realize that these pains and aches must not be neglected, for otherwise they will ultimately develop into full-blown arthritic conditions with their severe deformities and intense suffering.

## 15

## CONCLUSION

We are thinking of the millions of arthritis sufferers, with their deep pains and agonies and with the hopelessness in which they finally become engulfed as a result of their many failures to obtain help. Then, we cannot but think of the many persons who have discarded the conventional practices and succeeded in obtaining the help they were seeking.

We feel keenly on the question of disease and health, for we know that most of our diseases are of our own making, the results of improper habits of living and of health-destroying influences. We also know that as these health-destroying habits are eliminated and the restorative forces of Nature are given free rein, health can in the majority of cases again be restored.

We urge the readers of this section to realize that health is worth fighting for, and that while the task presented to them may seem difficult at first, the benefits in store for them are so great that the sacrifices required will appear infinitesimal by comparison. Health means life, laughter, beauty, joy, while disease means suffering, agony, torture, misery, and unhappiness. We should not have to stress what our choice should be!

It is now common knowledge that the various rheumatic diseases, to which arthritis belongs, are an outgrowth of a disordered metabolism. The various heart and blood vessel diseases—high blood pressure, hardening of the arteries, arteriosclerotic heart disease, rheumatic heart disease, and coronary heart disease—the diseases taking a terrific toll of human life and constantly on the increase—also develop because of disorders in our metabolism.

The next section in our encyclopedia explains the type

of care that is needed in these cases, to promote recovery and to save human life.

It furthermore explains the basic physiological principles that must be known to all people, whether healthy or sick, if they are to avoid the onset of these diseases.

# THE PREVENTION AND CONTROL OF HEART DISEASE

# PREFACE

It is amazing to note the many prevailing convictions and beliefs which, upon close examination, are unable to stand the light of day. Albert Schweitzer must have had this in mind when he stated in his *Out of My Life and Thoughts:* "The man of to-day is exposed to influences which are bent on robbing him of all confidence in his own thinking.... Over and over again convictions are forced upon him in the same way as by means of the electric advertisements which flare in the streets of every large town. Any company which has sufficient capital to get itself securely established, exercises pressure on him at every step he takes to induce him to buy their boot polish or their soup tablets."

It seems to us that many reasons could be advanced for the existence of these misconceptions and that the blame cannot be placed solely on one factor.

However, irrespective of the reasons, it should be apparent that only when we can free ourselves completely from the influence of these misconceptions can we examine each idea on its own merits, and arrive at the truth of any phenomenon.

An investigation of many of our concepts in the realm of health will reveal that here, too, many of the beliefs entertained by vast masses of people are contrary to reason or fact. One of the concepts almost universally accepted, which upon examination is found to be fallacious, is the almost blind belief that medicine provides the answer to disease and suffering.

For thousands of years we have clung to the idea that medicines heal the sick. The sick have multiplied and so have the medicines, which at first the medicinemen of ancient times, and more recently the profession of medicine, have been offering us in an ever-increasing stream.

Medicines come and go. Each time a new medicine is ushered into the world, it is heralded as the final answer to the sufferings of a large segment of our population. But disillusionment follows disillusionment, and the legions of the sick increase from year to year.

As a result of these failures, new concepts are constantly arising, challenging many of the outmoded ideas of the past and rolling up significant successes.

There are nuggets of gold hidden everywhere, but to be able to find them we must be willing to search, keeping our minds free from preconceived notions and beliefs, and be ready to accept values wherever they exist. Such an open-minded and dispassionate approach applied to the problems of health and disease will amply reward us.

We wish to express our deep appreciation to Jacob M. Leavitt, M.D., Fellow of the American College of Gastroenterology, who despite a very busy practice has given unstintingly of his time and effort to review all the phases covered in this section, and to check its contents for scientific accuracy. · Dr. Leavitt's suggestions have been of tremendous help.

We are also deeply grateful to Harry Sackren, M.D., M.P.H., who has devoted a great deal of research in the field of hygienic practice and has cooperated with us for many years in our work.

We are grateful to Dr. Stanley C. Weinsier, resident director of the Florida Spa, closely associated with us for the last twenty-five years, for his help in the assembling of this material, and wish to express our gratitude to Mr. Samuel Rosenbloom and Mr. David Holiday for the splendid job they have done in the editing and correcting of the manuscript.

Furthermore, to all scientists and research workers who are working unceasingly to effect a change in our approach to the diseases of the heart and circulatory system we express our gratitude.

MAX WARMBRAND, N.D., D.O.

# INTRODUCTION

In making this timely and well-authenticated plea to the public for a re-evaluation of our approach to the diseases of the heart and the circulatory system, Dr. Warmbrand is rendering a distinct public service.

Not only has he done an outstanding job of explaining in clear and concise form how these diseases develop; he has also presented a mass of solid and helpful information at a time when it is most needed.

Our approach to the treatment of the sick is in a constant state of flux, and changes with the prevailing concepts of the day. Both in theory and practice these changes continue, and what is considered sound practice at one time is often completely discarded at a later period.

However, irrespective of the practices that are being followed at any particular time, the point that must always be kept in mind is that, to aid the body in its recovery, the inherent recuperative powers of the patient must be permitted to function freely and unhampered.

The evolution of the school of homeopathy has to some degree proved the validity of this approach. Hahnemann's superior therapeutic results, as compared to those of his contemporaries in the eighteenth century, were attained because his inert medications were not powerful enough to interfere with the patient's recuperative powers and thus did not interfere with recovery.

By the end of the eighteenth century and during the early part of the nineteenth century, successful therapy was based largely on the application of Nature's physical forces through heat, electricity, muscular activities, hydrotherapy, massage, rest, climate, spa, diet, and other general hygienic measures.

This type of therapy, which arose as a reaction to the prevalent practice of the excessive use of drugs, also proved how superior results could be obtained when the body's recuperative functions are not obstructed.

From the end of the nineteenth century up to our time, medical research concentrated its attention on the specific causes of disease and, encouraged by its success in isolating bacterial agents as the apparent causative factors, broadened its vast fund of knowledge in the sciences of immunology, chemotherapy, antibiotics, hormones, corticoids, and vitamins in the hope that this would help unlock the door to cures for many of our baffling diseases. Thus, working in this direction, our attention was diverted from the simpler procedures of therapy, and this gave rise to a vast armamentarium of drugs which in most instances are interfering with the innate curative powers of the body and actually are defeating our purpose.

Dealing with the subject of health from a general point of view, we find that while the advance of civilization and the growth of science and technology have brought forth infinite life-enriching values, they have also given rise to practices that have proved highly detrimental to health. The devitaminizing and devitalizing of many of our foods to suit commercial interests and conveniences, the widespread use of the poisonous insecticides in agriculture, the continuous and progressive depletion of our soil, are some of the practices of today that exhaust the nutritinal potentialities of our land and ravage our bodies.

The pollution of the air we breathe, the overindulgences that come with our greater security and comfort, and the hectic life with its noise and bustle are all factors that ruthlessly shorten our lives.

The obligation of the physician to those who seek his advice and guidance should be above all to emphasize the need for avoiding, as far as possible, all influences that have a deleterious effect upon the body, and to stress an optimum nutritional program, plus those modifications and adjustments in our habits of living which will raise bodily resistance and fortify us against the impact of unavoidable tensions.

This is the basic thought that has motivated the author in his work, for which he has earned an enviable reputation.

It is now becoming clearly apparent that the trend in the healing professions is rapidly veering in this direction, and more and more physicians are now incorporating his approach into their practice.

We can find no quarrel with the author when he emphasizes that diseases of the heart and blood vessels do not develop suddenly, but arise gradually as a result of influences that lead to a premature wearing out of the organism and a breakdown of function. His thesis that the elimination of health-destroying habits and the substitution of a sensible way of living offer the best protection against these baffling diseases permits no serious contradiction. That these changes can be of material help in the correction of these diseases is also becoming every more evident.

With this presentation the author has made an important contribution to the literature of health. We physicians would do well to pause and reflect on his statement that only by following such a program can we obtain "the most of health and the best of life."

HARRY SACKREN, M.D.

## OUR GREATEST HEALTH HAZARD

The increase in heart and blood vessel diseases presents us with a challenge of major proportions, a challenge that must be met if millions of lives are to be saved from premature extinction. To highlight the seriousness of the situation, it should be sufficient to mention that well over ten million persons in the United States suffer from these diseases and that in 1960, 921,540 died from them—an all-time high.

One of the great tragedies in connection with this situation is that so many of those who suffer or die from heart disease are those in the younger age groups or in the very prime of life.

What is even more tragic is the fact that the number of sufferers from these diseases and the fatalities resulting from them have been mounting from year to year and are now at a peak, with no hope for relief in sight.

That the situation is critical is well known. *The New York Times* pointed out in an editorial (January 13, 1948) how serious the situation has become when it mentioned that while at the beginning of the century the mortality from the diseases of the heart and arteries in New York City amounted to 118.1 persons per 100,000 population, the number has risen steadily to the point where by 1947 it was 400.2 deaths per hundred thousand population.

In other words, mortality from diseases of the heart and arteries has multiplied almost fourfold in the City of New York in the last half century.

Dealing with another aspect of the problem, the Mutual Life Insurance Company in a report based upon a study of one million policy holders said that we have reached the point where 57 per cent of all deaths in all age groups result from diseases of the heart and blood vessels.

Scientists have long been aware of the seriousness of this problem and have been baffled by it. In the 1920's Dr.

Haven Emerson, Commissioner of Health of New York City, voiced his concern about the situation and wondered what could be done about it.

Only a few years later Dr. Donald H. Armstrong, Vice President of the Metropolitan Life Insurance Company, referred to the enormity of the problem when he pointed out that the mortality from these diseases in the whole of the United States had risen from 111.2 per hundred thousand population in 1900 to 184 per hundred thousand population in 1933.[1]

It was at about the same time that Dr. Jonathan C. Meakins, of Montreal, Canada, President of the College of Physicians, stated that "33 per cent of deaths of all ages and about one half of deaths at the age of 45 or beyond" were due to the disease of the heart and blood vessels."[2]

The problem has been growing more formidable with each year and has reached a state where, unless a solution is found, it will assume the nature of a major catastrophe.

That most of our health authorities are unable to tell how the inroads of heart disease may be checked or brought under control is apparent. "We are only at the beginning of advances in knowledge in the field of cardiovascular diseases," stated by Dr. Robert L. Levy, President of the New York Heart Association, only a few years ago[3] while Dr. Alfred E. Cohen, after discussing some of the theories advanced to explain the reason for the rise in these diseases, concluded "that pitifully little is known."[4] Dr. Irving H. Page, one of our leading heart specialists, and President of the American Heart Association, pointed out how far we were from a solution of the problem when he stated that "Medicine is still getting nowhere in its attack on heart and artery diseases (which cause more than half of all U.S. deaths)."[5] He also has said that "when it comes to arteriosclerosis knowledge lags fifty years behind the medical times."[6]

Dr. Paul Dudley White, noted heart specialist, was the latest to acknowledge that we are losing ground in our

[1] *American Medicine*, 1933.
[2] *The New York Times*, April 20, 1934.
[3] *The New York Times*, February 15, 1949.
[4] *The New York Times*, February 13, 1949.
[5] *Time*, April 19, 1954.
[6] *The New York Times*, Editorial, October 2, 1955.

fight against heart disease. He pointed out "that coronary thrombosis in the United States almost amounted to an 'epidemic.' "[7]

However, while the picture at this moment admittedly seems grim, there is no reason for despair, since more and more authorities are finally awakening to the realization that only by acquiring a clearer understanding of the underlying causes of these diseases can we come close to a solution for them.

When *The New York Times* in an editorial mentioned that "there is no certain information on the relation of occupation, stress and strain, diet, habits, the use of alcohol and tobacco to coronary thrombosis," and referred to the statement of Dr. White that "nobody as yet has made an adequate study of these various underlying factors," it indicated that our authorities are now finally beginning to realize the direction in which research has to be channeled if these diseases are to be brought under control.

While this involves a radical departure from the conventional approach, it should be of interest to learn that many authorities are now recognizing that only by a change in our habits of living can an adequate solution to this problem be found.

Dr. Edward L. Bortz,[8] Philadelphia's leading heart specialist and past President of the American Medical Association, has stressed the importance of these factors for a long time. He mentioned some time ago that the average person "eats too much of the wrong foods and generally overstuffs, passes up exercise and doesn't bother to relax" and that as a result wears out his body thirty years too soon.

He continued by stating that by correct living man "could live to be 100 easily."

That a change in our mode of living could save many lives and prolong the lives of others by many years is now being recognized to an ever greater extent. When Dr. A. A. Bogomoletz[9] of longevity serum fame stated that "a man of sixty or seventy is still young, he has lived only half of his natural life," it was not mere conjecture on his

[7] *The New York Times,* February 14, 1956.
[8] *Sunday Compass,* December 4, 1949.
[9] *The Prolongation of Life.*

part. His statement conformed to the observations of many scientists who, in search of a guide to what our life span could be, noted that animals in their natural state attain a life span of five to seven times the period required to reach maturity.

Since man reaches maturity at the age of twenty to twenty-five years, it seemed obvious that if we lived in accordance with the laws of nature our life span, too, could be extended to five to seven times our age of maturity, thus giving us a life span of from 100 to 150 years.

While Dr. Bogomoletz' serum failed to live up to its original promise and has long been forgotten (Bogomoletz himself died at the age of sixty-five from hardening of the arteries), the idea that our present-day life span of fifty to eighty is not Nature's limit, and could be considerably prolonged, should act as a challenge to all of us.

We are far from this goal. While we continue to boast of the progress we are making, we know that a great many of our people do not even reach the proverbial three score and ten, but die in their early forties, fifties, or sixties. What is even more tragic is that many of those who die prematurely suffer for many years from one or more of the many serious metabolic or degenerative diseases, that play havoc with our lives. Heart diseases and high blood pressure, cancer, diabetes, the various degenerative diseases of the nervous system, the diseases of the kidneys and the liver are found rampant, causing untold suffering and shortening the lives of millions of people.

While some of our readers may be skeptical as to whether our life span could really be extended to between one hundred and one hundred fifty years, we are certain that most of us would be interested if, by making a few simple readjustments in our habits of living, premature breakdown could be avoided and life could be prolonged.

It is unfortunate that the beginning of diseases are in most instances not easily recognized, and that we become aware that we are ill only when pain or other symptoms of discomfort set in. It is for this reason that the clear relationship between our habits of living and the diseased condition that ultimately makes its appearance is often overlooked. We fail to realize that these diseases are the outgrowth of abuses extending over a period of time, and that only when the abuses that have given rise to them are eliminated can these diseases be checked or modified.

The precious gift of life free from disease and pain is within our reach, but can only be attained when we learn to follow a sound program of living.

## 2

# THE FASCINATING STORY OF THE CIRCULATORY SYSTEM

One of the most fascinating stories of the body is that of the blood and its circulation. The role of the bloodstream, its composition, and its functioning has interested scientists for many ages. While the bloodstream is the medium through which oxygen and nutrition are carried to the cells and through which their waste products are eliminated, it performs many other valuable functions. It helps to regulate the heat of the body, distribute the secretions of the internal glands, maintain the acid-base balance of the system, and protect the body against what is commonly known as infection.

## The Blood

That the blood plays an important role in maintaining the health of the body was known long before Dr. Harvey's monumental discovery of the circulation of the blood. However, this discovery opened new vistas, helped to clear up many problems, and made possible a great deal of additional progress.

Today the importance of the blood and its effect upon our health and well-being are fully recognized, and it is now well known that any impairment in its composition or functioning will vitally affect the body as a whole.

When we talk of the blood, we talk of a vast world teeming with countless microscopic entities known as the blood cells. This enormous population confined within the blood vessels lives and functions in a sea of fluid known as the plasma. About half our blood is composed of plasma, while the other half is made up of the blood cells that live and work in it.

Two types of blood cells inhabit this strange world—the red and the white. The red blood cells pick up the oxygen in the lungs and carry it to all the cells of the body, while the white blood cells fight off "infection" or foreign matter.

For one to visualize the prolific life existing within our bloodstream it should be sufficient to mention that each cubic millimeter of blood in the average healthy human body contains about five million red blood cells and between seventy-five hundred and ten thousand white blood cells. The count of the red blood cells may vary somewhat with the individual. In women we may find about four and a half million, while in a newborn infant the count may run as high as six to eight million per cubic millimeter.

The count of the white blood cells increases considerably during so-called infection and falls back to normal when the infectious process clears up.

Since the average adult body contains about six to eight quarts of blood, we can readily visualize that the number of red and white blood cells living and working within the confines of our body reaches astronomical figures.

As is well known, the blood vessels are airtight to prevent air from coming in contact with the blood. In case of injury, the blood of a healthy person clots quickly when coming in contact with the air and this seals the wound. The blood contains such clotting substances as thrombin, prothrombin, thromboplastin, ionized calcium, and fibrinogen, which make it clot whenever it comes in contact with air. In case of injury this protects us against hemorrhage.

When some of these elements are not present in the blood in adequate amounts or when an imbalance exists, the blood may not be able to clot properly, and in case of injury we would be in danger of bleeding to death. On the other hand, under certain conditions the blood may tend to clot too quickly, and then we are in danger of blood clot formation. This is the condition that exists when clots form in the heart, the brain, or the extremities.

In the healthy body the clotting mechanism is in perfect balance and the problem of too rapid or incomplete clotting of the blood arises only when our health has become impaired sufficiently to upset this balance.

### The Heart: A Living Pump

The heart is a hollow muscular organ about the size of a

fist. The inner part of the heart is divided into four chambers, two on the right and two on the left side. The upper chambers are separated from the lower chambers by a partition each side of which contains a valve that opens downward. These valves open when the heart muscles relax, and close when contraction sets in, thus regulating the flow of blood to the body and to the lungs. This process continues without a stop throughout life.

Each side of the heart is completely separate from the other, and handles its own particular part of the circulation. Thus, the heart may be regarded as a dual pump, taking care of two separate but interrelated circulations.

The right side of the heart pumps the poison-laden and oxygen-deficient blood brought back from all over the body into the lungs, where carbon dioxide is given off and new oxygen is taken on. The left side of the heart receives the purified and oxygen-enriched blood from the lungs and then pumps it into the general circulation for distribution to all parts of the body.

Have you ever watched a pump at work, its piston moving up and down, up and down, at regular, rhythmic intervals? The heart has no piston but, like the pumping engine, keeps pumping steadily, contracting and relaxing its muscular tissue at regular, rhythmic intervals, forcing the flow of blood ever onward and forward.

Here is a step-by-step description of how the heart performs its work.

When the poison-laden and oxygen-depleted blood is brought back to the heart, it is first emptied into the upper right chamber. From there it is pumped into the lower right chamber, and then carried by two blood vessels (the pulmonic arteries) into the lungs.

After giving up its carbon dioxide and taking on a new supply of oxygen, it is then carried through an entirely different set of blood vessels, this time four in number, two from each lung, into the left upper chamber of the heart. From there it is pumped into the lower left chamber and then pumped into the general circulation for distribution to all parts of the body.

We have seen that each side of the heart is completely separated from the other. Occasionally, however, we are confronted with a case where an opening exists between the two sides of the heart. This is a mechanical abnormality of congenital origin and is dangerous to life since it permits the blood to seep through in the wrong direction, causing the blood of the two circulations to intermingle. Surgery is now being used in many of these cases as a corrective measure.[1]

The upper chambers of the heart fill with blood during their moment of relaxation and empty their content into the lower chambers during their moment of contraction, both sides performing their work simultaneously.

This work goes on continuously, each pumping beat of the heart, each lub-dub, taking about nine tenths of a second or about 72 times per minute. It is less when the body is at rest and more when the heart has more work to do

However, while the heart maintains its work continuously, it also has its periods of rest. It rests after each beat, and each interval of rest is about twice as long as the beat itself.

With each contraction, the heart pumps about three ounces of venous or oxygen-depleted blood into the lungs, and an equal amount of arterial or oxygen-enriched blood into the general circulation.

The total volume of blood in our body is about six to eight quarts. Since three ounces of blood pass through the heart with each beat and since each beat of the heart takes about nine tenths of a second, the total volume of blood passes through the heart and completes its cycle throughout the body in about one to one and a half minutes.

It is important to bear in mind that while each side of the heart handles its own specific part of the circulation, both sides work in unison. Both upper chambers of the heart fill with blood during their momentary state of expansion and empty their contents into the lower chambers during their moment of contraction.

The lower chambers of the heart also work in teamlike fashion. They fill during their momentary state of expan-

[1] Where this type of surgery is necessary, the importance of a carefully planned mode of living must be recognized since in addition to correcting the mechanical abnormality, the heart, as well as the rest of the body, must be strengthened so that the patient can come through the operation successfully and be protected against possible future breakdowns.

sion, and force the blood onward during their moment of contraction.

The rapidity or intensity with which the heart works is determined to a great extent by the demand placed upon it. When the heart has less work to do, it is more at ease and usually works at a slower pace. When a greater demand is made, it is forced to work at a faster pace and with greater intensity. When an organ is called upon to do more work, it must be supplied with more oxygen, and the heart must pump more blood to supply it. When we run or exercise, more oxygen is needed and the heart is forced to pump harder. The same is true when we eat. To digest food, the digestive organs require more oxygen and the heart is called upon to do more work.

More oxygen is required during illness, and this again increases the work of the heart. The same holds true in excitement, tension, overwork, or any type of emotional stress.

When the heart is in a healthy condition it possesses a great deal of power and strength that provide not only for the regular demands of the body, but also a great deal of reserve power to meet unforeseen or unexpected needs.

Whenever a demand for an increase in circulation arises anywhere in the body, this demand is transmitted with lightning speed to the pumping mechanism of the heart and when the heart is in good health, it unfailingly responds to this need.

It should be apparent, however, that whenever the heart is called upon to spend its reserve powers recklessly, it will ultimately become worn out, and its efficiency and power will become impaired.

These reserve powers should be husbanded carefully so that they may be at our disposal during periods of actual stress, as in the case of disease, accident, or shock, and it is the height of folly to squander them carelessly, thereby jeopardizing our health and our life.

That the normal heart possesses amazing functional and recuperative powers is well known. Scientific writers often overwhelm us with their description of the amount of work the heart can do and marvel at the precision with which it performs its functions. However, it is the rare scientist who points out that even this powerful organ can ultimately become weakened and worn out and that, to protect ourselves against this possibility, our reserve powers must not be needlessly drawn upon.

Since the heart too is composed of living tissue, it too must receive nutrition and oxygen if it is to keep well and be able to do its work. However, the nutrient elements and oxygen that the heart receives are not obtained by it from the blood that passes through it during its pumping operation, but from the blood supplied to it through a special set of arteries: the coronary arteries.

The coronary arteries are the first two arteries that branch off from the main arterial trunk as it emerges from the lower left chamber of the heart. They divide in many smaller branches and carry blood to all parts of the heart.

## The Arteries and Veins

While the work of the heart is to pump the blood and keep it in circulation, the work of the arteries is to carry the blood with its oxygen and other nutrient materials to every cell and part of the body.

The arteries are composed of soft, elastic muscle fibers and are powerful enough to take the full impact of the pumping heart. They expand to receive the blood that the heart pumps into them and contract to force it onward.

Since the arteries are composed of living tissue they also require food and oxygen, but, just as in the case of the heart, they obtain their nutrients not from the blood that flows through them, but from the blood brought to them by their own special arteries, the *vaso vasorum*. An intricate system of nerves plays an important part in regulating their functions.

Starting with the main artery, the aorta, which emerges from the lower left chamber of the heart, the arterial system branches into a vast network of large and small arteries, reaching out in every direction and carrying blood with its oxygen and other nutrient elements to every cell and part of the body. The large arteries subdivide first into smaller arteries, then into still smaller arteries, and finally into the minute, hairlike blood vessels known as the capillaries.

## The Capillaries

The actual interchange between the blood and the tissue cells takes place not in the larger arteries or their smaller subdivisions but in their smallest subdivisions, the capillaries. The capillaries are the minute, thin-walled hairlike channels stretching many thousands of miles, that reach into every nook and corner of the body, that transport food and oxygen to all the cells of the body and remove their waste products.

This interchange between the capillaries and the tissue cells takes place through the very thin walls of the capillaries and proceeds at billions of different points simultaneously.

This process of interchange is known as osmosis, and may be compared to the transposition that takes place when two liquids, one containing salt, the other sugar, are separated from one another by a thin, permeable membrane. A reciprocal exchange of the contents of both solutions takes place and the contents of both solutions become equalized. This is how the exchange between the cells and the blood takes place. The cells take the oxygen and other essential elements out of the blood, and in turn give up their waste products.

It is not always easy for the human mind to visualize the minuteness of a capillary. Kahn[2] states that each capillary is "fifty times finer than the finest human hair," and points out that it is so minute that about seven hundred capillaries could be packed into the space occupied by the thickness of a pin.

Through these microscopic blood vessels the blood corpuscles pass steadily in single file, carrying oxygen and other nutritive elements to the cells, and carrying off their toxins.

The capillaries, the smallest subdivision of the arteries, also form the beginning of the veins. Neighboring capillaries merge and form small veins, *venulea,* out of which by fusion the larger veins are formed.

[2] Fritz Kahn, *Man in Structure and Function.*

### The Veins

While the arteries carry the oxygen-enriched blood to the cells, the veins carry the oxygen-depleted and poison-laden blood back to the right side of the heart to be pumped into the lungs for purification and re-oxygenation. However, even though both types of blood vessels are part of the same circulatory system, they nevertheless show certain structural differences. The arteries, closer to the pumping heart and exposed to its full force, have a much heavier load to carry and because of this are more powerfully developed and possess a greater resiliency than the veins.

The veins, on the other hand, possess a unique feature not found in the arteries. They are covered with valves to prevent the blood from flowing back. The veins being farther away from the heart and not benefiting to the same degree as the arteries from its pumping force or "push," need this added protection.

### The Kidneys: Part of a Trinity

The kidneys, too, bear an important relationship to the heart and blood vessels. They are part of a trinity that together controls circulation and affects the health of the body. While the heart acts as the pump that maintains the circulation and the arteries provide the channels through which the blood circulates, the kidneys are the organs that filter the toxic wastes from the blood.

Another important function of the kidneys is to control the fluid content of the body. About two thirds of the human body is composed of fluids. The cells contain fluids and live in a fluid medium. The blood, too, is largely composed of fluids.

We take fluid into the system with our food and drink, and have to eliminate that which the body is unable to use. Some of it is expelled through the lungs in the form of vapor when we exhale. We excrete some through our sweat glands, but the greatest portion is usually eliminated through the kidneys.

The kidneys have an elaborate filter system composed of miles and miles of hair-sized filtering tubules. In one day many quarts of fluid pass through these filters, but the greatest amount is reabsorbed by the tubules and only about one to two quarts are actually eliminated through the kidneys.

When the kidneys become damaged, they are unable to filter out the wastes from the blood and the intricate mechanism that controls the fluid content of the body is unable to function efficiently. This upsets the equilibrium in the body and places an increased burden on the heart and the blood vessels.

How important the function of the kidneys is to the maintenance of health can be seen from the fact that approximately 20 per cent of all the blood pumped by the heart is carried to the kidneys.

When the heart is damaged, the kidneys fail to receive an adequate supply of blood and this in turn impairs the intricate filtering mechanism and upsets the fluid balance. As a result, fluids begin to accumulate in the system, appearing first in the area of poorest circulation, the feet and legs, and then, as the disease progresses, in the abdomen and chest. The retention of this fluid places an added load on an already overworked heart and may ultimately progress to the point where the patient virtually drowns in his own fluids.

It should be apparent from all this that the workings of the heart, the blood vessels, and the kidneys are closely interrelated, and that damage to one organ will adversely affect the function of the others.

## 3

# THE THREE MAJOR TYPES OF HEART DISEASE

The types of heart disease most prevalent and taking the greatest toll of human life may be grouped into three categories: hypertensive, coronary or arteriosclerotic, and valvular or rheumatic.

## 1. Hypertensive Heart Disease

Hypertensive heart disease is the type that develops as a result of or in connection with high blood pressure. When the blood pressure is high, the heart is forced to work harder to maintain the circulation. In order to cope with this added demand, the muscle of the heart is forced to enlarge.

While an enlargement of the heart is a characteristic sign in this type of heart disease, it must be remembered that a mere enlargement in the size of the heart is not in itself an indication of heart disease. Athletes or physically active persons often develop larger heart muscles as a result of their physical activities. However, a muscle that becomes larger because of normal physical exertion is a healthy muscle, while a muscle forced to enlarge when too much work is thrust upon it is sapped of its strength and ultimately becomes worn out and damaged.

### Arteriosclerosis or Hardening of the Arteries

Many factors contribute to the development of high blood pressure. Nervous tension, glandular disorders, certain types of kidney disease, and a change in the volume or consistency of the blood are among them. However, the factor that most often contributes to it is hardening of the arteries.

We have seen that the arteries in the healthy individual are soft and pliable and are able to expand and contract effectively. When the arteries become hard and brittle and the inner walls thicken and narrow, they are unable to do their work efficiently, and the heart is forced to pump much harder to maintain circulation.

Hardening of the arteries occurs in two forms. One, the pipestem or calcifying-type of hardening, is caused by the gradual deposit of calcium within the walls of the arteries. While this condition is found most frequently in older people, the young are not immune to it. The other, the cholesterol type of hardening, develops when cholesterol, a chemical substance of fatty origin, is deposited within the walls of the arteries.

When cholesterol accumulates in an artery, sores or ulcers develop at the site of deposit, and in time this is followed by hardening and thickening. This change narrows the channel through which the blood flows and ultimately leads to the formation of clots.

Since this type of hardening affects the younger age groups most frequently and takes the greatest toll of life from among them, this is the type of hardening of greatest concern to us.

## What Is Blood Pressure?

When we talk of blood pressure, we talk of the pressure exerted within the blood vessels by the circulating blood. The blood pressure is measured to determine the amount of effort exerted by the heart to maintain circulation and the amount of pressure that exists in the arteries when the heart is at rest.

When the heart is in action the pressure is known as the *systolic,* and is the higher of the two readings. The pressure when the heart is at rest is the *diastolic.* While both pressures are important, the diastolic is the more important as an index of normality since it indicates the degree of tension or strain existing in the circulatory system.

Blood pressure is measured by wrapping an airtight rubber cuff around the arm. The cuff is then inflated with air until the pulse at the wrist is completely obliterated. When this point is reached, the air is slowly released, permitting the flow of blood to return. The first pulse beat felt at the wrist or the first throbbing sound heard with a stethoscope at the large artery in the crook of the arm represents the systolic blood pressure.

As the air is gradually released, the sound again is obliterated. At this point we have what is known as the diastolic pressure.

The blood pressure fluctuates in accordance with the influences that affect the body as a whole. The same influences that affect the heart also affect the blood pressure. Nonetheless, it is of interest to know that blood pressure varies considerably in different parts of the body. It is higher in the arteries nearest the heart and diminishes as we get farther away from the heart. It is lower in the veins than in the arteries.

A mere fluctuation or a temporary rise in blood pressure need not cause alarm. It merely means that some tension or weakening influence has disturbed the normal rhythm and brought about a temporary rise or fall. To determine whether a given blood pressure is normal or not, the reading must be evaluated in relation to the other conditions in the body and to the influences that affect the heart and nervous system at the time the blood pressure is taken.

Authorities disagree as to what the normal blood pressure is. Some maintain that 100 plus age is normal. Others claim that the normal blood pressure is 100 plus age up to 20 years, and then one point for every two years.

Actually neither of these formulas is completely correct, not merely because the blood pressure varies with the individual and fluctuates in accordance with the many influences that affect the heart and the nervous system, but also because both of these formulas assume that blood pressure has to increase with age.

This is not true. While blood pressure tends to rise with age, this is not to be regarded as a normal condition. It occurs because as people grow older their blood vessels tend to lose some of their elasticity. This, however, need not happen since the blood vessels can be kept pliable and resilient, thus maintaining the blood pressure of the "younger age" range, even as the person grows older.

Dr. Harvey Kellogg, founder of the famous Battle Creek Sanitarium, had a blood pressure of 118/80 at the age of seventy-two and we have known many other persons who at a ripe old age have shown a similarly youthful type of blood pressure.

## When Clots Form

In the healthy person, the inner lining of the arteries is smooth and flexible, and the blood can flow through them easily. But, as already seen, when calcium or the fatlike substance, cholesterol, is deposited on the walls of the arteries, the arteries become hard and brittle, and the channel through which the blood flows becomes narrower. This slows down the circulation of the blood and in time may cause the formation of a clot, which will obstruct the circulation completely.

When this happens in the brain, we develop what is known as apoplexy, or a *stroke*. The affected part of the brain fails to receive its supply of blood and the part of the body controlled by this part of the brain becomes paralyzed. Whether and to what extent the paralysis clears up depends upon how rapidly and how thoroughly the clot can be reabsorbed. Where the clot fails to be reabsorbed quickly, the part of the brain that fails to get its needed oxygen and nourishment becomes damaged, and the paralysis becomes permanent.

When a clot forms in an artery in the leg, it causes severe cramplike pains and ultimately leads to a dying (necrosis) of the part deprived of its circulation. Gangrene often develops and amputation may become necessary.

## Coronary Thrombosis

When a clot forms in one of the arteries of the heart, we have a coronary thrombosis or coronary occlusion. In this condition, the affected part of the heart is deprived of its circulation, and failing to get its nourishment and oxygen, ceases to function. This is commonly known as a heart attack.

When the circulation to the kidneys becomes affected, their functions become seriously impaired. They are unable to eliminate the toxins effectively and the fluid balance in the body becomes upset. This in turn overtaxes the arteries and the heart and leads to their breakdown.

## 2. Coronary or Arteriosclerotic Heart Disease

While hypertensive heart disease arises from a general hardening of the arteries or high blood pressure, coronary or arteriosclerotic heart disease develops from a hardening of the coronary arteries, the arteries that supply the heart with its blood supply.

### Coronary Sclerosis

Coronary or arteriosclerotic heart disease begins with hardening of the coronary arteries. When the coronary arteries become hardened, the condition is known as coronary sclerosis. When this condition develops, the heart is unable to receive an adequate supply of oxygen and other essential nutritious elements and ultimately begins to break down. Since this condition usually develops slowly and insidiously, the early stages are often not easily recognized. However, as the disease progresses, certain warning symptoms or disturbances often begin to show up. Among these are heaviness or pressure on the chest or excruciating pains in which the chest feels as if it were tightly clamped in a vise, squeezing all life and strength from it.

During these attacks the pains often radiate into the left shoulder, sometimes into the right shoulder, occasionally into the abdomen.

These attacks, known as angina pectoris, occur when one of the coronary arteries is in spasm because of an insufficient supply of oxygen.

It is fortunate that these attacks last only for a short time, usually no longer than a few seconds, sometimes one or two minutes, rarely more than ten or fifteen minutes. Where they continue for more than a half hour, a coronary thrombosis or coronary occlusion must be seriously suspected.

### Coronary Artery Thrombosis

In coronary thrombosis complete obstruction of one of the branches of the coronary arteries has set in. This condition develps when a clot forms, blocking the circulation to the affected part of the heart.

A coronary thrombosis often sets in with catastrophic suddenness. In addition to the excruciating pains that persist without letup, some of the other symptoms are considerable difficulty in breathing and acute collapse. The face becomes bathed in sweat and turns ashen gray, and the afflicted person has a feeling of impending death.

The patient may in the words of Boyd[1] be "well one minute and in agony the next."

A point to bear in mind, however, is that while the attack may come on with dramatic suddenness, the disease itself does not develop suddenly, but builds up over a long period of time, and is the outgrowth of a blood vessel disease that has become continuously more severe.

The excruciating pains in coronary thrombosis are akin to those of a severe angina pectoris attack, with the only difference being that while in an angina attack they subside after a short period of time, in coronary thrombosis the pains persist continuously without a letup.

The sharp, excruciating pains that occur in coronary thrombosis or during an angina attack often radiate into the abdomen and may occasionally be mistaken for indigestion, a perforated ulcer, a gallbladder distress, or a diseased pancreas. "Under those circumstances, unless the possibility of coronary artery occlusion is kept in mind, it is easy to see how the abdomen may be opened with unfortunate consequences.'" Boyd warns.

While an attack of coronary thrombosis is of a grave nature, it should not be regarded as hopeless. Many sufferers recover from it and many return to a normal life. The seriousness of the case and the degree of recovery, however, depend upon the extent of involvement and the type of care the patient receives.

Where one of the smaller blood vessels is involved, a smaller area of the heart is affected and the danger is not too great. Where a larger blood vessel is affected, the attack is much more serious and may result in sudden death.

When an artery becomes obstructed, that part of the heart which fails to receive oxygen dies. However, as soon as this happens the body begins to marshal its forces in an

[1] Boyd, *Pathology of Internal Diseases.*

attempt to repair the damage. The dead tissue is softened and carried away and the damaged area fills up with scar tissue.

Of extreme interest at this point is the fact that new blood vessels shoot out from adjacent arteries to carry on the work of the damaged artery. This is known as collateral circulation, and plays an important role in repairing the damage.

Our task during this critical period is to provide that care which will enable the body to do an effective job of repairing and rebuilding the strength of the heart. However, even when this has been accomplished the job is not completed. The patient must be made to realize how the condition developed and the adjustments he must make to protect him against a reoccurrence.

Sufferers from coronary sclerosis [hardening of the arteries of the heart] are committing a grave error when they fail to recognize the seriousness of their condition and do not make an effort to make the necessary adjustments in their habits of living. They must realize that by neglecting to do this they fail to check the inroads of the disease, and actually expose themselves more readily to a coronary thrombosis. It is amazing to note that even many of those who have already suffered from an attack of coronary thrombosis will disregard these warnings and fail to make the changes that would protect them against a possible recurrence.

### 3. Valvular or Rheumatic Heart Disease

Valvular or rheumatic heart disease is another type of heart ailment that takes a terrific toll of human life. In it, the valves of the heart have become thickened and scarred and are unable to close or open completely. As a result, some of the blood leaks through or is pushed backward. This disrupts the normal circulation and places a great strain upon the heart. To cope with this condition, the heart is forced to enlarge and because of the added strain it ultimately becomes worn out.

Fortunately, a great deal of repair is possible in many cases. Proper care strengthens the heart and promotes the necessary readjustments which enables it to function better in spite of the damage.

While the damage in valvular or rheumatic heart disease can be readily discerned, the damage in hypertensive or coronary heart disease, especially during the earlier stages, is not always easily recognized. A physical examination will disclose the presence of an enlarged heart, but cannot always indicate how tired out the heart is or whether hardened or scar tissue exists.

Boyd describes this condition as follows: "Apart from this fibrosis (scar tissue) which may be minimal in degree, the heart muscle appears normal. The individual fibers are healthy and show no suggestion of degeneration."

And yet while apparently normal, in reality the heart does not possess its full strength and clearly shows the effects of wear and tear. Boyd aptly explains, "What seems to be a powerful muscle is unable to expel the blood from the heart with any vigor. The pathologist has to accept the fact that in the myocardium (heart muscle) morphological (structural) appearance does not necessarily correspond with functional capacity."

In other words, even though the heart appears normal it is actually unable to maintain an efficient circulation.

It is well to keep this fact in mind because many persons assume that once they have had their periodic health check-up and have been told that the heart is in good condition, they have nothing about which to be concerned. Many of us know of persons who were examined by heart specialists and were told that their hearts were in good condition who nonetheless died from heart attacks soon after.

In more advanced cases, the damage and worn-out condition is, of course, more easily recognized since by that time sufficient degenerative changes have already set in to make it apparent. Such changes as a wasting or shrinking of the heart muscle, advanced stages of fatty degeneration, or infiltration of fatty deposits in the heart muscle fibers are more easily recognized, and many abnormal symptoms such as difficult breathing, night asthma, rapid or slow pulse, swelling of the liver, fluid in the abdomen and chest, help one to make a correct diagnosis.

We are not often aware of this, but such mild disturbances as dizziness, blurred vision, or digestive distress often arise from minor heart damage. In some cases, several such areas of minor damage become confluent and cause a major defect, leading to so-called sudden death. While the sudden death in these cases is due to a major organic breakdown, it is really the outgrowth of a slow form of deterioration that has reached its peak.

## Heart Block

One of the conditions often found in the later stages of heart disease is known as heart block. We have seen that the function of the heart is in perfect balance. This balance or rhythm is maintained by the nervous system and a special control in the heart muscle, the sinus rhythm. When this special control becomes impaired, an imbalance between the upper and lower chambers of the heart develops. While the upper chambers function at a normal range, the lower chambers are unable to keep in step. This manifests itself in a slowing of the pulse.

However, a slow pulse is not necessarily a sign of a diseased heart. When a normal heart is at rest, its pulse too slows down, an indication that the heart is merely working at a slower rate and is conserving its energy.

## Failure Affects Both Sides of the Heart

When doctors discuss a heart case, they often mention left side failure or right side failure, implying that either one or the other side of the heart has broken down and is unable to do its work. In reality, no breakdown limits itself exclusively to one side of the heart. Failure in most cases begins with the left side but usually will affect the right side as well. When the left side of the heart is unable to pump the blood it receives from the lungs, the lungs cannot empty any more blood into it, and as a result there is a backing up to the right side of the heart. The engorgement that results causes a stretching or dilating of the heart, and causes trouble.

# 4

# METABOLISM: A FACTOR IN HEART DISEASE

While diseases of the heart and blood vessels have been increasing at an enormous rate, and while the search for the cause of these diseases and the reason for their continuous increase has been going on for a long time, our research workers, so far, have accomplished very little.

However, a profound change has recently taken place which, if carried to its logical conclusion, holds significant promise for the future. This change took place when our scientists began to realize that diseases of the heart and the circulation arise from an impairment in the metabolism of the body.

The term metabolism covers a wide field. It embraces all the known and unknown functions of the body and all the known and unknown chemical and physiological processes that break down our food and oxygen so that they can be utilized by the cells.

The living body is a complex mechanism; the digestion and assimilation of food, the secretion of the endocrine glands, the functions of the nervous system, the elimination of toxins, and the thousand and one chemical and physiologic changes that take place continuously within our organism are part of this complexity.

Anything that impairs these functions leads to a derangement in nutrition, affects the elimination of toxins, impairs glandular functions and causes a chemical imbalance. These are the impairments that exist and are part and parcel of our so-called metabolic diseases. Diabetes, arthritis, diseases of the kidneys and liver, the various degenerative nervous disorders, as well as the diseases of the heart and blood vessels, all belong in this category.

## Our Kidneys: A Vast Filtering System

We have mentioned that the function of our kidneys plays a vital role in the development of high blood pressure and heart disease. The type of kidney disease that contributes to the development of these diseases is known as glomerular nephritis. The glomeruli are the filters of the kidneys. Each kidney contains billions of these microscopic filters whose job it is to filter out the fluids and expel the waste products from the body.

When the kidneys become impaired, they are unable to function efficiently, and as a result, many of the toxins are retained in the system and the fluid balance in the body becomes disrupted. This places an added strain on the heart and raises the blood pressure.

The kidneys break down from overwork or when they have to rid the body of an excessive amount of noxious or irritating substances that have been taken into the system with food or drink, or in the form of drugs or chemicals.

In his discussion of the diseases of the liver, Boyd[1] expressed this point most vividly when, in explaining how the diseases of the liver arise, he states:

The cells of the liver are bathed in the blood brought by the portal vein from the gastro-intestinal tract, blood which may contain toxins known and unknown. The result of such toxic action may be the death of some or many of the cells of the liver lobule, it may be one or many of the lobules themselves. ... Among the numerous agents most diverse in character, which may cause degeneration and necrosis of liver cells may be mentioned chemicals, both organic and inorganic, certain drugs and tar-like substances (coal tar products), foreign proteins and products of protein decomposition, bacterial toxins, infections, and exposure to radiation.

Damage to any organ or tissues of the body results from overwork or is caused by toxins generated within the body or that find their way into the system from without—with our food or drink or in the form of drugs or chemicals.

It is highly gratifying to note that this concept is now gaining recognition in medical thnking. The credit for this belongs to Dr. Hans Selye, Director of the Institute of Experimental Medicine and Surgery at the University of

[1] Boyd, *Pathology of Internal Diseases.*

Montreal, the originator of the theory of stress. Dr. Selye has clearly demonstrated that stress and strain or, in other words, excessive wear and tear, caused by overwork or the accumulation of toxins or substances of an irritating nature that are generated within the system as a result of improper functioning or are taken into the system with improper food and drink or in the form of drugs or chemicals, cause disorders in metabolism that ultimately manifest themselves in one or other of our metabolic diseases, which include the diseases of the heart and blood vessels.

In other words, anything that overtaxes the organism impairs its functioning and brings about the onset of these diseases.

### Health Is Orderly, Harmonious Functioning

Health is an orderly, harmonious functioning of all the organs of the body, and this state of harmony continues as long as they are able to do their work efficiently. As an added protection against a disruption of this harmony, the body possesses a tremendous amount of reserve power, drawn upon in case of stress or difficulties. It is only when these reserve powers have become greatly depleted that the organs are unable to function efficiently and finally break down.

Selye demonstrated this most conclusively. He showed that whenever the body is subjected to stress of any sort, an alarm reaction immediately arouses the body's reserve powers, calling upon them to cope with the strain and restore the normal balance.

However, when the disruptive influences continue unabated or recur at frequent intervals, the reserve powers ultimately become exhausted, thus depleting the margin of safety that protects the body against deterioration and breakdown. Life becomes endangered when the body's reserve powers have become depleted and its ability to make lifesaving adjustments or adaptations has been lost.

That the body possesses the power to maintain normal harmonious functioning even under stress is not a new idea. Selye refers us to the work of the French physiologist, Claude Bernard, who called attention to the fact that the body maintains its own internal balance. Our own Walter Cannon called this the *homeostasis* (stability or equilibrium) of the body.

Selye has merely confirmed what other investigators have long suspected, namely, that the glands of internal secretion and the nervous system act as the balance wheels that maintain an equilibrium protecting us against collapse. He has demonstrated that when the body is exposed to stress it arouses an increase in the secretion of our glands; this counteracts the effects of stress and protects us against breakdown.

It is when stress continues over a long period of time or is greater than the body can safely handle that the ability of the glands to pour out these lifesaving secretions becomes impaired and the body is unable to make the necessary adjustments. When this happens, health and life are endangered.

## Heart Changes Are Part of This Adaptive Mechanism

The changes that take place in heart disease also develop when the body attempts to cope with conditions or influences that threaten life; as such, they are part of our defense mechanism. We have seen that when the heart has more work to do than it can safely handle, its muscle is forced to enlarge. This change allows the heart to cope with the increased amount of work and to protect it against collapse.

When the blood vessels become thickened and hardened or when scar tissue develops in the muscle or in and around the valves of the heart, these changes too arise from an attempt to repair an inflamed or damaged area, and to prevent the damage from spreading.

The ability of the body to make these repairs, even though they bring with them an alteration in structure, is instrumental in saving human life.

## Do We Live Longer?

While most authorities are profoundly concerned with the increase in the incidence of diseases of the heart and the arteries, some try to minimize the seriousness of the situation by telling us that since people live longer now than ever before, an increase in incidence and mortality from these diseases is to be expected.

Dr. Walter Modell is one of those who has stressed this view:

We have more heart disease today because our health is improving. It is paradoxical that we should seek to find comfort in the statement that more people than ever are dying of heart disease, but it is nevertheless a comforting fact to the physician. He knows that because of the dramatic reduction in deaths caused by infectious diseases, people are in general living much longer. Hardening of the arteries or arterio-sclerosis, the most frequent cause of heart disease, comes to more people today because it eventually comes to all who live long enough.[2]

At first glance this reasoning may seem plausible. Further examination, however, discloses how fallacious it is. Two major flaws exist in this type of thinking. One is the assumption that people in general live much longer than before. This is not true even though most persons have come to believe it.

The other is the assumption "that hardening of the arteries eventually comes to all who live long enough" and is, therefore, inevitable.

An examination of the facts will reveal that neither of these assumptions is true. The life span of our adult population, in spite of all propaganda to the contrary, has really not been considerably prolonged, while hardening of the arteries is not "inevitable" in the older population.

There is no question that the over-all life span of our population has been considerably extended in the last half century, but this does not mean that our adult population is living much longer than fifty years ago. We are not ungrateful even for little favors, but we really have not much to be grateful for insofar as this claim is concerned. An examination of the facts will reveal that the increase we boast of resulted primarily from a saving of infants' and children's lives, and not at all or only to a very

2 Walter Modell, "Straight Facts About Heart Disease," *Hygeia,* February, 1948.

limited degree from the prolongation of the life span of our adult population.

The weekly *U.S. News & World Report*[3] proved this clearly. Quoting the U.S. Public Health Service, this weekly disclosed that while the over-all life span in the last half century of an average boy at birth has increased by eighteen years, the life span of a man aged forty has increased by not more than three years.

The claim that our life span has been extensively prolonged has been repeated often, but many of our authorities have pointed out how baseless is this assumption.

Dr. I. Dublin,[4] former Chief Statistician of the Metropolitan Life Insurance Company, referred to this as early as 1928 when, in an address before the New York Academy of Medicine, he pointed out that while more people are living to an old age, "this has simply been due to the fact that we are saving more lives at younger ages. . . . A man has practically no more expectation of living beyond 70 now than he had in 1840," he said.

Somewhat later we find Alexis Carrel dealing with the same subject. In his book, *Man the Unknown*, he stated: "In spite of the progress achieved in heating, ventilation, and lighting of homes, of dietary hygiene, bathrooms and sports, or periodical medical examinations and increasing number of specialists, not even one day has been added to the span of life."

The Brookings Institute[5] also confirmed this point. The Institute disclosed that while the average death rate in the United States in the past 50 years has been reduced from 17.2 per thousand persons in 1900 to 9.4 per thousand persons in 1959, the greatest reduction has taken place in our infant and child population.

Elaborating further on their findings, the Brookings people pointed out that the death rate of infants under one year of age in 1900 was 162.4 per thousand live births, and that this has been reduced to 31.3 per thousand live births, or practically a fifth of what it was at the turn of the century. Continuing further, they say that this resulted primarily from a reduction in the mortality of infants

3 *U.S. News & World Report,* March 24, 1950.
4 *The New York Times,* October 2, 1928.
5 *The New York Times,* August 11, 1952.

and children, and only to an extremely limited degree was it due to an improvement in the life expectancy of the adult population.

## Hardening of the Arteries Not Inevitable

That hardening of the arteries is an inevitable process of aging and unavoidable has been repudiated by some of our most noted authorities.

Dealing with this subject, Dr. Joseph D. Wassersug stated, "It would be a mistake to believe that hardening of the arteries is simply a part of the general process of aging, and to accept it as such with resignation. On the contrary, scientists are quick to point out that many octogenarians and non-octogenarians die with a minimal amount of sclerosis in their blood vessels whereas fatal amounts are not infrequently noted in early youth and even childhood. To regard hardening of the arteries as a phenomenon inevitably associated with the process of growing old would be deplorable."

Dr. Irving H. Page stated, "Hypertension is certainly not merely a problem of aging. Nor is it a disease exclusively of the aged. It is not sufficiently realized by the public that it is sometimes found even in babies, and that young people in the twenties often have it. It increases in frequency from 30 years on, and is very common in the age period of greatest productivity and usefulness to society."[6]

A statement refuting this assertion was issued by Doctors Howard B. Burchell, Edgar V. Allen, and Frederick P. Moersch. In an article appearing in the *Journal of the American Medical Association,* these eminent physicians declared that they too desire to join in the crusade against the teaching of a close relationship between age and arteriosclerosis, which is either accepted or implied in past medical school curriculums.

"For the purposes of emphasis, let us make the provocative statement that while aging is relentless, arterio-

[6] Hypertension, A Manual for Patients with High Blood Pressure.

sclerosis is not necessarily a progressive nor irreversible process."[7]

What challenges this reasoning to an even greater degree is the fact that the number of cases of heart and circulatory disease has increased to a great extent not in the older population but in the younger age groups or those in the prime of life.

Dr. Paul Dudley White in the *Journal of the American Medical Association* June 28, 1952, discussed the progress made in the treatment of these diseases: "Despite all these advances, the incidence and mortality rates of cardio-vascular-renal diseases have increased enormously, far more than those of cancer. . . . Of all deaths in the United States, 51 per cent can be attributed to cardio-vascular-renal diseases."

He goes on to say that "the situation would not be so discouraging" if only our old persons died from these diseases. "Unfortunately, however, at present the increase in mortality from cardio-vascular disease does not occur only in old persons. There has been a great increase of the disease in young adults and those of middle age within the last half generation. There is actually a greater increase in these middle years between 30 and 60 than in the later ages."[8]

When Dr. White was called to attend President Eisenhower during his heart attack, he pointed out that these attacks are quite common by the time we reach fifty, but rightfully stated that they do not occur suddenly; rather they are the outgrowth of degenerative changes in the arteries that have gone on over many years.

We like to see health authorities emphasize moderation in diet, exercise, and the drive under which people work as precautions to be taken before a coronary attack develops for the fact that many come through to suffer subsequent attacks does not save those who succumb to it in the first instance.

[7] "Clinical Manifestations of Arterio-Sclerosis," *J.A.M.A.*, December 15, 1951.
[8] "Heart Disease Forty Years Ago and Now."

## Prevention Best

We cannot but commend the effort being made to counteract unreasoned fear, but the best way to accomplish this is not by pointing out that many of those who have heart attacks will recover, but by following a program of living that protects us against the onset of these attacks. James Reston[9] very wisely pointed out that while many recover, many others do not, and quoted Dr. Henry Kirkland, Chief Medical Director of the Prudential Insurance Company, who in a paper "Prognosis in Heart Disease," read only four months before President Eisenhower's attack, stated, "The occurrence of a documented acute coronary episode is of extremely serious moment. Sudden death is frequent. Death within a few months is common. It is only when the patient enters the third year that his chances of survival tend to brighten appreciably."

Dr. Ancel Keys, Director of the Laboratory of Physiological Hygiene, University of Minnesota, dealing with the same subject, pointed out that several thousand Americans had heart attacks on September 24, 1955, the day President Eisenhower was stricken, and that the President was merely one of the lucky ones, for "close to a thousand of his fellow citizens died of coronary heart disease that day."

"And it was a below average day. In recent years, the average daily toll from coronary deaths in the United States is considerably over 1,000," Dr. Keys continued.[10]

There is no reason why we should resign ourselves to the idea that a coronary attack at about fifty, or even sixty-five, is a normal expectation, for the right diet, correct eating habits, and moderation in living can keep our heart and arteries young and healthy even in the seventies and eighties.

That this disease does not show up suddenly but develops gradually over a period of time can be seen from our findings on the Korean battlefields, where the heart and coronary arteries of a number of young men who were killed in battle were analyzed. In "one series of 300

9 *The New York Times,* January 8, 1956.
10 *The Miami Herald,* February 12, 1956.

cases in which the average age was 22 years, the incidence of diseased coronary arteries was 77.3 per cent."[11]

*The New York Times,* on October 20, 1955, reported that a leading film actor, age forty-one, had "succumbed instantaneously of a coronary thrombosis" while shaving, and that his family physician stated that the actor "had been in good health and had no history of a heart condition."

Whenever confronted by a statement of this kind it is well to reflect on the statement by Dr. White, who pointed out that a coronary thrombosis usually does not develop suddenly but builds up over a period of years. This is true even though the attack occurs most unexpectedly, and even though the degenerative changes have not been recognized by either patient or doctor.

## How Children's Lives Have Been Saved

That the over-all life span of man has increased in the last fifty years is undeniable. We have seen, however, that the increase has resulted primarily from a saving in children's and infants' lives, not from a prolongation of the lives of the older population.

How has this saving in children's and infant's lives come about? An examination of the facts will disclose that the majority of deaths among our children and infants up to and during the early part of the century resulted from such serious diseases as tuberculosis, typhoid fever, dysentery, and pneumonia.

With the turn of the century, however, a significant reduction in the number of these diseases began to take place. The reason for this reduction has aroused some discussion. Some have tried to credit it to our newly discovered drugs, but it should not take much to see how fallacious this is since a significant reduction in these diseases began to manifest itself with the turn of the century, long before the introduction of these drugs. Most health authorities realize that extensive improvements in sanitation and hygiene, improved feeding practices, and generally ad-

[11] Major General Dan C. Ogle, "What Air Force Is Doing to Ease Heart Risks," *U.S. News & World Report,* October 14, 1955.

vances in our standard of living were primarily responsible for this change. Better housing conditions, and a growing appreciation of the benefits of the outdoors as well as sounder nutritional approach have contributed materially to improved child health and have brought about a reduction in these serious diseases among our children.

This was recognized by the Metropolitan Life Insurance Company when, in their bulletin, *A Century of Progress in Longevity*, they stated that the increase in the expectation of life at birth resulted because "we now enjoy a vastly higher standard of living—more abundant and better food, shelter, clothing, education and recreational facilities."[12]

That progress in hygiene and sanitation, an improved nutritional regimen, and advances in our standard of living have contributed materially to the improvement in the health of our children is unquestionable. Who doesn't remember the slum conditions which existed only thirty to forty years ago? It is not difficult to recall the relatively recent time when many parents kept the windows of their homes tightly shut for fear that their children might "catch cold."

Then again, it was comparatively recently when the main foods in a child's diet, in addition to milk, were refined cereals and white flour and white sugar products. Whole wheat bread and whole grain cereals were practically unknown in the average household, while fruits and vegetables were rarely if ever used.

Today most of this is considerably changed. While slum areas still exist in some of our large cities, the over-all improvements in housing conditions and our higher standard of living, plus the general improvement in hygiene and sanitation, have eradicated most of the so-called "infectious" diseases of children, and have contributed materially to the saving of infants' and children's lives.

People of all classes and walks of life are now aware that fresh air and sunshine are beneficial to health, and most parents realize the value of fresh fruits and vegetables.

Furthermore, we know that in many homes the use of white sugar and white flour products has been substantially reduced or even completely eliminated, and that sweet

[12] *A Century of Progress in Longevity*, Vol. 30, October, 1949.

fruits, raw sugar, honey, whole wheat bread, and whole grain cereals have been substituted in their stead.

## Adult Population Also Benefited

The tremendous strides in housing, the progress in sanitation and hygiene, the advances in nutrition, and the higher standard of living have also done much to improve the comfort and well-being of our adult population. Other factors that have contributed to their well-being are our vast technological and sociological advances that improved working conditions and reduced the hours of labor, thus providing more time for play, relaxation, and cultural pursuits.

It is, therefore, all the more depressing to realize that in spite of these advances the life span of our adult population has shown only a nominal increase, if any at all, while the many degenerative diseases have continued to multiply at a tremendous rate.

We fully agree with I. J. Rodale, editor of *Prevention*, a monthly magazine devoted to health, who said: "His [man's] body is ravaged by disease just as much as ever, in spite of the unconvincing mortality statisticians who, by their quirky, higher mathematics, measure death instead of health, who juggle day-old babies into the death averages. . . . I am fifty-four and am no longer a day-old babe. I want a mortality statistic tailored to my own needs and not to that of a baby."[13]

Our aim should not be to offer an excuse for the existence of these conditions, but to discover what the causes are and make an effort to correct them.

## Cholesterol Makes Its Appearance

Some years ago authorities thought that they were beginning to see daylight when they discovered that persons who were suffering from hardening of the arteries accumulated an excessive amount of cholesterol, a substance of fatty origin, in their blood, and that when this sub-

[13] *Prevention*, July, 1952.

stance was deposited within the confines of the arteries it caused sores or lesions, which were followed by hardening of the arteries.

Cholesterol is found in large quantities in the fatty foods of animal origin such as eggs, milk, butter, cream, as well as the fatty meats and fish. It seemed logical to assume that by controlling the intake of these foods hardening of the arteries could be eliminated or greatly lessened.

However, many of our authorities were not satisfied with this assumption. Although they were aware that a restriction in the intake of the cholesterol-rich foods benefited their patients, they were still confronted by questions that seemed baffling. For one thing, they noticed that many persons who consumed large quantities of the cholesterol-rich foods did not suffer from hardening of the arteries; for another, further research disclosed that not all types of cholesterol, but only a special type, giant cell cholesterol, caused damage.

Finally, they began to realize that hardening of the arteries does not develop merely from an intake of cholesterol-rich foods, but from a faulty utilization of them.

Research at many of our institutions confirmed this fact. *The U.S. News & World Report*[14] reported on the work done by scientists in different institutions, including the Heart Institute of the National Institute of Health in Washington, which proved that certain key substances (hormones) that normally break up our fat foods are lacking in persons suffering from these diseases. It further stated that our scientists are now working feverishly in the hope of discovering the missing element or elements so that where necessary they could be supplied to sufferers from these diseases, "artificially by pill or by injection."

We wish it were as simple as that! An examination of the results of hormone therapy in other metabolic diseases such as diabetes and arthritis will reveal how ineffective this type of treatment can be.

William S. Gailmor, discussing this subject, referred to the work of Dr. Wm. D. Kountz of the Washington University of Medicine, St. Louis, Mo., who based his work on the fundamental research of Dr. Timothy Leary of Tufts University and the so-called "anoxemia" (lack of oxygen) theory of Dr. Wilhelm C. Hueper, President of the American Society of Arteriosclerosis. Dr. Kountz demonstrated conclusively that "A thyroid hormone deficiency, by preventing metabolism or absorption of a fatty substance (cholesterol) into the tissues, allows it to accumulate in the arteries, ultimately causing the characteristic 'hardening.' "[15]

Stephen M. Spencer in an article in *The Saturday Evening Post* referred to the work of Dr. John Gofman, who demonstrated that "just as diabetics cannot handle sugar, so according to this theory, certain people cannot handle their butter and eggs as efficiently as the rest of us can."[16]

That the excessive accumulation of cholesterol in the blood is due to an impairment of metabolism, and that it is only one of the many changes which occur in the body as a result of this impairment, is now being recognized to an ever greater extent.

Waldemar D. Kaempffert, former science editor of *The New York Times*, referring to the work of Drs. Alfred Steiner, Forest E. Kendall, and James Q. L. Mathers of the Department of Medicine, Columbia University, says that the relative level of phospholipids and cholesterol may be as important in the development of arteriosclerosis as the increase in the level of cholesterol itself.[17]

Dr. Meyer Friedman, Dr. Ray Rosenman, and Dr. Sanford Byers of the Harold Brunn Institute of Mt. Zion Hospital, also challenging the idea that cholesterol is the sole cause of arteriosclerosis, mentioned that while it was thought that cholesterol caused an increase in phospholipids, research at the Brunn Institute disclosed that the increase in phospholipids "precedes and causes an increase in cholesterol" and as such "cholesterol is an effect, not a cause."[18]

"Deposits of cholesterol, a fatty alcohol, on the walls of the arteries, are not the primary cause of hardening of the arteries. First come mucoid proteins, then cholesterol, and large globules of fat—sometimes." This is another report by Waldemar D. Kaempffert. It is based on the work of

15 *Daily Compass*, June 6 ,1952.
16 "Are You Eating Your Way to Arteriosclerosis," October 21, 1950.
17 *The New York Times*, June 10, 1951.
18 *The New York Times*, February 14, 1956.

Drs. Henry D. Moon and James F. Rinehart of the University of California School of Medicine. "Moon and Rinehart saw cases of arteriosclerosis where there were no cholesterol deposits at all—only these mucoid proteins," Kaempffert continues.

Drs. Moon and Rinehart[19] did not overlook the presence of cholesterol deposits in these cases; they were merely not convinced that cholesterol was the primary cause of the hardening. They came to this conclusion by checking parts of arteries of persons who died suddenly, some from heart attacks, others from other causes. They checked samples of arteries of 250 persons ranging in age from four months to ninety years. They observed that the early changes in arteriosclerosis, especially in the coronary vessels of youngsters, showed slight thickenings of the innermost layer of the arteries, marked by an increase in the deposits of mucoprotein, by fibrous growths, and by breaks in the elastic tissue fibers, but not by deposits of cholesterol.

The second or later stage showed further accumulation of mucoprotein, the formation of hard, fibrous plaques in the walls of the arteries, and the presence of fat—but only sometimes cholesterol.

In the more advanced stages of arteriosclerosis parts of the arteries were hard and glossy looking, and deposits of large globules of fat (including cholesterol), and frequent deposits of calcium existed, causing narrowing of the arterial tubes and slowing down the flow of blood, which exposed the patients to the danger of the formation of fatal clots.

From all this, Drs. Moon and Rinehart concluded that *"fat metabolism becomes important only in the later stages of the disease and that the original trouble probably lies in how the body uses protein."*

That a diet rich in starches and sugars can lead to the accumulation of fats in the blood and predispose to hardening of the arteries and to heart disease is another point also reported recently by Dr. Edward H. Ahrens of the Rockefeller Institute. Appearing at a meeting of the Association of American Physicians he made it amply clear that

[19] *Time*, December 1, 1952.

dietary carbohydrate, not fat, is the thing to watch in guarding against those conditions."[20]

We are stressing all this to show that by pinpointing only one of the many changes that occur as part of the metabolic disorder we fail to obtain a true picture of what actually takes place.

It should not be difficult for us to agree with Dr. Herman T. Blumenthal[21] of the St. Louis Jewish Hospital, who concluded that "hardening of the arteries may not be one disease but many" and that even the "metabolic changes which have received so much attention, may be the *result* rather than the cause of the aging and hardening of the arteries."

The primary objective should be to obtain a clear picture of the many facets that contribute to the breakdown in metabolism and lead to the onset of these diseases; only in this way can we understand how this condition can be counteracted or prevented.


### Discovery of Hormone Likely


We have pointed out that many scientists working on this problem are endeavoring to discover the hormone or group of hormones presumably missing in the person suffering from diseases of the heart and blood vessels, so that they may be supplied by pill or injection.

It is likely that before long a particular hormone or group of hormones involved in these diseases may be discovered, and like insulin in diabetes or cortisone and ACTH in arthritis will be obtainable in the form of a pill or injection.

Furthermore, just as insulin in diabetes or cortisone and ACTH in arthritis, this new remedy may provide a certain measure of relief. It should, however, be evident that just as in diabetes and arthritis the relief will be only of a temporary nature, since only when the underlying causes of disease are removed or checked can thorough results be obtained.

For permanent and real correction, the factors that con-

[20] *The New York Times,* May 4, 1961.
[21] *Time,* December 14, 1953.

tribute to a breakdown or distortion of metabolism must be removed or corrected, and only such care as helps to restore normal functioning can be of value. These changes cannot be brought about through the supply of a particular hormone or set of hormones, but only through the removal or correction of all the influences that cause deficiencies, impair the functions of the glands, and create a chemical imbalance in the organism.

Even where the breakdown is already far advanced and complete correction is no longer possible, it is still imperative that these changes be instituted since only a program that removes the destructive influences and promotes rebuilding will arrest the progress of the disease and restore a measure of health and well-being.

## Merely a Link in the Chain

From all that we have stated, it should be clear that the heart and blood vessels are but part of the whole organism, and that the same causes that bring about their impairment simultaneously affect the body as a whole. In other words, the damage that shows up in the heart and blood vessels is merely a link in the chain of bodily derangements.

These influences usually operate over a long period of time and usually affect the other organs and functions of the body long before the heart and blood vessels begin to break down.

Furthermore, these abuses are usually cumulative in effect, and while the initial damage may at first not be apparent or recognizable, the ultimate effects are inevitable.

We have pointed out that these diseases are caused by toxins that originate within the body or are taken into the system with food and drink, or in the form of drugs or chemicals. Tobacco, alcohol, concentrated and processed foods, an excess of sweets, spices, and condiments, overeating, strained and frayed nerves, and various harrying emotional conflicts, as well as the health-sapping and exhausting tempo of present-day living, all contribute to a depletion of our energies, upset the chemical balance of the body and give rise to the diseases of metabolism, the diseases of the heart and blood vessels included.

## Low Blood Pressure

While high blood pressure is of greatest concern, it is well to mention that low blood pressure too must not be neglected since this also may be a warning that our health is not in best condition.

Low blood pressure may result from extreme debility, weakened arteries, a bad heart, an impoverished blood supply, poor quality of the blood, or a disorder of the glandular system. While it is not well known, a stroke or coronary thrombosis or other abnormal clotting phenomenon may develop in cases of low blood pressure, and may result from a weakened heart or a poor circulatory condition.

The question as to whether the blood pressure is high or low can be determined in many instances only when all the factors related to it are taken into consideration. We have pointed out that blood pressure does not have to rise with age and that a person of seventy can have as normal a blood pressure as one of twenty.

It is also well to remember that the range of blood pressure is subject to variation, depending upon influences that affect the heart and nervous system, and that a blood pressure of 90/60 is often found in persons of normal health.

Too, blood pressure is often influenced to a considerable degree by the food we eat. Rich, spicy foods will increase blood pressure, while a simple bland diet will often show a reduction in blood pressure of about 15 to 20 points within a few days.

However, a rapid drop in blood pressure coupled with a weak pulse must be carefully investigated, since it could indicate heart muscle damage or weakness.

While an abnormally low blood pressure can temporarily be elevated with certain medicines or treatments, it should be apparent that only when the underlying weaknesses or disorders are overcome or brought under control can the condition be permanently corrected or improved.

## 5

## THE ROLE OF NUTRITION

That nutrition plays an important role in the treatment of diseases of the heart and blood vessels is now well known. That unwholesome or careless nutritional habits contribute to the development of these diseases is, however, unfortunately not yet fully recognized.

While some authorities in their approach to these diseases stress the importance of limiting the cholesterol-rich foods such as eggs, butter, milk, cream, cheese, and fat meats and fish, and while some prohibit the use of salt and others restrict the intake of protein, it is essential to point out that these modifications are only a few of the changes that must be made if we are to obtain optimum results.

To restore good health, an all-around healthful, well-balanced nutritional regimen is imperative. Such a program will embody the use of simple natural foods such as raw and stewed fruits, raw, steamed, and baked vegetables, and moderate amounts of easily digestible proteins and carbohydrates.

It will exclude the use of refined and denatured foods, control the intake of sweets, restrict the consumption of rich and highly concentrated foods, and eliminate the use of sharp and irritating spices and condiments, as well as coffee, tea, and all other stimulants.

### Why Fat Foods Should Be Excluded

The reason for limiting the use of eggs, cream, butter, milk and fat meats and fish as well as other cholesterol-rich foods should be clear. However, a point worth stressing is that even fatty foods of vegetable origin such as nuts, avocado, and the various oils must be used in moderate quantities or even entirely omitted until positive results have been attained. All fat foods are difficult to digest, and as a result can impair the heart and the blood vessels.

## Why Table Salt Should Be Excluded

Table salt is excluded in heart disease, hardening of the arteries, high blood pressure, and in the diseases of the kidneys, because sodium, one of the elements of table salt, is eliminated through the kidneys and can be a burden to them.

Furthermore, when the kidneys are damaged or weakened they are unable to eliminate all the sodium, and when it is retained in the body it often causes the accumulation of fluid.

Some authorities insist that even the foods that contain sodium in organic form, among them fruits and vegetables, should be excluded from the diet. This is not only unnecessary but in the long run actually may be harmful, since it deprives the body of many valuable nutritional elements. The authorities who exclude the sodium-containing foods fail to realize that many of the sodium-containing foods are essential for good nutrition, while table salt is not a food but a load on the kidneys.

## On the Question of Protein

The question of protein has been the subject of controversy for a long time. While currently many doctors advocate the intake of large quantities of protein, this is contrary to the findings of some of our most outstanding nutrition authorities.

Sherman of Columbia, Hindhede of Denmark, Chittenden of Yale, Clive McCay of Johns Hopkins, to name only a few world renowned authorities, have proved conclusively that the intake of an excessive amount of protein can do great harm to the body.

### Denmark During World War I

Some of our observations during World Wars I and II have demonstrated this fact. Denmark during World War I is a case in point. The Danish people at that time were not self-sufficient, and had to import part of their food supply from other countries. A blockade by the Allies made it impossible for them to import the food they needed, and a severe drought made the situation even more critical.

To cope with this problem, the Danish government under the enlightened guidance of Dr. Michael Hindhede, their Minister of Health, embarked upon a program that involved a considerable reduction in their livestock and the conversion of all arable lands to the raising of grains and vegetables. While this program reduced the available meat supply to a mere trifle, it not only saved the Danish people from the threatened famine, but also helped improve the health of the nation. Such diseases as diabetes, heart disease, arthritis, as well as many of the other chronic and degenerative diseases were significantly reduced during that period, and the general level of health was raised considerably.

Harold Westergaard, Professor of the Copenhagen University, in his English summary of the report[1] dealing with this period, pointed out that while "the average death during the last five years before the war was, for the whole of the country, 12.9 per thousand . . . the death rate during the first year of restriction from October 1, 1917, to October 1, 1918 had only been 10.4 per thousand," and then concluded by stating that "never in any European country had there been such a low death rate."

In another part of the report, Professor Westergaard pointed out that whereas in Copenhagen "during the five most favorable years before the war, 1910-14, the yearly number of deaths for persons over twenty-five was 4543 (2205 men and 2338 women), the number of deaths in the year of restrictions was lower by 1016 (665 and 351) than it would have been, in case the death rate had been the same as 1910-14, or in other words, a decrease of 30 per cent for men and 15 per cent for women."

In all fairness, we wish to point out that this phenomenal improvement resulted not merely from a restriction in the consumption of meat, but from a complete readjustment in the living habits of the population which, ac-

[1] *Beretning Til Indenrigsministeriet on Rationeringens Indvirkning Paa Sundhedstilstanden ved M. Hindhede.*

cording to Professor Westergaard, embraced among other things:

"1. A reduction of the quantity of protein, generally speaking, but in particular of animal protein in favor of vegetable protein.

"2. A large reduction of the consumption of fat.

"3. A very large reduction of the consumption of alcohol.

"4. A general reduction of the quantity of food."

## Great Britain and World War II

The more recent experiences of the British people during World War II, one of the most difficult periods in their history, also illustrates this point. We know that the meat rations of the English during World War II were drastically reduced. Yet despite the grueling difficulties experienced by them during that harrowing period the health of the English people not only was maintained, but actually improved.

To illustrate how meager the meat rations of the English were during the war, it should be sufficient to mention that Ernest O. Hauser in an article in the *Saturday Evening Post* pointed out that even as recently as January, 1951 the *weekly* meat ration in England was eleven cents' worth per person, and that a year later it was raised to the grand total of sixteen cents' worth per week.

Two eggs and one ounce of cheese a week were the only other concentrated protein foods allowed. Yet "in spite of rationing," Mr. Hauser reports, "physicians claim that the English people are healthier than ever."[2]

Mr. Hauser's observations are in line with the statement of Sir Wilson Jameson, Chief Medical Officer of the Health Ministry of Great Britain that "the general health of this country (England) showed an improvement despite nearly four years of war" and emphasized that "one important factor in this improvement was the simple but excellent diet imposed by the exigencies of war."[3]

In view of this authoritative statement, we wonder whether it would not have been more exact for Mr.

[2] "It's No Fun to Be an Englishman," July 5, 1952.
[3] *The New York Times.*

Hauser to state that the English people were healthier *because* of food rationing and not *in spite* of it.

## Our Experiences During the War Years

Our own experiences during those fateful years were also illuminating. Most of us still remember the long queues in front of meat shops, and the disappointments of many of our people when they were unable to obtain a sufficient supply of meat for their table. Owing to its high cost, many persons were forced to go without meat altogether, while those who could afford the high prices were able to purchase only small quantities of it. Yet, none were any the worse off.

It was during those years that our government as well as many of our scientists pointed out that the protein we need for complete nourishment could be obtained from foods other than meat, and that we could be well nourished even if meat were completely omitted from our diet. *The Journal of the American Medical Association* declared: "Dietary protein derived in proportions of one half to two thirds from plant origin is entirely adequate in quality to meet all protein needs for normal growth, development, reproduction, and lactation."[4]

Howard B. Lewis of the Department of Biological Chemistry, Medical School, University of Michigan, in the September 18, 1948 issue of the *Journal* stated that "both animal and vegetable foodstuffs are good sources of protein, provided that they supply adequate amounts of the essential amino acids."

This is in line with a statement by Dr. Theodore R. Van Dellen, who at an earlier date wrote that "since the substances in meat are not superior to those of milk, eggs, and cheese, we do not need to worry as long as dairy products are available."[5]

It was during those years that the so-called Oxford experiments were released proving that a diet containing fifty grams of protein provides ample protein, and that of this amount only 10 to 15 per cent of the so-called com-

[4] "Nutritional Contributions of Wheat," November 27, 1948.
[5] "Now You Don't Have To Eat Meat; Study Your Protein!" *Daily News*, October 25, 1946.

plete protein, obtainable in meat, eggs, cheese, or milk, was necessary.

A fact often overlooked is that the green leafy vegetables such as spinach, green peas, string beans, kale, broccoli, supply the finest type of complete protein, although not in concentrated form. Our lowly potato also offers a fine type of easily digestible protein, although in small quantities.

While the protein foods are the tissue-building materials and, therefore, essential to life, an excess can easily cause a great deal of harm. Protein is essential for growth and for the replenishment of the worn-out tissues. Adults need it primarily to replace wear and tear. While starches and sugars can be stored up in the body in the form of fat, our body is not equipped to store up protein. It can use only what it needs and the excess must be eliminated. Most of it is eliminated through the colon where, when the intake is excessive, it undergoes putrefactive changes and is capable of creating a host of harmful waste products.

Bogomoletz was right when he stated that, if meat is used, it should be used sparingly. He wrote: "Although meat is predominantly protein foodstuff, it is also responsible for the formation of waste products that are not only unwholesome but even harmful, when functions of the liver and kidneys are impaired."[6]

Lautman, too, pointed out that meat gives rise to harmful waste products. In his discussion of meat soups and beef broths, he stated: "Soup is actually a concentrated essence of meat, low in protein substance, but rich in extractives. Since it contains only those elements of the meat which are supposed to be harmful, without retaining any of the qualities of the protein, soup as a regular article of diet would not be especially helpful."[7]

That a nonmeat regimen can do much to protect us against heart and blood vessel diseases has been confirmed only recently. A cross-country study conducted by Dr. Richard Walden, Assistant Professor of Preventive Medicine at the College of Medical Evangelists, in cooperation with Dr. Louis Shaefer of Mt. Sinai Hospital of New York, Dr. Frank R. Lemon of the College of Medical

[6] *The Prolongation of Life.*
[7] Maurice F. Lautman, *Arthritis and Rheumatic Disease.*

Evangelists, Dr. Abraham Sunshine of New York University, and Dr. Ernest L. Wynder of the Sloan-Kettering Institute for Cancer Research, among Seventh-Day Adventists, many of whom follow a vegetarian diet and abstain from the use of tobacco, alcoholic beverages, and coffee, disclosed that the blood cholesterol levels "could be lowered drastically within two weeks by taking a special diet."

Seventh-Day Adventists as a group show 40 per cent less heart and blood vessel diseases than the general public, and the research workers participating in this study are convinced that the meatless regimen followed by these people has much to do with it.

Nevertheless, we applaud Dr. Walden for stating that "other factors—tobacco, alcohol, caffeine, and possibly stress—obviously must also be investigated to complete this part of the picture."[8]

The *Journal of the American Medical Association*, June 3, 1961, also called attention to the fact that a vegetarian or nonmeat regimen can do much to protect us against the diseases of the heart and blood vessels. In an editorial entitled "Diet and Stress in Vascular Disease," it quotes Dr. W. A. Thomas *et al.*, who in a report published in the January 1960 issue of the *American Journal of Cardiology* pointed out that after comparing thromboembolic disease in Negroes in St. Louis and in Uganda, they came to the conclusion "that a vegetarian diet can prevent 90 per cent of our thromboembolic disease and 97 per cent of our coronary occlusions."

## Diet and Stress

This editorial marks a milestone in medical thinking and is highly significant. It stresses without equivocation that, contrary to popular opinion, faulty diet and not stress is the major cause of heart and blood vessel diseases.

"Diet is certainly the main factor in achieving protection or in predisposing to early disability or death from clots in veins and from clots and plaques in arteries," the editorial states.

The editorial does not minimize the effect of stress in

[8] *New York Herald Tribune,* May 18, 1961.

these diseases. It makes it clear, however, that while stress can cause a great deal of damage to those whose diet is "rich in saturated fat, cholesterol, and alcohol," it "has little or no effect if the diet is poor in animal fat."

Continuing further, the editorial points out that stress hastens the use of ascorbic acid (depleting the system of this essential vitamin), that it lowers resistance to infection, and that it leads to the accumulation of cholesterol and other fatty substance that damage the walls of the blood vessels and cause the formation of clots in the veins and arteries.

"It accelerates the progress of a disorder, it may make the difference between latent and lethal [deadly] manifestations of many diseases, but it is not the cause of any of them," is the way the editorial finally puts it. "It should be some consolation to those who like their work and its rewards more than they do ice-cream, butter, and eggs, that frustration may do them no harm if they can learn to live on fish, lean meat, fruit and the low calorie vegetables. . . . For those who have or who dread heart disease, it would seem that avoiding food which nature provides for infants, calves, and embryonic birds might be far more effective than tranquilizers, or 'slinking out of the race, unexercised and unbreathed' in an attempt to avoid frustrations."

This merely confirms that a well-regulated, wholesome nutritional program is the prime requisite for protection against heart and blood vessel diseases. It does not condone or minimize the effect of stress; nor does it write off the effect of any of the other harmful influences such as the use of tobacco, alcoholic beverages, etc. It leaves no doubt, however, as to the role that nutrition plays in the onset of these diseases.

## The Classical Rice Diet

In recent years the use of a rice diet in the treatment of diseases of the heart and blood pressure has gained considerable attention.

This diet, originally introduced in 1940 by Dr. W. Kempner at Duke University School of Medicine, demonstrated anew the value of a modified nutritional program.

Dr. Kempner discovered this diet when he observed that the people living in countries where rice is the main staple of food had a low incidence of heart and blood vessel diseases.

This diet is very simple. The main food is rice cooked in plain water or fruit juice, with the addition of some fruit.

Spectacular results have been obtained with this diet. A marked drop in blood pressure, a reduction in the size of the heart, absorption of hemorrhages in the eye, a change in the reading of the electrocardiogram, and a clearing up of edema or swellings were some of the changes observed following its use.

A point that should be stressed is that the phenomenal benefits derived from this diet result not because of any special quality inherent in rice but because of the limitations imposed in connection with the diet.

The classical rice diet eliminates the use of all salt, reduces the fat intake to no more than five grams a day, restricts the use of protein to twenty grams a day, and provides a total food intake of no more than 2000 calories per day. Furthermore, it excludes most of the so-called conventional foods, including spices and the stimulants, which overtax digestion, lead to the formation of irritating toxins, and are conducive to damage to the heart, the arteries, and the kidneys.

These restrictions are the real factors that contribute to improvement in heart and circulatory diseases, and it is imperative that we recognize this fact if continuous healthful results are really desired. The sufferer from these diseases needs a suitable diet, worked out to satisfy his permanent needs, and not one that serves merely as a temporary expedient.

The rice diet itself presents many disadvantages that preclude its use for more than short periods of time. One of its disadvantages is its extreme monotony. Another is the exclusion of many fruits and vegetables merely because of their sodium content. While it is true that table salt can be extremely harmful in these cases and therefore must be excluded, this does not hold true with regard to fruits and vegetables that contain sodium. The element sodium is essential to health, and it is well to bear in mind that the sodium in fruits and vegetables affects the body differently from the sodium present in concentrated form in table salt.

While those who prescribe the classical rice diet try to guard against deficiencies by the addition of concentrated "supplements," it is well to bear in mind that the vitamins and minerals obtained in supplements can never take the place of the vitamins and minerals obtainable in foods in their natural form.

One of the major fallacies of the rice diet is that it fails to take into consideration the need for an all-around flexible nutritional program, and that as a result many of its followers sooner or later return to most of their original harmful habits of eating.

### Other Nutritional Requirements

While it is imperative that the necessity of a rounded, well-balanced nutritional program be recognized, Dr. Kempner deserves credit nevertheless for making large sections of the medical profession acutely aware of the importance of a modified dietary regimen in these cases. In his *Radical Dietary Treatment of Hypertensive and Arteriosclerotic Vascular Disease, Heart and Kidney Disease, and Vascular Retinopathy,* Dr. Kempner stated that while in the past he advocated the use of the rice diet in all serious heart, artery, and kidney diseases that did not "respond to the customary treatment with salt restriction and drugs" and in all uncomplicated cases where "a more liberal regimen has failed," he now recognizes that "treatment should be more aggressive and uncompromising and should be started as soon as the diagnosis is certain."[9]

He continued further, "Loss of time is as unjustifiable as it would be in cancer or tuberculosis, and the inconveniences involved are no excuse for delaying optimal dietary treatment until the more unpleasant and often irreversible complications have appeared."

We fully subscribe to this statement, and because we are also concerned with prevention, we favor a careful dietary program before any of these diseases show up.

[9] *G.P.,* March, 1954.

## Complete Nutritional Program Essential

While we enthusiastically subscribe to the modifications inherent in the rice diet, such as the restriction or exclusion of the cholesterol and other fat-containing foods, the elimination of table salt, the reduction in the intake of protein, and the limitation in the total amount of food eaten, these are only some of the steps that must be taken if maximum and lasting benefits are to be attained.

For optimum as well as permanent results, we must plan a nutritional program that includes a liberal supply of the protective foods such as raw and steamed vegetables, raw and stewed fruits, plus a moderate amount of easily digestible proteins and starches, and excludes refined and processed foods, as well as foods of a stimulating and irritating nature. A diet worked out along these lines can give us meals of a most enjoyable nature, and at the same time provide all the health- and body-building benefits on a much more prolonged basis.

That nutrition plays a vital role in diseases of the heart and blood vessels is now universally recognized. When Drs. Otto Saphir and Leonard Ohringer of Michael Reese Hospital, Chicago, Ill., mentioned that diet may be responsible for the increase in heart disease "in persons younger than 50"[10] they had in mind primarily the large increase in the consumption of fat in the American diet. However, it is imperative to realize that if we are really to do an effective job, all factors that enter into the formation of a wholesome nutritional program must be taken into consideration. This involves not only the use of foods that are easily digestible and provide optimum value from the standpoint of health, but also the drastic elimination of the denatured and processed foods, as well as those foods which are difficult to digest.

### Uncooked Foods Superior in Health-Giving Qualities

Uncooked foods are living foods, foods which in addition to their easily digested protein and easily digestible carbohydrates are also rich sources of valuable minerals, vita-

[10] *Orlando Sentinel*, April 8, 1955.

mins, and enzymes. However, those who for one reason or another cannot eat them in their raw state should prepare them in such a way that only a minimum of the valuable protective elements such as the vitamins, minerals, and enzymes be lost. They may be steamed or baked but should not be fried or overcooked. No irritating spices or condiments should be added.

## Dr. Pottenger's Feeding Experiment

Dr. Pottenger's[11] feeding experiments with cats, subsequently tried on rats, "to determine the effect of heat-treated foods upon growth and development," is of interest at this point.

The experiments were conducted with cats, used for experimental purposes at the Pottenger Sanitarium. The animals were fed meat scraps from the sanitarium, together with raw milk and cod liver oil, but had proved "poor operative risks although the (operative) technique was good."

In time, the sanitarium had more cats than they were able to feed, and to supply the food needs of the extra cats they placed an order for raw meat scraps at the market where the sanitarium meat was bought. These scraps included muscle, bone, and viscera, and were fed each day to the same cats.

Before long, a phenomenal change in the health of the cats became noticeable. They "survived the operations, the unoperated cats appeared in better health, and the kittens born were vigorous," Dr. Pottenger recorded. He wrote: "The contrast in apparent health between the cats in the pens fed on raw meat scraps and those fed on the cooked meat scraps was so startling that we decided to do a feeding experiment."

This experiment was conducted over a period of ten years on approximately nine hundred cats. All cats were fed alike, except that one group was fed cooked meat while the other was kept exclusively on raw meat. Both

[11] Francis M. Pottenger, Jr., "The Effect of Heat Processed Foods and Metabolized Vitamin D Milk on the Dento-Facial Structures of Experimental Animals," *American Journal of Orthodontics & Oral Surgery*, August, 1946.

groups were fed two-thirds meat, one-third raw milk, plus cod-liver oil. The results were dramatic:

"The cats receiving raw meat and raw milk reproduced in homogeneity from one generation to the next. Abortion was uncommon ... and the mother cats nursed their young in a normal manner. The cats in these pens had good resistence to vermin, infections, and parasites.

"They possessed excellent equilibrium; they behaved in a predictable manner. Their organic development was complete and functioned normally," Dr. Pottenger stated.

Cats receiving the cooked meat scraps presented an entirely different picture:

[They] reproduced a heterogeneous strain of kittens, each kitten of the litter being different in skeletal pattern. Abortion in these cats was common, running about 25 per cent in the first generation to about 70 per cent in the second generation. Deliveries were in general difficult, many cats dying in labor. Mortality rates of the kittens were high, frequently due to the failure of the mother to lactate. The kittens were often too frail to nurse. At times the mother would steadily decline in health following the birth of the kittens, dying from some obscure tissue exhaustion about three months after delivery. Others experienced increasing difficulty with subsequent pregnancies. Some failed to become pregnant.

Cooked-meat-fed cats were irritable. The females were dangerous to handle, occasionally viciously biting the keeper. The males were more docile, often to the point of being unaggressive. Sex interest was slack or perverted. Vermin and intestinal parasites abounded. Skin lesions and allergies were frequent, being progressively worse from one generation to the next.

Pneumonia, empyema, diarrhea, osteomyelitis, cardiac lesions, hyperopia and myopia (eye diseases), thyroid diseases, nephritis, orchitis, oophoritis, hepatitis (liver inflammation), paralysis, meningitis, cystitis (bladder inflammation), arthritis, and many other degenerative diseases "familiar in human medicine," took a heavy toll among these cats.

Unhealthy conditions of mouth and teeth, degenerative

skeletal changes, and malalignment of teeth were found in most of them.

"In autopsy, cooked-meat females frequently presented the picture of ovarian atrophy and uterine congestion, whereas the males often showed failure in the development of active spermatogenesis." The bones of these cats showed "evidence of less calcium" and they generally showed signs of shriveling or wasting or became overly fat with distended abdomens. Dr. Pottenger reported:

"In the third generation of cooked-meat-fed animals, some of the bones became as soft as rubber and a true condition of osteogenesis imperfecta [imperfect bone structure from birth] was present. . . . Of the cats maintained entirely on the cooked meat diet, with raw milk, the kittens of the third generation were so degenerated that none of them survived the sixth month of life, thereby terminating the strain."

When these experiments were later repeated on rats, essentially the same results were obtained.

An interesting point in connection with these experiments is the fact that when raw metabolized vitamin D milk, pasteurized milk, evaporated milk, or sweetened condensed milk was substituted for the plain raw milk, bony disorders and deficiencies began to manifest themselves. Most marked deficiencies, however, occurred in the cats fed sweetened condensed milk, and Dr. Pottenger believed "that the excessive carbohydrate in the milk was responsible for much of this heavy damage."

"What vital elements were destroyed in the heat processing of the food fed the cats?" Dr. Pottenger asks. His reply is that the precise factors are not known. Ordinary cooking precipitates proteins, rendering them less easily digested. Probably certain albuminoids and globulins are physiologically destroyed. All tissue enzymes are heat labile and would be materially reduced or destroyed. Vitamin C and some members of the B complex are injured by the process of cooking. . . . Minerals are rendered less soluble by altering their physicochemical state. "It is possible that the alteration of the physicochemical state of the foods may be all that is necessary to render them imperfect foods for the maintenance of health. It is our impression that the denaturing of protein by heat is one factor responsible."

Dr. Jacob M. Leavitt summed up the situation very succinctly when he stated: "Living food contains an element which we have not as yet been able to crystallize. There is more to food than calories, enzymes, and vitamins. There is a living energy, a form of solar energy which is not available to us except as we obtain it through viable or vital foods in their uncooked state."

While the nutritional value of uncooked food is vastly superior to cooked food, it is well to repeat that in certain digestive or nervous disorders the patient may not be able to handle uncooked foods. When this is the case, we must make sure that the food is prepared in such a way that only a minimum of the valuable protective elements be lost. Our main objective, in these cases, however, should be to overcome the affliction so that uncooked foods can again be used without difficulty.

That nutrition is a major factor in the control of our chronic and degenerative diseases and plays a vital role in diseases of the heart and circulation can be seen from the report presented by Dr. Charles Glen King, Professor of Chemistry, Columbia University, and Scientific Director of the Nutrition Foundation, to the New York State Joint Legislative Committee on Problems of the Aging.

## Rockefeller Foundation Experiments

That faulty nutrition plays a major role in the production of many of our diseases has been demonstrated by some of our most outstanding investigators. Dr. Victor G. Heiser of the Rockefeller Foundation, in a talk before the American Association for the Advancement of Science, pointed out that large-scale animal feeding experiments in India, in which the diets eaten by various sections of India's millions of people were fed to large colonies of animals, reproduced at the will of the research workers the same state of health and well-being and the same types of disease observed in the human population.

Among the parts of the body which developed various types of serious diseases in the animals fed the faulty diet were the chest, ear, nose, upper respiratory passages, the eye, gastrointestinal and urinary tract. The skin, blood, lymph and glands, nerves, heart and teeth.

The diseases included stomach ulcers and two cases of cancer of the stomach, sinusitis, adenoids, inflammations of the eye, infections of the middle ear, pneumonia and bronchiectasis, loss of hair, skin diseases, pernicious anemia, seven types of diseases of the kidney and bladder including several types of kidney stones, goiter, enlarged adrenal glands, polyneuritis, various types of heart disease, and even mal-occlusion of the teeth and a large percentage of tooth decay.

On the other hand, the animals getting the diet eaten by some of the people of northern India developed no illness of any kind for two and a half years, corresponding to forty to fifty years in the life of man. Furthermore, none died during that period from natural causes ... and there was no infant mortality.[12]

Now what were the diets that produced such varied results?

This health diet, eaten by the animals and the human beings in some parts of northern India, consisted of whole wheat flour, unleavened bread lightly smeared with fresh butter, sprouted Bengal gram (legume), fresh raw carrots and cabbage ad libitum, unboiled whole milk, a small ration of raw meat with bones, once a week, and an abundance of water for drinking and washing purposes.

The ill-balanced diet fed to the animals that developed the thirty-nine varieties of diseases common among the human beings eating the same type of food consisted mostly of cereal grains, vegetable fats, with little or no milk or butter or fresh vegetables.

The experiments by Dr. Pottenger, the large-scale investigations carried on by the Rockefeller Foundation, and research carried on at many of our universities have conclusively demonstrated the importance of nutrition in the prevention and control of heart and blood vessel diseases.

They also proved the superior value of uncooked foods

[12] "Big Feeding Tests Give Disease Clue," *The New York Times,* June 21, 1939.

over cooked foods and have amply demonstrated the importance of including a liberal amount of raw fruits and raw vegetables in our diet, proving furthermore the superiority of natural, unrefined food products over refined denatured foods.

So far as the findings of Drs. Pottenger and Heiser in relation to meat are concerned, we do not wish to imply that meat be eaten raw, but their findings are clear. If meat be eaten, it is best eaten raw.

## The Importance of Small Meals

Next to knowing what to eat is the question of how much to eat. Small meals are now considered advisable in cases of heart disease. Dr. King's statement that we should eat "simple good food, but less total food" if we wish to stay well and live a long life, deserves special emphasis.

James Rorty in "The Thin Rats Bury The Fat Rats" pointed out that studies conducted over a period of twenty-five years by Clive McCay and associates at Cornell University demonstrated "that it is possible to double the normal life span of the rat; to delay the onset of the degenerative diseases that rats—and human beings—normally die of . . . simply by keeping . . . on an excellent diet which is low in calories . . ."[13]

It should be clear why this is so important in diseases of the heart and blood vessels. Large meals overburden the digestion and this in turn overtaxes the heart, while small meals lessen the work of the heart and help in more rapid recovery.

Next to eating small meals, other habits of eating need watching. We must make sure not to eat too fast, chew our food thoroughly, eat only when hungry, and not eat when mentally disturbed or emotionally upset, for all this miliates against good health.

## The Benefits Derived from the Omission of Food

"I saw few die of hunger . . . of eating, a hundred thousand," said Benjamin Franklin.

[13] *Harpers Magazine*, May, 1949.

We cannot stress too strongly the benefits derived from small meals. In line with this, complete abstinence from food for limited periods of time in some cases can be even more beneficial. When food is eliminated for a day or two or even longer, our organs of digestion are given a chance to rest, and the kidneys as well as all other organs of elimination are able to catch up with their work of eliminating the accumulated toxins from the system. The experiments reported by Cutter and the benefits derived from the Karrell diet (mentioned in another part of this book) illustrate how effective such therapy can be.

This does not mean that one can abstain from food indiscriminately or resort to this procedure in a haphazard manner. A fast must be carefully supervised and should not be extended beyond the point physiologically advisable in the individual case.

A point worth stressing in connection with total abstinence from food is that, except where an emergency exists, the patient should be properly prepared for it physiologically as well as psychologically.

A change to a better diet and a tapering off to less food, plus plenty of sleep and rest, are advisable for a few days or even longer before a fast is undertaken. A program of this kind can be highly beneficial not only in case of disease but also as a measure of prevention.

However, it is important to bear in mind that while such a regimen can be highly beneficial, its benefits can be quickly dissipated by a return to a conventional way of eating or by overeating.

# 6

## CHEMICAL ADDITIVES IN OUR FOOD

The necessity of avoiding all chemically preserved foods and foods to which chemicals have been added cannot be stressed too strongly.

The era in which we live has rightly been called the era of chemistry. The chemical industry has grown by leaps and bounds, and influences our existence in many ways. Practically every other industry is dependent upon it, and the food industry is no exception. However while its contributions to industry as a whole have been of tremendous value, its use in the food industry has turned out to be a menace to health and life.

Congressman James J. Delaney, Chairman of the House Selective Committee to Investigate the Use of Food Products, pointed out that 704 chemicals are now being used in the food industry "of which 428 are known to be safe.[1] In other words, Congressman Delaney pointed out, "276 are unknown and untested, and some of them may be slowly poisoning us!"

There is strong support for Congressman Delaney's conclusion. It was not so very long ago that the papers were filled with the story of agene (nitrogen trichloride),[2] a chemical used to bleach the flour used in the baking of our bread and cakes. Research workers suddenly discovered that when this chemical was fed to animals it induced various nervous reactions, including fits of an epileptic-like nature; as a result of these findings the Food and Drug Administration finally prohibited its use.

Agene had been in use in the baking industry for over a quarter of a century, and 95 per cent of all breads and cakes sold commercially were prepared from flour containing it. Although some of our foremost nutritionists had

[1] "Peril on Your Food Shelf," *American Magazine*, July, 1952.
[2] See Silver *et al.*, "Agene Toxicity," *J.A.M.A.*, November 22, 1947.

warned against the use of this chemical, the baking industry continued to use it without restraint until it was actually banned by the Food and Drug Administration.

We cannot help wondering how many cases of heart disease or other diseases of a degenerative nature may have had their inception or may have become intensified as a result of this dangerous chemical.

Not too long afterward, another chemical, lithium chloride, used as a salt substitute in cases of heart and kidney diseases and high blood pressure, was found injurious to health and was ordered withdrawn from use.

Fortunately lithium chloride was not in use for very long, but even for the short time that it was used, a number of fatalities were reported.[3]

More recently a group of chemicals used as bread softeners in the baking industry, polyoxyethylene monostearate and related compounds, were ordered discontinued by the Food and Drug Administration, which explained that the ban became necessary because these chemicals "could deceive consumers as to the age of the bread—and because they had not been tested adequately for their safety as ingredients of bread."[4]

Another reason, according to Commissioner Charles W. Crawford of the Food and Drug Administration, was that "these compounds were derived in part from ethylene oxide, a stranger in the food world."

While being grateful for the discontinuance of these chemicals, we cannot but wonder why similar and probably equally questionable bread softeners are still being permitted.

From the report[4] of the Food and Drug Administration, it is apparent "that about 80% of all bread and rolls manufactured commercially contain emulsifiers (bread softeners)" and that only about a third of the bread and rolls baked commercially were affected by this ruling. Since one of the reasons for the prohibition of the use of the polyoxyethylene monostearate and related compounds was because they "could deceive consumers as to the age of the bread," in what way are the other emulsi-

---

[3] Corcoran, Taylor, and Page, Lithium Poisoning from the Use of Salt Substitute, *J.A.M.A.*, March 12, 1949.
[4] *The New York Times*, May 15, 1952.

fiers, still in use in about two thirds of the bread and cakes baked commercially, any less deceiving?

Furthermore, does the fact that the other emulsifiers are still being permitted mean that they have been found to be harmless, or must we as with agene wait a quarter of a century before the detrimental effects of these chemicals are recognized and steps are taken to outlaw them?

Dr. Robert Riley,[5] Director of the Maryland Department of Health, in a report presented at the 97th annual convention of the American Medical Association, referred to a number of chemicals being used in bread and cakes baked commercially. Among them he mentioned "potassium bromate which is used to make the flour easier to handle and produce loaves of greater volume," also sodium bicarbonate, calcium phosphate, and sodium acid pyrophosphate, each used for a different purpose. While some of these chemicals, according to Dr. Riley, may be harmless or innocuous, what tests have been made to determine their long-range effects? Furthermore, is their use any less deceiving?

That arsenic sprays used in agriculture are harmful has been known for a long time, but unfortunately nothing has been done so far to prohibit their use. As a matter of fact, the use of these compounds has grown tremendously in the past thirty years, and Dr. Riley points out that "the danger to the consumer (of receiving a toxic amount of arsenic) is thus constantly increasing."

While Dr. Riley is hopeful that "insecticides free from toxicity to human beings will in time replace the present dangerous substance," the insecticides introduced most recently, according to recent health investigators, are actually even more dangerous.

We can think back to the time when, many years ago, Alfred W. McCann, Sr., in the *New York Globe*, conducted his one-man crusade against the use of these dangerous sprays, and when Dr. I. Sirovich, then Congressman from New York, in a series of articles published in the *Daily Mirror* emphasized the harmful effects of these chemicals. Since then, the use of these chemicals has be-

[5] "The Health Department and The Food of The People," *J.A.M.A.*, October 2, 1948.

come only much more widespread and nothing is being done to discontinue their use.

Congressman Delaney referred to the synthetic hormone stilbestrol which is used by poultry breeders to "add weight quickly and increase the market value of their products," and pointed out that in Canada its use had been outlawed because it can lead to sterility in the young.

A point often overlooked in connection with this hormone is that it is seriously suspected as a carcinogenic (cancer-producing) agent.

With regard to phosphoric acid, a chemical used by the soft drink industry, Congressman Delaney referred to the experiments at the Naval Medical Research Institute that "have shown that a human tooth put in soft drinks containing phosphoric acid lost its enamel and became soft in 24 hours."

DDT is now being used extensively as an insecticide and fungicide in and around barns. Congressman Delaney mentioned that DDT accumulates in the body fat of the animal and gets into our bodies through the meat we eat, and that this "can eventually have a cumulative and serious effect on the liver."

He continued further "that people suffering . . . from Virus X exhibited the same set of symptoms as those suffering from DDT poisoning."

Chlordane, an insecticide introduced in 1947 and now used extensively on fruits and vegetables is, according to the statement of Dr. A. J. Lehman, Director of Food and Drug Administration's Pharmacology Division, "four or five times more poisonous than DDT."

In a report published in the *Journal of the American Medical Association,* Dr. O. Bruce Lemmon and Commander Wilmot F. Pierce stated that their investigation disclosed that "Continuous administration of chlordane to laboratory animals caused focal hepatic necrosis [liver degeneration], edema [swelling], congestion and exudates in the lungs and degenerative changes in intestinal submucosa and in the convoluted tubules of the kidneys."[6]

Dealing with the same subject, Dr. Paul Lensky and Dr. Howard Evans in the same issue of the *Journal* described a case of poisoning of a fifteen-month-old child owing to

[6] "Intoxication Due to Chlordane," *J.A.M.A.,* August 2, 1952.

accidental swallowing of "probably not more than a mouthful" of a mild chlordane solution, and stated that "the insecticide enters the body by absorption through the intact skin, by inhalation of dusts or sprays, and by ingestion."[7]

*U.S. News & World Report* reported that the Committee on Pesticides of the American Medical Association issued "A fresh warning against the dangers of poisoning through improper use and careless handling of chlordane." It cautions against using chlordane in areas frequented by children, in waxes and polishes that touch the skin, and slow liberation of fumes—especially in closed, heated rooms.[8]

One can well understand why Dr. Lehman stated that he "would hesitate to eat any food that had any chlordane residue on it."

Congressman Delaney, reflecting on the "growing number of mental diseases," wondered "if there is not some connection between the increase in mental diseases and the many new chemicals used in our foods."

We, too, have often wondered about this, and also have wondered how much of a connection there is between the increase in the diseases of the heart and blood vessels and the use of these chemicals in our foods. We have seen how dangerous some of these chemicals can be, and we cannot refrain from asking, why no steps are being taken to check the use of these dangerous chemicals?

In explaining the reason for their use in food processing, Congressman Delaney said "they are relatively cheap, easy, and work 'wonders' as preservers, blenders, softeners, bleachers, emulsifiers, insect and fungus killers, and crop stimulators."

While the food industry is adamant about its right to use chemicals in the manufacture of its products until or unless they are proved harmful, it should be evident that the only way to serve the interests of the public is to establish rigid controls and not permit the use of any chemical in the food industry before its long-range effects have been fully tested and evaluated.

The immediate question is, as far as the consumer is

[7] "Human Poisoning by Chlordane," *Ibid.*
[8] "News You Can Use," September 2, 1955.

concerned, What can we do to protect ourselves against this mass danger? For one thing, we urge that whenever possible packaged and manufactured foods be avoided, since many of these foods are processed and contain chemical preservatives.

Where such foods are used it is important that all the printed matter on the label, including the small print, be carefully read, to find out what has been added. While the law requires that all ingredients be listed on the label, the chemicals and preservatives added are usually printed in the smallest type, often barely legible to the naked eye.

In an endeavor to avoid the use of foods grown with chemical fertilizers or chemically treated or sprayed, some health-conscious people are turning to the use of organically grown fruits and vegetables. These foods, grown on soil that is organically fertilized and without the use of chemical conditioners or the various chemical pesticides or insecticides, are infinitely richer in taste, flavor, and quality. We urge our readers to become more familiar with this type of farming and, whenever possible, to use fruits and vegetables that are grown this way.

Those who raise fruits and vegetables organically employ special farming methods that put back into the soil in organic form, and not through the addition of chemicals, the elements that are taken out of it. This type of farming keeps the soil properly conditioned and enables it to maintain its own immunity against the insects and pests that otherwise menace the crop.

This is very much in line with the immunity that exists in the body when we are in a healthy state. It is well known that our best protection against dangerous bacteria and viruses and harmful foreign substances is found in the immunity of our own body, and the same holds true with regard to the soil.

For those who are not in position to obtain organically grown, insecticide-free fruits and vegetables, the use of diluted hydrochloric acid to wash off the poisonous sprays used in agriculture is being suggested by leaders in the health field. The *Journal of the American Medical Association,* in reply to an inquiry, mentioned that one ounce of concentrated hydrochloric acid diluted with three quarts of water will remove "the commonly used inorganic insecticides such as lead arsenate, Paris green, and cryolite" and "remove most of an organic insecticide such as DDT."[9] A washing for five minutes in this solution will remove the residue of most if not all of the poisonous insecticides, according to this reply.

The editor also stated that Public Law 518, passed on July 22, 1954 as an amendment to the Federal Food, Drug, and Cosmetic Act "requires that residues of pesticides on fruits and vegetables not exceed a tolerance that is regarded as safe food." However, it should be apparent that this is far from providing the protection we need. For one thing, it is well known that the tolerance of individuals for chemicals and drugs varies. For another, we must always bear in mind that chemicals as well as drugs tend to accumulate in the body, and that as a result their harmful effects may not show up for some time.

At this point, we wish to utter a word of warning. While it is sound policy to use every precaution to obtain wholesome and poison-free foods, and to do everything possible to wash away or remove the poisonous sprays from our foods, it is extremely unwise to permit ourselves to become so panicked about the foods we eat that we lose our balance or peace of mind. While we deplore the existence of this hazardous situation and while we should try to do everything we can to counteract or eliminate the harm that can arise from it, we would endanger our health only the more if we started to worry every time we sat down to eat a meal.

Let us follow a sensible routine of using only the best of foods (best from the standpoint of nutrition and selection), and of preparing them in the best way possible, and then let us be content in the knowledge that we are doing everything possible to avoid the pitfalls that confront us.

[9] *J.A.M.A.*, February 18, 1956.

## 7

## THE SMOKING QUESTION

No one has to be told that smoking is harmful. While recent reports in the press have dealt primarily with the effect of smoking on the lungs, its detrimental effects on the heart and circulatory system, although not as extensively publicized, have been known for a long time.

Dr. Alton Ochsner, Chairman of the Department of Surgery, Tulane University, School of Medicine, in a talk before the Greater New York Dental Society, pointed out that medical men are ". . . extremely concerned about the possibility that the male population of the United States will be decimated by cancer of the lung in another fifty years if cigarette smoking increases as it has in the past, unless some steps are taken to remove the cancer-producing factor in tobacco."

He added, sardonically: "Smoking may have at least one virtue, by smoking heavily a man may have a heart attack: then he would not live long enough to develop lung cancer."[1]

At a meeting of the Public Health Cancer Association, an organization related to the American Public Health Association, a resolution was adopted urging the discontinuance of smoking as a protection against cancer of the lungs. One participant stressed the fact that there was good reason to believe that smoking causes "cancer in body sites other than the lungs and the oral areas" while another stated "that the now suspected relationship between smoking and heart disease might eventually prove to be more significant than the present relation between smoking and lung cancer."[2]

Dr. Theodore R. Van Dellen, in one of his syndicated articles, stated that cancer of the lungs, as well as

[1] "Cancer Rise Laid to Smoking," *The New York Times,* December 9, 1953.
[2] *The New York Times,* September 12, 1954.

smoker's throat and smoker's bronchitis is caused by the tars and other combustible materials in tobacco. He then quoted Dr. Grace Roth of the Mayo Foundation, University of Minnesota, who pointed out that 2.5 to 3 milligrams of nicotine is absorbed into the blood from one standard cigarette, and that while some individuals are more sensitive to the chemical than others, "The blood vessels suffer most; nicotine causes them to constrict."[3]

Dr. Roth, who has done a great deal of research on the effects of smoking, pointed out at the 29th annual meeting of the Greater New York Dental Society that nicotine causes an increase in blood pressure and pulse and a decrease in skin temperature. Dr. Irving S. Wright of the Cornell University Medical College stated that "the use of tobacco may mean the difference between life and death for persons with diseases of the circulation."[4]

Dr. Morton L. Levin, Assistant Commissioner of Medical Services of the Health Department of the State of New York, dealing specifically with the effect of smoking on the lungs, stated "that the relative incidence of lung cancer among men who smoke twenty or more cigarettes a day was ten times that of non-smokers," and "those who smoked less than one pack a day had five times as much lung cancer as non-smokers."[5]

Dr. Charles Cameron, Medical and Scientific Director of the American Cancer Society, himself a smoker, was at first reluctant to admit that smoking is harmful. He acknowledged "that the smoking picture, based on large segments of population, was admittedly grim."[6]

Dr. Harry J. Johnson, head of the Life Extension Examiners, a nationwide group of physicians specializing in physical examinations for industry, only confirmed what other scientists are finally beginning to recognize. Studies covering 2,000 men disclosed that "smokers complained of cough 300 per cent more often than non-smokers, of irritation of nose and throat 167 per cent more often, of heart spasms 50 per cent more often, of shortness of

[3] *Daily News,* November 3, 1953.
[4] "Cancer Rise Laid to Smoking," *The New York Times,* December 9, 1953, *op. cit.*
[5] "Ten Times More Lung Cancer Among Pack-a-Day Smokers," *New York Herald Tribune,* March 15, 1954.
[6] *The New York Times,* June 22, 1954.

breath 140 per cent more often, and of heartburn 100 per cent more often."[7]

The N.Y. Academy of Medicine, entering into the discussion on the effects of smoking, pointed out that it was well known in medical circles that moderate smokers died sooner than nonsmokers and that heavier smokers had an even shorter life expectancy. The Academy called attention to the findings of Dr. Raymond Pearl of the Johns Hopkins Department of Biology who sixteen years ago disclosed that "Deaths would start occurring among heavy smokers at age 35 and would continue to outnumber the deaths of non-smokers and light smokers all the way to age 70 at which time mortality rates tend to level off."[8]

The findings of Dr. Raymond Pearl were known in medical and scientific circles, and as we were reading this report from the Academy of Medicine we couldn't but wonder why responsible medical organizations failed to stress this point before, and why some of them even went out of their way to minimize or deride it.

## Why Do Doctors Condone Smoking?

Occasionally we are asked why, if smoking is really harmful, do doctors condone it? Dr. Martin Gumpert[9] has answered this question lucidly and unequivocally: "It is, of course, an open secret that medical prohibition or tolerance of tobacco depends a great deal on the physician's own smoking habits."

Dr. Gumpert, once a heavy smoker, was forced to give up smoking because of a heart attack. He was aware of many warning signals preceding the heart attack, but like the many others who are addicted to smoking, disregarded them. "My pulse rate had for some time been definitely higher than it should have been; yet the extra beats were merely considered by me as of no consequence."

He went on to say that it took a heart attack to make him realize the dangers of smoking.

Dr. Alton Ochsner has confirmed Dr. Gumpert's expla-

[7] New York World Telegram, June 26, 1954.
[8] New York World Telegram, June 23, 1954.
[9] Martin Gumpert, "The Dangers of Smoking," Tomorrow, April, 1934.

nation. He stated: "Unfortunately many physicians, probably because they themselves smoke, are unwilling to admit that there is a causal relationship between smoking and cancer of the lungs, in spite of the overwhelming statistical evidence."[10]

In the past many doctors who condoned smoking maintained that no direct relationship had been found to exist between smoking and heart disease. This argument certainly does not hold water. What difference does it make whether the harm is caused directly or indirectly?

Dr. Lemmon Johnson, dealing with the subject of smoking in the British Medical Journal, *Lancet,* after mentioning that "tobacco contains a number of poisons such as nicotine, pyridine bases, carbon monoxide and arsenic" went on to say that smoking becomes "a general analgesia against life's little, or even big, stresses and vexations."

Once one masters this habit, he will find an "accession of high spirits, energy, appetite and sexual potency, with recession of coughing," Dr. Johnson pointed out. However, before we can expect the public at large to accept this idea, doctors must set the example, he said.

"About 80% of us are smokers," he estimated, "and we behave collectively like an addict. Radical cure of tobacco smoking lies in its prevention and tobacco smoking is no more difficult to prevent than opium smoking. Our duty is plain."

The economic aspect also enters in. Tobacco is an immense industry, and large sections of our population depend upon it for their existence. It is evident that millions of people would suffer economically if a vast segment of our population ceased smoking.

Our government too has a financial stake in the industry. According to the *New York World Telegram,* taxes collected by the federal government from this industry amount to about $1,600,000,000 annually, while the states collect an additional 488 million yearly.

However, as Dr. E. Cuyler Hammond of the American Cancer Society pertinently pointed out, there should be much more to this question than economics, since our government also has "a stake in the welfare of our people, and in this instance the stake is the more than 20,000

[10] "The Case Against Smoking," *The Nation,* May 23, 1953.

deaths from lung cancer a year with an ever mounting toll."

While Dr. Hammond failed to mention it, in addition to the 20,000 or more deaths from cancer of the lungs, we must also think of the hundreds of thousands of deaths from heart and circulatory diseases as well as other diseases of a degenerative nature in which smoking plays a part. We are in complete agreement with Dr. Clarence Williams Lieb, who in his book *Safer Smoking* mentioned that if he had his way every pack of cigarettes would be inscribed with a skull and crossbones.

That smoking disturbs the fat metabolism and raises the fat level of the blood to a point where it becomes a contributing factor in the development of heart disease has been demonstrated by Dr. John W. Gofman, Professor of Medical Physics at the University of California in Berkeley. In the course of a research project financed by the United States Atomic Energy Commission, Dr. Gofman demonstrated that twenty or more cigarettes increased the fat level of the blood in male subjects sufficiently "to raise the over-all coronary heart disease death rate by 40 per cent."[11]

While Dr. Gofman asserted that "the process by which giant particles in the blood are increased by smoking" and "the mechanism by which large fat particles (including cholesterol) contribute to heart and artery affliction" are not known, and while he recognized the fact that the "lipoprotein elevation resulting from cigarette smoking may not be entirely responsible" for the higher incidence of coronary disease mortality, his statement that "it must account for an appreciable portion of it" was significant.

### How to Stop Smoking

Once you have reached the point where you realize that smoking is harmful and that it is best that you discontinue it, the question naturally arises, how to go about it. We are not going to pretend that it is always easy to break

[11] "Cigarette Linked to Heart Disease," *The New York Times*, September 6, 1955.

this habit. While some do it with relative ease, others find it a most exacting task.

The more firmly an addiction is rooted, the more difficult it is to break away from it. However, we can help ourselves considerably by approaching the problem with the right point of view. To begin with, it is well to start by keeping constantly in mind the fact that smoking is harmful. When you do this, you will not feel too sorry for yourself for trying to give it up. Then you must realize that it is a habit like any other habit, and that habits can be broken just as they can be acquired. Others have succeeded in doing it, and why shouldn't you?

Modern man is enslaved by many bad habits, and it is well to keep in mind that one stimulating habit only begets another one. To conquer the habit of smoking, it would be tremendously helpful if all other stimulating habits were discarded. Coffee, tea, alcohol, spices, condiments, sweets, and rich sauces all keep the body in a constant state of stimulation, each stimulant keeping awake the desire for the others. One stimulating habit often only chains us to all the others.

The experience of one man who succeeded in giving up smoking is worth relating at this point. The man was making plans to take his customary summer vacation, but this time decided to spend it at a resort where nutrition and careful living were stressed.

Since he was a confirmed smoker, he brought along two cartons of cigarettes and a box of cigars. "No Smoking" signs in the living and dining rooms caught his attention. To comply with this rule, he made it a practice to pick himself up after each meal and go outdoors for his habitual smoke.

This seemed necessary to him during the first few days of his stay, but as time went on he found that his need to smoke became less urgent and before very long, actually dispensable. The eating of simple, unseasoned food plus the relaxed atmosphere apparently diminished his desire to smoke. It did not take long for him to lose his craving and give up smoking altogether: "It seemed natural to smoke after a steak dinner with French fried potatoes, coffee, and cake; but I just had no desire for it after one of the simple vegetable meals served at this resort," he commented afterward.

This doesn't mean that it will work as easily in all cases. Individuals differ in temperament and will power, and the adjustment in some cases is much more difficult than in others. However, even where real difficulties exist it must still be done if health is to be rebuilt.

Always remember that with each smoke, you only keep adding to your difficulties. Also bear in mind that there is no such thing as "can't" when we are really determined to accomplish something. Others have done it, and so can you! Your life and health are certainly much more important than the momentary pleasure you derive from smoking. And what is even more important is that as you conquer this habit, you acquire an entirely new outlook on life and a variety of wholesome new pleasures.

In many cases, the "day-to-day method" has proved successful. We start this by making the patient feel that he is giving up smoking only for one day. A day later, he is urged to do it for one more day. It may seem difficult, but after all it is only one more day, and come hell or high water, he decides to stick it out! The third day comes along; well, since he has been able to do it for two days, why not one more day?

By then the sharp edges of the craving have in many cases begun to wear thin, and the person begins to realize that the battle is, after all, not as difficult as it seemed at the start.

In many cases the confirmed smoker may at first become extremely restless or irritable, even as the dope addict is miserable when he is deprived of drugs. He sometimes feels as though he is ready to "jump out of his skin." This, however, wears off before long, and what a joy he experiences when he finally realizes that he has conquered his enslaving habit and is now master over himself!

Once this stage is reached, it would be a serious mistake to test oneself by taking even a single puff, for this may undo all the good that has been done, since it may reawaken the old craving all over again.

Once you have gained control over this habit, persist in carrying on, and you will be able to boast of the fact that you too have gained mastery over yourself. You can do it, just as the many others have done it. Get started, be persistent, and as time goes on, you will feel happy and gratified at a good deed well done!

Some persons insist that they are unable to stop smoking, but what they really mean is that they have not as yet made up their minds to do it.

A habit is nothing more than something we have done for so long that it has become part of us. A good habit enriches our life, while a bad habit harms us. Any habit is developed by doing a certain thing constantly, a harmful habit just the same as a good habit. Replace your harmful habits by good habits and you will be the happier for it.

Those who persist in smoking despite all this evidence might well ponder the words of Dr. Peter J. Steincrohn who stated: "When I look back over the years, and think of the thromboangiitis cases who would not give up smoking after warnings, and actually lost two legs by amputation; when I think of coronary patients who persisted in smoking two and three packages a day in spite of warning and who died prematurely, I marvel how intelligent individuals calmly go about killing themselves."

# 8

## EFFECTS OF ALCOHOL

While the healing professions are now awakening to the dangers of smoking this cannot be said with regard to their attitude toward liquor. Most of them still regard it as a harmless indulgence, while some even encourage it on the assumption that if used moderately it will counteract nervous tension or help digestion. Some recommend it because it promotes a happier frame of mind and greater sociability.

We do not deny that, like smoking, liquor will produce some of these immediate effects. However, close observation will disclose that its long-term effects are entirely different.

Lichtwitz pointed out that alcohol destroys the thiamin (vitamin) reserve in the liver, and that as a result the liver is forced to take these vitamins from the nerves. The final result is that the liver, "like the gastro-intestinal mucosa and the salivary glands exhibits atrophy and cellular degeneration."[1]

MacCallum has declared that alcohol is "the commonest of poisons that affect human beings and that protracted habitual use seems to give rise to many anatomical changes in the organs."[2]

Henry H. Rusby asserted that "small quantities of alcohol, properly diluted when taken into the stomach, produce an agreeable sensation of warmth" and hasten the digestion and absorption of food. He went on to say, "The continued recourse to this artificial aid to digestion tends to necessitate it, and in increasing degree. Larger and larger amounts are apt to be required, and the natural powers of digestion become permanently and seriously impaired, and at length may be almost completely lost."[3]

[1] *Functional Pathology.*
[2] *A Textbook of Pathology.*
[3] *Reference Handbook of the Medical Sciences.*

He pointed out that its effects are like "those of a drug which for a very brief period stimulates, then depresses the tissues upon which it acts." It is "wholly depressing" upon the nervous system, weakens the will power and the higher functions of coordination, damages the liver, frequently induces Bright's disease, and affects the functioning of the heart and circulation.

Alcohol is often prescribed as a remedy in angina attacks because it supposedly dilates the blood vessels. Three respected research scientists, Dr. Henry I. Russek, Charles F. Naegels, and Frederick D. Regan of the U.S. Marine Hospital, Staten Island, New York,[4] pointed out that the relief obtained in angina pectoris through the use of alcohol is obtained primarily from its sedative effects, and not from the dilation of the blood vessels.

They concluded that, while the "sedative effects might be good for a patient with an angina attack, it could so thoroughly mask the pain with a false sense of fitness that the patient would not know what ailed him until it was too late."

Alcohol is injurious not only when taken in excess, but even in small doses, and don't let anybody tell you differently! The quarterly *Journal of Studies on Alcohol,* published at Yale University,[5] referred to the work of Dr. Kjell Bjerver and Dr. Leonard Goldberg of the Karolinska Institute in Stockholm who, by testing 37 skilled drivers between the ages of twenty-five and forty-five who were accustomed to drinking moderate amounts of alcohol, proved that two to three pints of 3.2 beer or three ounces of eighty-proof spirits impaired their driving ability by 25 to 30 per cent, even though they otherwise showed no obvious symptoms of intoxication.

"The usually careful drivers became careless, judgment was impaired, self-confidence and casualness were increased and they pretended not to notice the commissions of an obvious error," the two scientists noted. They concluded that even "a small amount of alcohol causes a sharp decline in the driving ability of normally expert drivers."

That drinking and smoking complement each other and

[4] "No Alcohol for Angina," *Newsweek,* June 12, 1950.
[5] *The New York Times,* March 15, 1950.

intensify the harm done to tlhe body was attested to by Dr. Sully Charles Marcel Ledermann, chief of the section of economic studies of the French National Institute of Demographic Study, Paris, who in a report presented to the United Nations Conference on Population stated that the risks of alcohol and tobacco "seem not merely to add up but to multiply one another."[6]

In taking note of man's many profound achievements, one cannot but wonder what greater heights might have been attained had he been free from the debilitating effects of tobacco and alcohol.

Tobacco and alcohol are accepted as part of our normal social amenities. Many persons are aware of their harmful effects but are unwilling to stop indulging for fear of appearing different from the others.

If you really wish to discontinue these habits, the problem is really not as difficult as it seems. You simply offer your apologies, and are done with it.

If you are fearful of offending or are unwilling to attract attention, you can do it more tactfully. If offered a cocktail, accept it graciously, if necessary even place it to your lips, but do not drink. A cigar may be put in one's pocket "for later use."

But it really isn't too difficult to say "No, thank you" and how often people will remark, "how smart you are; I wish I could do the same!"

[6] *The New York Times.*

## 9

## DANGERS OF OBESITY

"One of the common complications of obesity is damage to the cardiovascular system," according to Drs. Morris B. Green and Max Beckman.[1] They point out that abnormal electrocardiographic changes in their obese patients with hardening of the arteries were eight times as frequent as in their nonobese with hardening of the arteries.

Studies carried on by life insurance companies over an extensive period of time have proved conclusively that excess weight is not only dangerous to the heart and the vascular system, but also to all other vital organs of the body and is, therefore, a menace to health from every point of view.

Dr. Louis I. Dublin, Chief Statistician of the Metropolitan Life Insurance Company, in one of his reports on the subject, said: "A recent study among employees of the Metropolitan Life Insurance Company showed that elevation of the blood pressure was more than twice as frequent at ages 45 to 54 and three times as frequent at the ages of 35 to 44 among those of heavy build as among those of light build."[2]

You will notice that excess weight is considerably more dangerous in the thirty-five to forty-four than in the forty-five to fifty-four age groups. This is clearly in line with the greater increase in mortality from heart and vascular diseases in these age groups, and undoubtedly one of the factors responsible for it.

One Metropolitan study, which included 50,000 men and women, showed that mortality from diseases of the heart and vascular system were 50 per cent higher in men and 75 per cent higher in women who were obese over those who were not.

[1] "Obesity and Hypertension," *N.Y. State Journal of Medicine,* June 1, 1948.
[2] "Overweight—America's No. 1 Health Problem," *Today's Health,* September, 1952.

Dr. Dublin reported that another study, based on a sample of 74,000 industrial workers, showed at every age and among both men and women a steady increase in the average blood pressure with increase in weight. He noted also that "Among Army Officers, a group of men who were initially carefully selected and on whom careful medical observation was continued as long as they were in service, the rate of development of high blood pressure was about two and a half times as high in those who were overweight as in those who were not."

But high blood pressure is not the only penalty of obesity. Dr. Dublin pointed out that four fifths of those who develop diabetes after forty are overweight, that gallbladder disease is found more frequently among the overweight, and that obesity is "an important contributing factor in the development of degenerative arthritis, one of the most commom diseases of middle and later life."

Dr. W. H. Sebrell, Jr., Director of the National Institute of Health, is another of the many who emphasize that obesity is the number one nutrition problem in the United States. He points out that the "significance of this is apparent from the fact that mortality rates for the obese are well above average at every age, and rise steadily with increasing weight."[3]

James Rorty, referring to insurance company findings, pointed out that persons who are but 10 per cent overweight have a 20 per cent greater chance of dying prematurely than those whose weights are normal. If one is 15 to 25 per cent overweight, his chance of dying prematurely is 44 per cent greater than the average. And, above 25 per cent overweight, one's chances of living as long as one's normal contemporaries are only one in four.[4]

Dealing with the effect of overweight in cardiovascular diseases, Rorty mentioned that life insurance companies have proved that "overweight increases the mortality by 62 per cent"; and continued by quoting Dr. Stieglitz, author of The Second Forty Years who "believes that more than half the cases of heart exhaustion in later years are due to obesity."

[3] "Obesity Is Termed No. 1 Nutrition Ill," The New York Times, December 9, 1952.
[4] "The Thin Rats Bury The Fat Rats," Harpers, May 1949.

## Doctors Should Set an Example

Strange as it may seem, doctors as a class are more overweight than persons engaged in most other professions. Dr. Donald B. Armstrong, Vice-President of the Metropolitan Life Insurance Company, reported this fact at the convention of the American Medical Association, June 12, 1951, and belabored his obese colleagues for failing to do something about it.

Some years ago, a physician connected with one of the life insurance companies came into our office and, noticing a scale in the corner, stepped on it to weigh himself. He tipped the scale at 200 pounds.

"Doctor, why don't you reduce?" we asked him.

"I don't seem to be able to do it," he replied almost apologetically.

"It's simple; all you have to do is eat less."

He hemmed and hawed, and finally came up with the answer that he was working too hard and therefore "could not control his appetite."

Dr. Edward L. Bortz must have had a doctor like this one in mind when he remarked that "we're going to have to take off the kid gloves in dealing with people who are wallowing in their own grease."

One of the most interesting cases of overweight that we remember was that of a physician who weighed about 280 to 290 pounds, and who, because of his weight, was dubbed by his friends "The Man Mountain."

The first time we met the "man mountain" was at a restaurant. When we ordered a fruit salad, he ordered the same, but he later confessed that in all his life he had never thought of ordering a fruit salad.

We would frequently visit patients together, and once, while on a trip, we stopped the car to buy some fruit. He was, at that time, "dieting," for it was obvious, even to himself, that he was getting sicker by the day.

He too stepped out of the car, ostensibly to make a telephone call. But when he returned from the store, mustard was dripping from his lips. Evidently the telephone call was but an excuse for grabbing a hot dog on the run.

Once he became very ill. He could hardly breathe and his legs swelled up like balloons. He knew that his heart and kidneys were in bad shape. We pleaded with him. "Doctor, why don't you control your appetite?"

This time he pledged that from now on he would really be careful. He decided to go on a juice diet, and assured us that this time he would do a real job.

About two or three days later, he came to see us again. Because we were busy with a patient, he had to wait in the anteroom. Quite by accident, as we looked out the window, we noticed that our good doctor was crossing the street to buy an ice cream from a "Good Humor" man who was just then passing by. Somewhat later, the following dialogue took place between us:

"How is your dieting coming along?"

"Oh, fine!"

"Is ice cream part of your diet?"

He realized that we must have seen him through the window, and turning red, he mumbled, "a portion of ice cream is the equivalent of two glasses of orange juice."

This wonderful physician died at the age of fifty-three. He was a great friend, and beloved by everybody who knew him. He had a keen mind and was willing to do anything that would help his patients, but was not strong enough to conquer his own appetite, and so shortened his life by many years.

## Mountains of Flesh Can Melt

However, for each one who fails to do a good job, there is another one who succeeds and who benefits from it.

We can think of another case much the same as the one just mentioned. This man was twenty-eight. He wasn't really ill, he said, but he realized that he had to reduce.

We smiled when he said he wasn't ill. He was puffing and wheezing and dragging his load before him. He suffered from frequent heartburn, and a sour stomach made him very uncomfortable.

He was an accountant, and every afternoon while working over his books he would find himself getting so drowsy that he was unable to stay awake.

He was planning to be married and he felt he owed it

to his future wife to reduce. At any rate he realized that his present life was not very pleasant, and he was determined to change.

And it wasn't so hard. He watched with a sense of satisfaction the shrinking of his waistline, and he was jubilant when at last he could announce that clothes that he had had to discard years earlier because of his increased weight were again usable and comfortable to wear.

At first he didn't think that he had been sick, but he was pleasantly surprised when, after losing about sixty pounds, he found that his puffing and wheezing and all othr abnormal symptoms had completely disappeared.

His drowsiness by then was a thing of the past. He was as alert and awake as anyone. There was a new buoyancy in his steps. And when people complimented him upon the change in his appearance, he became really proud of his accomplishment.

### "Eating for Two" and Other Superstitions

There are many misconceptions about weight, and the sooner these misconceptions are recognized, the better it will be for all concerned.

Years back, pregnant women were under the impression that they had to "eat for two" if they wanted to stay well when pregnant, and have a healthy baby.

Recently, a man told us that when he married his wife she was a slim, petite, beautiful girl, weighing 109 pounds, but because of this mistaken idea she had permitted her weight to climb to 149 pounds during pregnancy. The more she spread out, the more of her charm and youthfulness were lost, and before long she was just another ordinary, middle-aged housewife. This old superstition is gradually fading away, but there are still many who cling to it.

Another superstition that still lingers among many mothers is the idea that the heavier their children are, the healthier they are. This leads to constant stuffing and overfeeding, which not only makes their children fat but also lays the foundation for many diseases.

The well-known humorist Sam Levenson, himself rather heavy, once mentioned that his mother believed that children had to eat plenty to grow big and healthy, and that as a result his brother had become so healthy that "he couldn't even walk."

His mother, who herself was heavy, was persuaded at one time to go on a diet. She was happy at first, but couldn't overcome her fear that she might be hurting herself. She would keep looking into the mirror, repeating again and again that she was beginning to look like "skin and bones."

Many persons realize that excess weight is harmful but lack the will to control appetite, and therefore keep looking for short cuts. Many doctors will still prescribe thyroid extracts, which often cause great harm, and others prescribe other hormones, or laxatives of various kinds; it is well known that none of these remedies accomplishes its objective.

At a meeting of the American Medical Association at which the question of obesity arose, Dr. Stromont stated that the drug dinitrophenol, at one time used for reducing, raises body temperature so that "the obese are literally frying in their own fat."

Some believe that long walks or heavy exercises will work off their excess weight. As a matter of fact, long walks and strenuous exercise only increase the appetite and invariably induce overeating. They also overtire the body, which may actually require rest rather than increased activity to rebuild normal glandular functioning.

While more rest may be necessary, this does not mean that exercise or activities are to be omitted. It merely means that we must guard against an indulgence in exercises or activities that overtire the body and weaken the functions of the glands still further.

We were told about one woman who was young and beautiful, but extremely overweight. She ate constantly, and never knew when to stop. Finally she decided to go on a diet.

One time, while on a trip with some of her friends, she suddenly remembered that she had to make a telephone call. We'll never know whether she actually had to make the call, but those who were with her in the car had no doubt that her real reason for going into the candy store was to gulp down several pieces of candy.

Many fool themselves this way, and then keep on complaining that they do not know why they are not reducing.

They are just not honest with themselves. The most important factor in reducing is to eat less. Begin by cutting your food intake in half, and eating very little or none of the foods you crave most. Discontinue white bread, white cereals, cakes, cookies, candy, creams of all kinds, sauces, and use more of raw and stewed fruits and raw and steamed vegetables along with a small quantity of your favorite protein, once daily.

Exclude all sugars and all fat foods. Discard the use of condiments and spices. Table salt tends to put weight on by retaining fluid in the system, and should therefore be eliminated from the diet. Furthermore, do not be afraid to go without a meal or two. An eliminative regimen for a day or two, or even several days at a time, will work wonders. It will hasten the reducing process and benefit you immensely. Our task is not only to reduce weight but to rebuild the body to the point where the glands and the digestive organs function normally. After the correct weight is attained, this program of living must be continued if you are to maintain your gain or, to say it otherwise, to hold down what you have lost.

When a person says that he cannot reduce, he merely means that he hasn't yet reached the point where he is willing to try hard enough. In almost all cases, results are attainable if we are willing to apply ourselves diligently to the job. The problem is merely how to go about it most efficaciously. Determination is the surest way to surmount this problem.

People often eat too much without realizing it. Others eat too much because they have too much time on their hands and don't know what to do with it. For some, eating is an emotional outlet.

If you have too much time on your hands, find something of interest to do to divert your mind from food. Perhaps a hobby or some such outlet as music, literature, gardening, the outdoors, or some social interest, anything that diverts the mind and counteracts boredom is helpful.

When confronted with a problem, some fall into the habit of "compulsive" eating, but it is well to realize that not only does this not solve any problem, but it adds another one. Analyze your problem, discuss it if need be with one who may be able to advise you properly, and make the necessary adjustments. But do not seek an escape in overeating.

Some persons claim that they hardly eat anything, and yet keep on gaining weight. If they would only make a list of what and how much they eat, what a surprise it would be to them! They simply do not realize how much they eat.

By following the suggestions on diet outlined in this encyclopedia, and by cutting down to half the quantity of food usually eaten, effective and lasting reduction will be inevitable.

And make all these changes cheerfully! Don't act the martyr, and don't feel as though you are doing somebody a favor or making a great sacrifice. You are doing the only thing that will help you gain renewed helath, increased strength, new vigor, and with it, a new "look," as well as an entirely new outlook on life. Aim high and do it graciously, joyously, and under your own power. Your rewards will be commensurate with your efforts.

## 10

## NERVOUS TENSION

In this world of tension, very few persons learn how to lead a serene and contented life. From very infancy, all through childhood, and well into adulthood we are trained to strive, to conquer, to succeed.

In business, as well as in social and cultural endeavors we desire to excel and win acclaim, and this competitive existence leads to constant tension and ultimately becomes a permanent pattern and vicious cycle.

This is the reason so few persons know how to relax or how to take life more at ease. Most persons blame their heart and blood vessel diseases on their high-strung, keyed-up existences, but are unwilling to recognize the fact that their ways of life can be altered. They are simply unwilling to make the changes necessary to alter their pattern of living. It should hardly be necessary to point out that this is an immature approach, and will not solve anything.

There is no question but that nervous tension and the difficulties of our present-day existence affect our health, but we delude ourselves when we place the blame exclusively on these factors and refuse to recognize the many other causes that contribute to our breakdown.

Because the majority of people are unwilling to concede that most of the influences responsible for their breakdowns are within their control, many of them seek to shift the blame onto factors for which they cannot be held responsible. To those persons we would like to say that a cursory examination will reveal that our life today is in reality much less difficult than it was in years past, and that this excuse is offered merely as a cloak to cover up an indifference or unwillingness to give up some of the unwholesome habits of living.

Who doesn't remember the depression years with their hopelessness and despair, with millions of people deprived of the very necessities of living, with nothing to look forward to? Who doesn't remember the poverty and insecurity of the sweatshop era, when people were slaving fourteen to sixteen hours a day in unhygienic, unclean workshops, and then, after work, spending the remaining few hours of the day in squalid, unsanitary tenement homes? Then, what about the war and postwar problems that took a great deal out of us?

When some of us begin talking of the "good ol' times" and start blaming the increase in many of our chronic and degenerative diseases merely on the stress and strain of present-day existence, let us not forget the difficulties and hardships of the past.

When confronted by problems, it is actually a matter of self-preservation to sit back and reappraise them so that we may discern how best to deal with them. Have you ever heard of "the richest man in the cemetery?" The forty-odd-year-old executive who decides to slow down, even though this means doing less business, is perforce a wise man indeed. Life is too valuable to be squandered in the chase for a few more dollars or a little additional glory, nor should it be thrown away by indulgence in unnecessary, health-destroying habits.

Each of us must pause and think seriously of how best to readjust our way of doing things, for no matter how close we get to our goal, whether it be in striving for wealth or in the attainment of any other possessions, if our health is sacrificed in the process our life is a failure.

The man in his prime who is suddenly forced to give up his business because of a heart attack has managed his life poorly. Even though he has amassed a fortune he has failed to make the most of life. He hasn't accomplished very much, whatever his achievements, if in attaining his objective he has brought about his premature collapse.

## How Life's Problems Should Be Handled

This does not mean that we should disregard our problems or be indifferent to our needs. We must learn to approach and deal with our problems with calmness and understanding, since this is the only way to cope with them adequately. Furthermore, we must make sure to follow a sound and well-regulated program of living, for only this will enable us to maintain a high standard of health and endow us with the strength and vitality we need if we are to handle our problems efficiently and make life a success.

Always keep this in mind: healthy individuals do not succumb when confronted with difficult problems or faced with hardships. Those who possess the stamina and endurance that goes with sound health do not break down during periods of stress, but face their problems with equanimity, and handle them in the most effective way possible. We saw many examples of this during the depression years when millions of people were stripped of their possessions in a matter of minutes. Those with strong bodies and healthy nerves were able to take their reverses in stride and start life all over again, while those with shattered nerves and depleted bodies were unable to bear the brunt of the burden and went to pieces altogether, often dragging their families along with them.

## Emotional Problems

The points we have made regarding our every-day problems of life apply with equal force to our emotions. Tension, fear, greed, hatred, jealousy, resentment, insecurity, gnaw into our vitals and destroy our heart as well as the rest of our body. Composure and self-control, on the other hand, keep us free from these harmful emotions, and protect us against their deleterious effects.

Emotional imbalance and instability are really signs of immaturity, and harm the individual who gives way to them. Life cannot be fashioned in patterns of our own choosing, and when adversities arise we must make sure that we are mentally and physically equipped to cope with them.

Calmness, composure, patience, and understanding are traits that are easily developed by the healthy person; these qualities enable us to cope with our difficulties and help to make life a joy instead of a torment. Some persons are more sensitive than others and react more keenly to their surroundings or their problems, but this need not create unhappiness. As a matter of fact, this type of temperament can actually enrich life, provided we understand how to direct our emotions into the proper channels. Persons with this type of temperament possess a much greater appreciation for the things that make life more beautiful, such as the arts, literature, music, and have a great capacity for love, compassion, and understanding. It is only when these sensitive qualities are misdirected or uncontrolled that they give rise to suffering.

If you are one of those sensitive individuals, what a world of beauty and warmth can open up for you, provided you learn how to readjust your outlook and how to handle your problems intelligently. This may not always be easy, but many compensations will come your way, once you achieve it. Beauty, love, kindness, understanding, joy, compassion, are some of the great qualities within your reach, and are the attributes conducive to tranquility.

An easy way to make this adjustment is to choose a favorable time of the day when you withdraw to a quiet room, and while relaxing in a comfortable chair or in a reclining position, retrace all your actions and thoughts of the day, freely recognizing your shortcomings, and picturing how you would handle simliar situations or problems in the future. After having done this, continue in your calm and relaxed position, picturing yourself as the person you would like to be, with the strength that you wish to possess, and the weaknesses that you are determined to overcome. In other words, visualize the person you wish to be, and keep on visualizing it daily until it becomes a part of you.

## 11

## RHEUMATIC FEVER

Various acute diseases place a strain upon the heart and often leave their imprint upon it. One of the acute diseases often followed by heart damage is rheumatic fever, a disease that most often affects the young. About 75 per cent of all who suffer from rheumatic fever are below the age of twenty.

This disease takes a terrific toll of human life. About 50,000 children are known to die from it yearly, and many of those who survive are left with permanently damaged hearts.

Those who recover from their first attack are always in danger of recurrent attacks, and each succeeding attack is usually of a much more serious nature.

At least one third of all adult heart diseases arise as an aftermath of rheumatic fever, while 90 per cent of all heart diseases in children are of this type.

Rheumatic fever was originally regarded as an acute rheumatic disease of the joints. However, since many of these cases are followed by heart damage, many authorities now classify it as a disease of the heart.

E. C. Laseque once described this disease as the disease that "licks the joints and bites the heart," However, this disease frequently affects other parts of the body as well. The kidneys, the nerves, as well as many other parts of the body may be affected by it. When the nerves are affected, it gives rise to the condition known as chorea or St. Vitus Dance. Another point worth mentioning is that in many cases of rheumatic fever the joints may be completely free from pain.

No permanent heart damage need result from rheumatic fever. The type of treatment employed will often determine whether the patient is left with permanent heart damage or comes through unscathed.

## Aspirin, Cortisone, and ACTH

The conventional treatment in rheumatic fever is rest in bed, the application of heat, plenty of "good" food, and the use of aspirin. Aspirin is regarded as a specific in this disease, and is part of the armamentarium of the average physician.

While there is no question that rest in bed and the application of heat are of great help, physicians would do well to re-evaluate the effects of aspirin as well as the conventional type of feeding in the light of our new concepts of disease and the more modern findings of nutrition. They would soon realize that a change from the conventional approach is imperative if permanent heart damage is to be avoided.

Let us begin by examining how aspirin affects a rheumatic fever patient. We can do no better than turn to Dr. Paul Dudley White, who said that because "the possibility of long continued salicylate (aspirin) therapy may depress the production rate of immune bodies in the organism, it makes one hesitate to recommend such chronic treatment unreservedly." He continued: "It is of considerable importance to recognize that evidence of the persistent activity of the rheumatic infection may be masked by the long continued use of salicylates, which abolishes temporary symptoms and signs including fever and leucocytosis."[1]

In other words, long-continued use of aspirin suppresses or masks the rheumatic infection, and actually interferes with the immunizing powers of the body. It should not take much to see how this can permanently damage the affected parts of the body.

Looking further, we find Graham and Parker saying: "Sodium salicylate (a salt of aspirin) is widely used in the treatment of acute rheumatic fever and the more chronic forms of rheumatism. While there may be disagreements as to its precise value in the therapy of various rheumatic conditions there is general agreement that it is a toxic substance giving rise to a variety of untoward and even alarm-

[1] Paul Dudley White, *Heart Disease.*

ing symptoms which may interfere with its administration."[2]

The *United States Dispensatory* (20th Edition) states the following about aspirin: "Overdoses of acetylsalicylic acid (aspirin) commonly produces ringing in the ears as do the inorganic salicylates. Frequently, however, even in quantities not excessive, it produces a very different type of intoxication. Among the most common symptoms are profuse sweating, cold extremities, either with or without a fall in body temperature, rapid or irregular pulse and occasionally albuminuria [albumin in the urine].

"In many reported cases there has been marked facial edema involving not only the skin but the mucous membrane of the mouth and throat."

In addition to aspirin, other drugs have been used in the treatment of rheumatic fever. Cortisone and ACTH are the drugs which have been tried most recently. Results of a three-year study undertaken by the American, British, and Canadian Heart Association, "to determine whether ACTH, cortisone or aspirin is most effective in alleviating the symptoms of rheumatic fever," while so far inconclusive has, nevertheless, demonstrated "that there is little difference in the efficacy" of these remedies and that the dangers of side reaction with aspirin are much less.[3]

In discussing the relative merits of these remedies, a well-known physician pointed out that cortisone and ACTH are in reality more dangerous than aspirin because they are much more potent and have to be much more closely watched for side reactions affecting the pituitary, the adrenal, the thyroid, the pancreas, the kidneys, as well as the psyche (mind).

Now if these drugs are not the treatments of choice, what is the ideal treatment in these cases?

## How Rheumatic Fever Develops

Before answering this question, it might be well to see whether we could not at first determine how this disease develops.

[2] *Quarterly Journal of Medicine*, April, 1948.
[3] *The New York Times*, April 11, 1953.

If you should ask your doctor what causes rheumatic fever, he may in all sincerity tell you that he doesn't know, and that while a germ has been suspected, this is a mere guess. Here is how Levine puts it: "The exact etiology [cause] of this disease is not known although a streptococcus is thought by many to be the cause. The evidence, however, is very conflicting and the question is best regarded for the present as unanswered."[4]

MacCallum explains: "Although for years many investigators have attempted to show that it is caused by one sort of bacteria or other, generally some type of streptococcus—there is no convincing evidence that any of the different bacteria occasionally found in the blood or respiratory passages have any importance as its cause."[5]

We can see from all this that the question of a germ being the cause is mere conjecture. Now, if the disease cannot be blamed on a germ, how does it develop? The answer is not so mysterious as it seems. Medical literature asserts that many predisposing factors play a role in its development. Dr. Paul Dudley White states:

An important factor in the occurrence of the rheumatic infection and of rheumatic heart disease appears to be the social and economic status of the individual. These diseases are much more common, by several times at least, among the crowded poor than among the well-to-do inhabitants of almost every community. In the large American private shools, rheumatic fever, chorea, and rheumatic heart disease are uncommon, while in the large public schools they are relatively very common.

Crowding, exposure to cold and wet without sufficient protection, malnutrition and fatigue are probably all factors in producing this contrast.[6]

Dealing with the same subject, Dr. Norman L. Moore[7] of the School of Nutrition, Cornell University, observed that the incidence of rheumatic recurrence was four times as high in a poor environment as in a good one.

4 Levine, Samuel: *Clinical Heart Disease.*
5 MacCallum, *A Textbook of Pathology.*
6 Paul Dudley White, *Heart Disease.*
7 "A New Approach to the Rheumatic Fever Problem," *New York State Journal of Medicine,* January 1, 1949.

"It has long been suggested that economic, sociologic, and dietary factors are concerned in some way in the etiology and recurrence of the disease. The above study gives emphasis to that point."

Here then, in clear and unequivocal terms, is an indication of why rheumatic fever develops. Malnutrition or poor dietary factors, fatigue, poor environment, or any of the influences that lower the resistance of the body play an important role in the development of this disease. The reason we have a preponderance of rheumatic fever among the poor is simply because these unfavorable factors predominate in the homes of the poor.

However, since unfavorable influences are not limited exclusively to the poor and since children in well-to-do homes are often improperly nourished and exposed to influences that lead to overfatigue, they are not altogether immune to it.

Improper food, excessive indulgence in sweets, the use of rich concentrated foods or refined foods, overeating, exhaustion, and excessive emotional influences are among the many factors that affect the children of all classes.

Dr. Moore made this point clear when he stated that studies have given "positive evidence of the relationship between adequacy of diet and the susceptibility of the host of rheumatic fever." He specified that "one of the three factors in the genesis of the rheumatic state is conditioning of the host by a poor diet."

Dr. Moore further referred to the contribution of Jackson, Kelly, Rohret, and Duane, who have proved that "the degree of deficiency of the diet was related to the incidence and degree of heart damage" and that "an excellent diet plus wholesome living conditions will practically eliminate the chances of recurrence with carditis [inflammation of the heart]."

Dr. Moore concluded by pointing out that observations have demonstrated conclusively that an incomplete or deficient diet plays an important role in the development of this disease, and that a well-balanced diet plus wholesome living conditions will not only help toward rapid recovery but will protect the heart against damage.

## The Best Treatment for Rheumatic Fever

It should not be difficult to conclude what the most logical approach in these cases should be: certainly not the use of suppressants, but the type of care that helps overcome the inflammatory process and aids in rebuilding the debilitated body. Rest, warmth, the use of hot baths, and the application of moist heat packs to the affected joints, plus good nursing and a carefully regulated nutritional program, make up an ideal approach in these cases.

How effective such a program is can be seen from the following case histories.

### A Case History: IRA S.

Ira S. was eight years old when he became sick with rheumatic fever. The onset was sudden with high fever and excruciating pains and swelling in his legs and wrists.

The family physician who was called in and the specialist who joined him in consultation suggested conventional treatment: aspirin at regular intervals, complete rest in bed, the application of heat to the inflamed joints, and what is usually considered "good, nourishing food." The physician was to see him daily to watch his progress and check his heart.

We need not describe the fear with which the parents received the information that their child was suffering from rheumatic fever. Most people know the dangers associated with this disease, and are terribly frightened by it. This may have been the reason for Ira's parents' refusal to go along with the conventional treatments, and for their having turned to the hygienic methods.

Now followed an interesting period, which was closely watched by family and friends. To the parents these were fearful days; the other members of the family doubtfully shook their heads. Some even berated the parents for rejecting the standard type of treatment.

The treatments employed were simple. At first, plain lukewarm cleansing enemas followed by hot epsom salt baths were given twice daily. Following the bath, the boy was wrapped in sheets and rolled in blankets to induce perspiration.

The food during the first few days was limited to freshly squeezed orange and grapefruit juice, as well as other fruit juices.

For local relief, hot moist compresses were applied to the swollen and painful joints. Tepid spongings every two hours, to make the boy more comfortable, completed the routine.

Noticeable improvement became apparent within a few days. The temperature began to drop about the second or third day, and the swellings began to diminish materially. The pain lessened and sleep became more relaxed, less fitful.

After the first few days, the enemas and baths were reduced to one daily, and more substantial food was gradually introduced.

We began with small amounts of raw fruit. Then small meals of raw and steamed vegetables and raw and stewed fruit were gradually introduced. A baked potato was added a few days later.

Each day brought further improvement, and after about three or four weeks, the boy was completely well.

During this time, no medication of any sort was used. The doctor who had first examined the boy and who was a close friend of the family watched the boy's progress closely, even though he was not officially in charge of the case. He knew that no medication was used, and while at first he had predicted all kinds of dire consequences, he ultimately was amazed to note how rapidly the boy recovered.

Neither he nor the specialist who re-examined the boy after he had completely recovered could discover any signs of heart disease.

Years later when Ira was inducted into the army cadet flying corps, a rigid checkup only confirmed that he was in excellent health.

*A Case History:* LYDIA C.

Here is another illustration of the effectiveness of this type of treatment:

Lydia C., four years old, came down with rheumatic fever. In checking over the child's history, we found that she had been suffering from asthma and other allergic conditions since birth, and that only a short time before her rheumatic attack had been subjected to a series of injections for these conditions.

Lydia was not suffering from painful joints but the examination left no doubt in the mind of the doctors that Lydia was suffering from a severe case of rheumatic fever.

The treatments in this case were practically a repetition of the other, with some minor modifications. Eliminative treatments and hydrotherapy (water applications) were used. Natural mineral and vitamin-rich fruit juices were used during the first two or three days after which small meals of raw and stewed fruit, raw and steamed vegetables, and baked or steamed potatoes were introduced.

All other foods were at first completely excluded but the dairy products and small portions of chicken and lean meat were later permitted as the child improved.

It took over three weeks before the fever and heart symptoms were under complete control, and altogether about three months before the child had fully recovered. A cardiologist (heart specialist) called in to recheck the patient found her in excellent condition!

It is interesting to note that not only did the patient recover from her rheumatic fever, but also that all former signs and symptoms of her allergic condition completely disappeared.

"You will never realize how frightened we were when the doctors told us how seriously ill Lydia was, and we will never forget what this rational regimen has done for her," her father said.

These are only a few of many cases of rheumatic fever that have been treated with these simple rational measures and that have proved how easily such cases can be brought under control. In a practice extending over a period of 40-odd years, we have had occasion to observe many cases of rheumatic fever, and in none of the cases treated by these conservative reconstructive methods from their inception could any evidence of heart disease be detected as an aftermath of the acute condition.

The reason these methods are so successful is because they permit effective elimination of the deleterious substances by enabling the kidneys, the skin, as well as all other organs of elimination to function efficiently, give the body a chance to organize its own defenses, and bring about a reversal of the disease processes as rapidly as possible. Nothing is done to interfere with or suppress the body's restorative efforts.

## A Case History: LUCY C.

In cases where the heart is already damaged, the problem is, of course, more difficult. However, even in such cases a discontinuance of the suppressive treatments and a change to the hygienic regimen often produces dramatic results.

In this type of heart disease, the damage primarily affects the valves of the heart. Scars form on and around the valves and prevent their closing or opening completely. If you remember, the valves of the heart open to empty the blood from the upper chamber into the lower chamber and then close to prevent the blood from flowing back. When the valves are damaged they are unable to close or open completely and as a result the blood either fails to flow through entirely or some of it is forced back. This places a great strain on the heart and forces it to enlarge.

Lucy C., ten years old, is a case in point. Lucy had a history of frequent colds and recurrent attacks of tonsilitis.

Her tonsils were finally removed but soon after, rheumatic fever developed. For months conventional treatments were employed, but Lucy only continued to grow worse.

On several occasions, friends tried to induce Lucy's parents to discontinue the conventional treatments and turn to hygienic methods, but because of the dangers associated with this disease and the seriousness of Lucy's condition they were afraid to try anything new. However, when the doctor in charge of the case mentioned that Lucy was "very low" and that he was "surprised that she hadn't died 24 hours ago," the parents finally realized that they had nothing to lose and decided to make the change.

By that time, Lucy's heart was already badly damaged and greatly enlarged. Cor bovinum (ox heart), doctors call this type of heart. What was even more serious was that in addition to the enlarged and badly damaged heart, she was also suffering from a severe congestion of the lungs and showed all the signs of impending circulatory failure.

An examination by the physician revealed a low grade

fever and a rapid pulse that was barely perceptible. Respiration was 46 per minute. No wonder the new physician too regarded the case as critical and couldn't hold out much hope!

Eliminative treatments were immediately instituted. All medication was discontinued. Warm cleansing enemas, mild hydrotherapy in the form of packs and hot foot baths, and a bland, vitamin- and mineral-rich diet was prescribed, which was later supplemented by meals that provided all essential nutritional needs of the body in easily digestible form.

It took about three weeks before we felt that we were on safe ground in this case. It is worth noting that at first Lucy's temperature began to rise, reaching as high as 103½, while her pulse slowed down and became much stronger, and her respiration grew much deeper and more regular.

The first ten days were days of extreme uncertainty, but after that we began to feel more confident. Another ten days or so and the temperature, pulse, and respiration were normal. From then on it was just a matter of continued rest in bed, adequate nutrition, and good nursing care.

It took about four months before Lucy had completely recovered, and before she was permitted to leave her bed.

The last few weeks were rather difficult, for with the return of her health and strength came the desire to get out of bed, and we had considerable difficult to keep her at rest until we were sure that it was safe enough to permit her to get up.

Lucy was seen again about 19 years later. She was then twenty-nine years old, married, and the mother of a child.

While the defects of the heart could not be completely erased, the heart had become considerably smaller than it was at the time of her illness and had grown sufficiently strong to enable her to lead a normal life.


## The Question of Allergy in Rheumatic Fever

In discussing the factors that predispose the body to acute rheumatic fever, the question of allergy is often brought up. Some maintain that acute rheumatic fever is an allergic disease and arises from the intake of foods or exposure to substances to which the body has become oversensitive.

The *Journal of the American Medical Association,* July 17, 1948,[8] commented editorially on the work done by Vaubel and Kling, and later substantiated by Hall and Anderson, Rich and Gregory, as well as Moore and Associates at the University of Southern California, which proved "that rheumatic fever is a reaction to parenteral contact with foreign protein to which tissues previously had been sensitized" and that the human rheumatic heart, by the same token, also arises from "parenteral contact with foreign protein to which the cardiac tissues have been previously sensitized."

In other words, rheumatic fever affecting the heart as well as the other organs and parts of the body, arises from an allergy to a foreign protein, which, getting into the body by ways other than the digestive system, irritates the tissues or parts of the body that have become sensitive to it.

The first question that naturally arises in connection with this is, What causes an allergic condition? If we re-read the reports of Heiser, Pottenger, *et al.,* we will find that incorrect nutrition plays a vital role in the development of allergy.

Another question then follows: Assuming the body has become sensitized (allergic), what are the foreign proteins that will set the vicious circle in motion? To obtain the answer to this, it is well to bear in mind that vaccines and serums are foreign proteins. Thus, isn't it possible that Lydia's attack of rheumatic fever, following the multiple injections in the treatment of her "allergic" conditions, actually contributed to the onset of this disease?

While the editorial quoted above tries to make a case for the streptococcus, since the streptococcus too is a foreign protein, we wonder whether a much stronger case could not be made against the use of vaccines and serums which are much more dangerous than is generally recognized.

8 "Allergic Carditis."

## 12

# HOW ABOUT THE DRUGS USED IN HEART DISEASE?

At this point, two questions naturally arise: What can be done for a person whose heart is already damaged? Are the drugs applied in these cases of any help?

We wish to reiterate what we have stated before, namely, that no drugs actually restore health, they merely modify or suppress the symptoms of disease. This holds true with equal force to the drugs used in heart disease. While it is true that in an emergency, one may feel that there is no alternative but to resort to these drugs, it is well to bear in mind that while these drugs may provide temporary relief, they can also cause a great deal of harm, and that because of this a well-regulated program of care along the lines outlined in this encyclopedia offers the only sound approach.

The drugs most often used in heart disease are digitalis, the mercurial diuretics, and the nitrites (Amyl Nitrate and nitroglycerine).

## The Effect of Digitalis

A sick heart is a weak and damaged heart. The heart does not possess the strength to contract fully and as a result is unable to maintain a healthy circulation. In an effort to make up for its shortcomings, it is often forced to work much faster, and pump many extra times each minute. This prevents it from getting enough rest between beats, and in time causes it to become completely worn out.

Digitalis causes an increase in the contraction of the heart, and slows down the number of heartbeats per minute. This improves the circulation and provides the heart with greater intervals of rest.

Needless to say, digitalis often provides dramatic relief. However, it is well to bear in mind that the relief is only of a temporary nature, and that no permanent correction is possible unless the muscle of the heart is strengthened and rebuilt.

There is another aspect that must be considered in connection with digitalis. What are its permanent effects on the heart when used over an extended period of time?

An investigation will reveal that digitalis is a poison, and if not stopped in time can cause a great deal of damage to the heart.

In an article, "Digitoxin Intoxication," Dr. Arthur M. Master quoted von Jacksch who in his book on poisons stated, "Digitalin and digitoxin (digitalis preparations) are frightful cardiac (heart) poisons. Their use at the bedside necessitates the greatest care. A single excessive dose of these glycosides invariably results in death from cardiac paralysis in a short time."[9]

Paul D. White, who considers digitalis one of the most valuable drugs in heart disease, nevertheless pointed out:

Auricular paralysis, auricular fibrillation, various high grades of heart-block, a coupled rhythm due to ventricular premature beats every second beat, idioventricular rhythm, ventricular paroxysmal tachycardia, and ventricular fibrillation have all been induced in man or in animals by massive doses of digitalis. . . . When any of these disorders of cardiac mechanism are found to result from the digitalis given and not primarily from other factors, the drug should be discontinued, for a high percentage (50% to 90%) of the lethal dose has probably been given by the time such disorders are found."[10]

Levine states, "While the therapeutic doses of digitalis produce no pathological changes in the heart muscles, toxic doses do cause definite necrosis (death, degeneration) of the heart muscle fibers and inflammatory changes and also changes in brain cells."[11]

Doctors know that digitalis is a poison, but nonetheless consider it a most valuable remedy for those who suffer from congestive heart failure. To avoid the damage that may result from its use, they prescribe it in therapeutic

[9] *J.A.M.A.*, June 5, 1948.
[10] White, *Heart Disease*.
[11] Levine: *Clinical Heart Disease*.

doses which, according to Levine, average "about 35 to 40 per cent of the lethal (deadly) dose."

The basic fallacy in this explanation is that digitalis, like most other drugs, tends to accumulate in the system, and that its damaging effects are usually not recognized in the early stages.

*The U.S. Dispensatory* points out that "at times when the drug is being used continuously, no evidence of its action may be manifest for several days and then suddenly symptoms of toxic effects come on. This is what is meant by the term cumulative action."

When a physician is confronted with a heart case, he is often in a great dilemma. He must do something to help the patient and when digitalis is indicated he will resort to it as the best possible remedy at his disposal even though he knows that it is toxic. In his effort to be as careful as possible, he may use one digitalis preparation in preference to another on the assumption that it may be less poisonous. However, this precaution is delusory, since the degree of effectiveness of a digitalis preparation is directly proportionate to its degree of toxicity, and a digitalis preparation is less poisonous only when the body fails to absorb it.

And White emphasized this fact by stating; "The toxic and therapeutic effects of various preparations of digitalis or of other drugs of the digitalis series are parallel; a preparation that can be taken in large dosage without toxic effects is apt likewise to be therapeutically inactive and a preparation that is very active therapeutically tends quickly to cause toxic symptoms."

Because of the poisonous effect of the digitalis preparations, some authorities have in recent years become more partial to the preparation known as digitoxin, on the assumption that this preparation is less poisonous. That this is an illusion is affirmed by Masters, who pointed out that "the symptoms of digitoxin poisoning ... do not differ from poisoning with other types of digitalis." Furthermore, "since digitoxin has a definite cumulative action, the toxicity persists longer than after other preparations of digitalis."

It is true that when used in moderate doses the degenerative effects of this drug may not be apparent for some time. Its cumulative effect, however, is unavoidable and when used over a period of time can easily lead to an increase in the degenerative changes in the heart.

Furthermore, its effect varies with the individual case. David P. Barr,[12] pointed out that the age of the patient, the degree of the heart failure, and the use of other medications in the case make the heart "more susceptible to the action of the drug," and are also to a great degree implicated in "the variable responsiveness" that takes place.

One can well understand why the cautious physician reduces the dosage of this drug to a mere "maintenance dose" as rapidly as possible, and dispenses with its use as soon as he can.

## The Mercurial Diuretics

In congestive heart failure the heart is unable to keep up with its work and this often causes the feet to swell and the abdomen and lungs to fill up with fluid. Salyrgan, Mercuhydrin, or mercupurin is then injected into the body. They are diuretics, drugs that force the explusion of large quantities of fluid through the kidneys. This relieves the heart of the added strain and protects it against the danger of collapse.

However, here too it is important to bear in mind that these remedies can be dangerous, and often cause additional damage or even collapse.

Dr. Leon Merkin, from the Cardiac Clinic of the City Hospital of New York, dealing with this subject, stated; "With the rapid growth in the number of cases in which mercurial diuretics have been administered, we find in the literature an increasing number of reports of untoward effects resulting from the parenteral administration of these drugs. Among the side reactions the most important is the death of the patient shortly after the injection."

Dr. Merkin then gave, as illustrations of how dangerous these drugs can be, two case histories in which collapse followed the use of this remedy.[13]

---

[12] "Hazards of Modern Diagnosis and Therapy—The Price We Pay," *J.A.M.A.*, December 10, 1955.
[13] "Untoward Effects of Treatment with Mercurial Diuretics," *N.Y. State Journal of Medicine,* October 15, 1949.

Tetany, uremia, and in some cases stupor are some of the serious side reactions that occur from the use of these drugs.

"One may wonder why these side-reactions and death . . . are comparatively rare even though the number of injections reaches thousands per day," Dr. Merkin asks. His own reply is that "Side-reactions are much more frequent than doctors suspect. Very often these reactions are transient, and at the same time the clinical picture is obscured by other signs and symptoms arising from the heart failure."

Dr. Merkin pointed out that the administration of the mercurials leads to the excretion of many other essential elements, to a diminution of the alkalinity of the body, and to a disturbance in the balance between sodium and potassium that leads to a preponderance of potassium in the system.

On this point, Dr. Merkins writes that "potassium intoxication results in widespread impairment of neuro-muscular function" and that the "accumulation of potassium in the body causes mortality and morbidity."

An editorial in the *Journal of the American Medical Association,* November 17, 1951, stressed that "although congestive failure itself predisposes to thrombosis (a closing of a blood vessel) there is some evidence that this tendency is aggravated by currently accepted therapy for congestive failure and particularly by the injudicious use of mercurial diuretics" and March and Pere, Russel and Zohuam, as well as the more recent findings of Marvel and Shullenberger, are cited to prove this fact.[14]

Henry A. Schroeder, in a report read before the intern session of the American Medical Association, asserted that the mercurial diuretics are of great value. Nonetheless, he pointed out, their use may lead to an excessive elimination of sodium chloride as well as other essential elements and that "this can lead to serious consequences if not recognized." He stated further that this drug is sometimes excreted rather slowly, and said that "the rather slow excretion of mercury can lead in certain subjects to the accumulation of toxic amounts."[15]

[14] "Thromboembolism Following Diureses."
[15] *J.A.M.A.,* November 17, 1951.

Flaxman, referring to the mercurial diuretics used in heart disease pointed out that "cases of sudden death due to the use of these drugs and fatal mercurialism continue to be reported."[16]

Boyd's remark in his chapter on "Necrosis of the Liver" that "the introduction of the newer diuretics, such as the organic mercury compounds in association with ammonium chloride, has diminished the dangers of ascites (swelling) as a cause of death, only to bring into greater prominence that of hemorrhage" is rather significant in connection with this point.

## The Nitrites

The nitrites (nitroglycerin and amyl nitrite) relieve severe angina attacks most dramatically. You just place a pellet of nitroglycerin under your tongue or break one of the tablets of amyl nitrite in your handkerchief and breathe it, and presto, the attack subsides.

How do these remedies provide relief? They force the heart to work harder and help to dilate the arteries, and this lowers the blood pressure and relieves the attack.

However, it is imperative that we realize that no matter how welcome the relief may be, the basic condition has not changed. Furthermore, it is important to mention that as the use of these remedies is continued, the attacks often recur with more frequency and greater severity.

We have seen many sufferers from angina who started with one nitroglycerin tablet occasionally, but who ultimately ended up by taking them as often as every 15 minutes. Doctors know that nitrites will combine with the body's oxygen, and reduce its availability for functional use. Thus, a vicious circle is established.

Now, if these drugs are inadvisable, what should be done to obviate the need for them? Our first objective is to improve circulation to the heart, and to overcome the periodic spasms that cause these attacks. While there is no single or stereotyped program that can be applied in all cases alike, we wish to point out that a program that embodies the use of simple, natural, easily digestible foods, and a restricted dietary regimen, even complete abstinence

[16] "Drug Fatalities," *J.A.M.A.*, September 29, 1951.

from food for limited periods of time when necessary, plus plenty of rest, often works wonders in these cases.

This is a sound approach and should be followed in all types of heart disease. In those cases where digitalis and the mercurial diuretics have been used routinely and where, because of the condition of the patient, cannot be discontinued immediately or completely, this basic approach will help to strengthen and rebuild the damaged and weakened heart and reduce the need for them, and, in many cases, may ultimately make their use entirely unnecessary.

We have seen many cases where mercurial diuretics were used as often as two or three times a week but where by eliminating food for short periods of time and reducing the fluid intake, plus the application of the nursing care outlined in this section, the need for them was considerably reduced or the patient was enabled to do without them altogether.

## Drugs That Influence the Blood Clotting Mechanism

In coronary thrombosis or any other condition in which the blood congeals and forms clots, dicoumarol and heparin are used to thin the thickened blood. These drugs accomplish this by reducing the production of the blood-clotting elements or by interfering with their normal effects on the blood.

That such methods are dangerous is well known. They can cause various blood derangements, lead to hemorrhage, and have caused many deaths. Flaxman[17] pointed out that dicoumarol has accounted for 32 fatal hemorrhages. These fatalities resulted even where there was careful laboratory control "and despite long prior use without serious complications."

He further pointed out that many cases of nonfatal reactions have been reported from the use of this drug, and quoted Link, the developer of this drug, to the effect that "the briefest meditation on the strictly theoretical aspects of the clotting phenomena leaves one with the appalling feeling that tampering with the coagulability of the blood is hazardous business."

[17] "Drug Fatalities," *J.A.M.A.*, September 29, 1951.

The *Journal of the American Medical Association,* April 22, 1961, in an editorial entitled "Possible Risks in Anticoagulation Treatment of Cerebral Vascular Disease," reporting the findings of neurologists in nine Veterans Administration hospitals covering the observations of 155 patients, in half of whom anticoagulant drugs were used for an average period of about nine months, states: "Not only was the incidence of recurrent cerebral infarction apparently unaltered by anticoagulation, but treated patients had a higher mortality than controls (those who did not receive anticoagulant drugs). The increase in deaths was due partly to the occurrence of cerebral hemorrhage, a complication which has been observed in other studies and which is regarded as a major risk of this therapy."

Of course, it is important that to obtain results the thickened blood be thinned, but it is one thing when this is accomplished by following a regimen that helps bring about this change and quite another when it is done with a remedy that tampers with the coagulability of the blood.

Some years ago, Dr. Ernest Klein, a physician from Europe who was connected with the New York University, Bellevue Medical Center, disclosed that a diet of orange juice diluted in water will help thin thickened blood.[18] Dr. Klein was subsequently discharged from his position in the hospital, apparently because he published the results of his findings without obtaining prior approval from his medical colleagues.

Levine stated that "diet during the early days (of an attack) should be confined to liquids, gradually returning to more ordinary food in small amounts," and then mentioned that "it has been advised that a low calory diet (500 to 800 calories a day) should be used in acute coronary thrombosis and in fact, is being advocated in the treatment of many severe or stubborn cases of congestive heart failure." He points out that this semi-starvation diet diminishes the work of the heart, and produces other favorable effects on the circulatory dynamics.[19]

If in addition to a low calory intake we also make sure that the food is easily digestible and provides the body with its much needed minerals, vitamins, and enzymes, and

[18] *New York Medicine,* May, 1949.
[19] *Clinical Heart Disease.*

when, in addition to this, we have provided the other care that helps to restore normal functioning, we have done everything possible to counteract the progress of the disease and thin the thickened blood.

Abstinence from food for short periods of time and restriction of the fluid intake are of great help in these cases. Many physicians are acquainted with the dramatic results obtained by the Karell diet, which consists of seven ounces of milk used four times a day.

Levine, in discussing the efficacy of the Karell diet, explains that "semi-starvation produces a fall in blood pressure, in pulse rate, and in the basal metabolic rate," and that "this may diminish the work of the heart and may thereby improve the circulation when failure is present."

Continuing on the same subject, he quotes Proger, who suggested "that patients suffering from severe heart failure be kept on a diet containing adequate protein but only 500 to 800 total calories," and that such diets be continued for months, possibly indefinitely.

Dr. Irving C. Cutter in one of his syndicated articles related that J. Hatsilver, after trying numerous types of management, finally decided to place forty-eight of his high blood pressure cases on a bold starvation program. Each patient was kept on nothing but fruit juices, tomato juice, hot lemonade, or vegetable broth for six days. On the seventh day, he was given a normal diet. This program was repeated each week as long as the symptoms improved, or until the blood pressure was reduced to normal.

Relief of symptoms in 90 per cent of the cases was "dramatic," Dr. Cutter wrote. "Headaches and sleeplessness disappeared within three days, and dizziness, shortness of breath, and other symptoms were usually relieved by the end of the first week. In certain instances, the period of reduced pressure was fairly extensive and a number of otherwise incapacitated patients returned to full or part time employment."[20]

We have demonstrated the efficacy of this approach in some of the most difficult cases. In describing them, we do not mean to imply that no recoveries occur in standard practice, but merely how much more complete the results would be if sound physiological methods were employed.

[20] *Daily News,* October 8, 1935.

## 13

## STORIES THAT TELL THE STORY

*A Case History:* MR. JOHN S.

Mr. John S. was fifty-nine years old. He had been sick for a long time, but the family decided to resort to the hygienic treatments only when the doctors who attended his case held out no hope for his recovery and said that death was merely a matter of days away.

As soon as we stepped into the sick room, we realized that we were dealing with a very sick man. Mr. S. was all propped up with pillows, gasping for breath, his face flushed to a deep bluish hue. An examination revealed an extremely enlarged and damaged heart and extensive ciruclatory damage. His legs were badly swollen and his abdomen and part of his chest were filled with fluid. He had great difficulty in passing his urine, voiding only small quantities at a time.

A physician who was connected with one of New York's large hospitals, an excellent heart man, performed the examination.

"What do you think of his chances for recovery?" we asked the physician after he had completed his examination and we had stepped into another room. "This man may die within the next 24 hours, but whether he dies tonight or tomorrow, there isn't much that can be done for him," he replied.

Because of this seemingly hopeless situation, and because all that could possibly have been done by medicine had been tried, this physician was willing to try the rational approach.

We started by eliminating all food and by discontinuing all medication. All that we permitted for the first three days was about two ounces of freshly squeezed orange or grapefruit juice every two or three hours. Warm cleansing enemas and hot mustard foot baths were used twice daily.

To keep a check on how his kidneys were functioning,

we left instructions that the family collect his urine and keep a record of his daily output.

We need not mention that the first few days were most trying. The first hopeful sign came when the patient began to pass large quantities of urine, many times the amount of liquid he was taking in.

Before long, several significant changes became noticeable. His breathing became easier, deeper, and more regular. His face and skin began to lose its bluish hue, changing to a paler, healthier color. He was able to rest more comfortably and sleep much better.

As these improvements continued, our patient began to clamor for food. We began with small servings of grapefruit and oranges, but later added other fruits in small quantities.

A few days later we started with small meals, served at regular intervals: grapefruit and raw grated apple or stewed prunes for breakfast, lettuce and tomato salad with a small portion of a plain steamed vegetable for lunch, and a similar meal for dinner.

A few days later, we added other raw vegetables to his salad and also increased his meals by adding small portions of cottage or pot cheese for lunch and a baked potato for dinner.

An orange or section of grapefruit were permitted between meals when he was hungry.

Later, some rye krisp or shredded wheat was added to his breakfast, and small servings of chicken, lamp chop, or fish twice or three times a week were permitted in place of the cheese.

It took about four weeks before Mr. S. was able to get out of bed. We first sat him up in bed for short periods of time with his feet dangling down. A few days later he was able to get into a chair. He sat up a half hour at first, and gradually increased the time each day. Later we encouraged him to take a few steps, and increased the distance each day. Finally, he was strong enough to move about from one room into the other.

His treatments had commenced about the middle of March. He lived on a top floor, and by the time warm weather set in he was able to walk up to the roof for fresh air and sunshine, where he remained, at first for about an hour, and then for gradually increasing periods of time.

His progress was slow but steady. He continued to grow stronger and after six or seven months he had recovered sufficiently to be able to return to work.

About eight years later, we were again called to see him, this time because he had suffered a mild stroke. He was then about sixty-seven years old. He had continued at his work since his original recovery until then. After about two and a half or three months of the same type of care, Mr. S. was again able to return to his job.

We were called to see him once more when he was about seventy-two years old, about 14 years after we had first treated him for his congestive heart failure. Again we found him suffering from difficult breathing, swollen legs and abdomen, and again he had difficulty passing his urine.

Members of his family expressed the opinion that worry because of the induction of his grandson into the Armed Forces had contributed to his breakdown this time.

A short fast followed by a carefully regulated program, plus good nursing care and rest in bed, brought about sufficient improvement to enable him to get out of bed and finally go outdoors for short periods of time, but could not completely clear up the swelling of his ankles and feet.

The family, hoping that medical care might bring added improvement, then decided to call in a physician who administered a variety of drugs. Results were disappointing, however, and the patient died a few months later. By that time the family accepted his death as a welcome relief, since they felt that his lingering existence caused him a great deal of misery.

"Frankly we expected him to die years ago and never thought that he would have so many more years of good life." was his wife's comment at that time.

The question is not merely one of controlling the food intake or of providing enough rest, but of making sure that every little detail that enters into the management of a case of this kind be carefully controlled.

*A Case History*: DWIGHT D. EISENHOWER

Consciously or unconsciously many persons go on deceiving themselves. That way seems easier, and like the proverbial ostrich, they persist in ignoring realities. Our nation was greatly upset by the report of the then President Eisenhower's heart attack. To most persons this came as a terrific shock, since the then President had had regular checkups and was always reported to be in fine condition. The *U.S. News & World Report* in its September 23, 1955, issue stated that while the numerous reports "about the President's good appearance and robust health" made some persons wonder whether these reports might not have been deliberately exaggerated, the fact was that President Eisenhower was "in peak condition." *The New York Times,* September 27, 1955, pointed out that a check-up on August 1, 1955, "failed to detect any hint of arterial disease."

And yet, a coronary attack like Mr. Eisenhower's does not develop suddenly. We keep building up to it, and a superficial appearance of what is usually regarded as robust health is not an indication that a heart condition may not be developing.

Dr. Paul Dudley White, called in consultation on the President's case, said rightly that though it is not always easy to diagnose the thickening of a coronary artery before an attack," that thickening "may occur years before the thrombosis."

This disease is "about the commonest important illness that besets a middle-aged man in this country today," Dr. White pointed out and added that "the average age is about fifty in this condition." Since the President's age was nearing sixty-five, he was "fifteen years ahead of the game from the standpoint of that type of illness."

We were pleased to note that Dr. White, in discussing causes of the disease, specified stress and strain, diet, alcohol, and tobacco among the factors that might contribute on this development. However, we couldn't but wonder why, if the onset of this disease is to be controlled or checked, these factors aren't stressed ahead of time, as a measure of prevention?

Because of the President's illness, coronary artery disease became a subject of wide discussion, and scientific writers quoted authorities to the effect that the disease is not nearly as dangerous now as it was in the past, and that a greater number of sufferers recover now than formerly.

We should all be grateful for this. However, an investigation will disclose that whatever progress has been made has taken place not because of any new remedies, but because there has been a vast improvement in the handling of these cases, which are now treated very much more in line with the approach advocated in this volume.

We note that the President took no food except orange juice for the first few days, and then was kept on a very careful diet. The use of oxygen is, of course, standard procedure and was necessary in the President's case. But we still ask, why weren't the factors enumerated by Dr. White as possible causes of hardening checked before the attack occurred to make certain that the President's case would not progress to the point where an attack became unavoidable?

## *A Case History:* NICK N., the Man Who Wanted to Die

Hardening of the arteries often leads to loss of vision. Nick N. was only forty years old when he lost his sight. His illness began with sharp pains in his head and in his extremities, which persisted without relief for several months.

While under the care of his doctors, Nick began to notice that his vision was gradually growing dimmer, becoming increasingly worse with time. At the suggestion of the doctors, he agreed to go to a hospital where, a few days later, he lost his sight completely.

Repeated checkups disclosed that he was suffering from a condition known as acute toxic neuroretinitis, which was brought on by hardening of the arteries and, possibly, kidney damage.

Members of the family were told by the doctors that though Nick was still relatively young, the damage to his eyes resulted from deteriorations in his body equaling those found in a seventy-year-old man, and that no hope for the recovery of his vision could be held out.

In search for help, the family brought Nick to New York. He was taken to a private hospital where a well-known New York physician only confirmed the previous findings. An eye specialist called in to examine his eyes reported the loss of almost the entire vision of his left eye, and loss of the greater part, especially the central part, of his right eye.

Since neither the general practitioner nor the eye specialist was able to offer any concrete help, these doctors had no objection to the use of the nonorthodox methods, even though they were clearly skeptical of results.

As a first step, all food and all drugs were eliminated. Nick was put to bed and was fed nothing but a few mouthfuls of orange juice or grapefruit juice several times a day.

In addition, warm cleansing enemas and hot baths were ordered twice daily, after which he was wrapped in wet sheets to induce sweating. His eyes were kept covered to exclude all light while the room was darkened for further protection.

This program was carried through for about a week. Then some solid food was introduced: first, sliced orange and grapefruit; later, small meals of fresh fruits and raw vegetables. The enemas and hot baths were reduced to once a day.

Hospitals as a rule are not suitable places to put such regimen into operation since it is usually impossible to obtain the food we order and since the nurses and other members of the staff are not trained to handle this kind of routine. One may wonder, therefore, how we were able to put this regimen into operation for Nick N.

As a matter of fact, none of the workers in the hospital were aware of what was actually going on. The enemas and the baths were administered upon doctor's orders. Nothing was mentioned in the chart about his diet. The nurse would bring in his tray, and when she left the room one of his relatives, who was always with him during the day, ate the food. The fruit juices and the other foods that he was to eat were brought in by the family from the outside.

It is only proper to mention that we had no way of telling how badly damaged his eyes were and therefore could not tell how much we could accomplish. In cases of this kind, recovery is always limited by the degree of damage and only the tissues not fully destroyed have a chance of being restored to health. Where reabsorption of the hemorrhage or the exudates is delayed or where the inflammatory condition persists over an extended period of time, degenerative changes may progress to the point where it reversible damage sets in, precluding all chances of recovery.

At the start, Nick was terribly despondent. He had never been seriously ill before, and the thought that he might never see again was almost unbearable to him. If he couldn't see again, life wasn't worth living and he would rather die!

Over and over again, the patient would ask whether he would ever see again. We could not be sure, but telling him this would have been like pronouncing his death sentence. So while the members of his family were apprised of our doubts, the patient was constantly assured that everything would come out all right.

So far as his general condition was concerned, improvement began to show almost immediately. His blood pressure began to drop almost from the start of the treatment and continued to drop until it reached a normal level. As far as his sight was concerned, however, no discernible improvement was apparent during the first ten days or two weeks.

Nick reached the depth of despair. We kept telling him that he must have patience, but so far as he was concerned, life was not worth living. Life without his sight was worthless. Unless he regained his eyesight, he would kill himself!

Then, early one morning as he awakened from sleep and opened his eyes, he seemed to notice the shadow of two horses reflected from the street on the wall opposite his bed. Unbelievingly he turned to look at other things. So, it was not a trick of the imagination—he was actually able to see again. Exultantly, he began to shout, "I can see! I can see!"

At first his vision was dim and blurred. He was able to distinguish only outlines, but this change was enough to imbue him with new hope. Now he knew that his sight was coming back!

Improvement continued with each day. About a week later, Nick left the hospital and was taken to his sister's home where he stayed until he had fully recovered.

We need not mention how surprised the eye specialist was when upon re-examination a few weeks later, he found that the condition had completely cleared up. The following is a copy of his final report on the case:

Mr. Nick N. shows almost complete regression of the neuroretinitis. His vision is R. 20/25, L. 20/30 and he accepts no correction. The tension is normal, lenses and media are clear. The fundi show minute whitish soft retinal exudates, mostly in the posterior poles. There are also some radiating yellowish lines in the macular region which are probably the remains of the retinal edema, surrounding the macula. No hemorrhages are present; the disc margins are sharp and the color of the disc is normal except for a slight yellowish pallor temporally. The retinal spots are more numerous in the left than in the right eye. On examining his left fundus with a binocular Gullstrand ophthalmoscope, the whitish exudates appeared to be in the nerve fibre layers of the retina.

The peripheral fields were normal. The blind spots showed slight enlargement which, however, is of no consequence. There were no other scotomata present.

When we compare this report with the one of only a few weeks earlier which stated that the examination revealed the loss of almost the entire vision of his left eye and the greater part, especially the central part, of his right eye, we can see how remarkable his recovery was.

Nick continued his treatment for another three months, and then returned to his home town and resumed his former work.

An interesting highlight in connection with Nick's recovery was the fact that while before his illness he was nearsighted and had to wear glasses, the examination by the eye specialist revealed that his vision had been restored practically to normal, and that he was able to discard his glasses completely.

Unfortunately, not all cases respond alike. As already stated the results depend upon the extent of the damage, and in cases where the exudates and hemorrhages are not quickly absorbed and the inflammatory condition is not quickly eliminated, the damage may be irreversible. This is the reason it is important that no suppressive treatments be used and that the measures employed in these cases help to normalize function and repair the damage as rapidly as possible.

## A Case History: The Progress of MRS. M. G.

Even in cases where a great deal of the damage is irreversible, much can be done to stem the progress of the disease and to bring about improvement in health.

The case of Mrs. M. G. is a case in point. We will let Mr. G. tell the story of his wife in his own way:

My wife suffered from stomach trouble even before we were married. Soon after our marriage she developed high blood pressure. Not long after, she began to complain of severe headaches and dizziness and pains all over her body. Doctors told us that this was due to hardening of the arteries.

Following the suggestion of doctors, we took her to Saratoga Springs where the baths, plenty of rest, and the invigorating air made her feel much better. Encouraged by this, we returned to Saratoga Springs several seasons in succession.

Then, a few weeks after our return from a trip to Saratoga Springs, her cousin died suddenly, and the shock of this made a ghost of her. She was then forty-eight years old and her blood pressure soared to 260, from where it could not be budged.

We had to wait upon her hand and foot, and we kept a woman in constant attendance to take care of her.

At that time somebody suggested that a change in diet might help her, and a doctor who specialized in this type of care prescribed a new regimen for her and taught her how to relax. From then on, an entirely new life began for her. She began to feel like a new woman. Her pains began to lessen almost immediately and in time disappeared altogether. Her appetite and digestion returned to normal. She became much stronger, and her blood pressure showed a gradual reduction.

At one time her vision had become so bad that she couldn't cross the street without help. She thought she was losing her sight and became terribly frightened. The practitioner's encouragement and patient guidance helped her immeasurably at that time. Her vision gradually improved and she was able to resume her former activities.

Because of the many years that she suffered from high blood pressure, her heart had become badly damaged, but the program she followed strengthened the heart sufficiently to enable her to carry on her normal activities.

On several occasions, especially during the latter years of her life, her heart would sometimes give way. Whenever this happened, this doctor's instructions helped to bring her around in quick order.

My wife followed these instructions for the rest of her life. Before these treatments were started, no doctor could hold any hope for her. This care and the patient guidance of her doctor not only relieved her pains but prolonged her life by many years.

She finally passed away at the age of seventy as a result of a heart attack, and we know that this new way of living gave her many years of comfort and happiness.


To elaborate on this case, we wish to mention that the care in Mrs. G.'s case was similar in most respects to the care in the other cases we have mentioned. A careful nutritional regime, composed primarily of fresh fruits and vegetables, with small portions of easily digestible proteins; and simple natural treatments, gradually reduced her blood pressure from a high of about 250/140 to about 170/100.

Some years later, when for at time her vision became badly affected, complete rest and an especially restricted diet, in addition to simple natural care, restored her sight sufficiently to enable her to lead a fairly normal life again.

## 14

# WHY THESE MEASURES ARE HELPFUL

As you follow our approach in these cases, many questions will naturally arise, and among them will be some as to why the various methods that we have described are used.

## The Usefulness of the Cleansing Enema

You will notice that in almost every case the warm, cleansing enema was used. The enema is practically a routine measure since it helps to eliminate the pressure and strain caused by gas and constipation.

Even a cursory examination will disclose that most sufferers from heart disease are constipated and suffer from gas pressure, and this condition exists even among those who have daily evacuations.

Dr. Harvey J. Kellogg of the Battle Creek Sanitarium pointed out that people who eat three meals a day and have only one evacuation daily suffer from intestinal stasis or sluggishness. Dr. C. Ward Crampton, Chairman of Geriatrics, Medical Society of New York County, stated that "colonic delay of a week is possible for one with daily evacuation."[1]

When this condition exists, the patient is not only bothered with gas that presses up against the heart and aggravates the palpitation as well as the various heart symptoms, but often suffers from other physical disorders such as protruding abdomen, prolapsed organs, or mechanical pressure that affects the adjacent organs and hampers the circulation of the blood. It should be obvious that this throws an added burden upon the heart.

Careful use of the enema helps to remove the accumulations in the colon and relieves the heart of the extra load caused by this condition.

[1] "Young at Any Age," *Yearbook of N.Y. State Joint Legislative Committee on Problems of the Aging.*

## The Reason for the Hot Baths

The full hot bath or the partial foot bath is used to promote elimination through the skin and kidneys, to improve circulation, and to promote relaxation.

Incidentally, different hot and cold applications can be used to great advantage to relieve many of the discomforts of heart disease. A cold compress applied over the heart goes a long way to check palpitation, while heat applied to the upper part of the back or between the shoulder blades counteracts pain in the chest and is of great help in heart and blood vessel spasms.

At this point we wish to stress the importance of keeping the feet warm. A hot water bottle, electric pad, or the wearing of socks will be helpful for this purpose.

You will notice that we mention the hot full bath or hot foot bath frequently in our case histories. Baths and compresses can be of great help when properly used. However, when used improperly or at the wrong time, they can overstimulate and increase debility. Make sure that the type of bath or application used in the case be carefully determined by the doctor or practitioner in charge.

## Why Control of Food Intake Is Helpful

We recomment partial or even complete abstinence from food for limited periods of time to rest the organs of digestion and give the organs of elimination a chance to catch up with their work of eliminating the undesirable by-products of metabolism from the body.

The value of small meals or abstemious eating is now generally recognized. It lessens the work of the digestive organs and reduces the work of the heart. We conserve the energies of the body when the work of all the organs of the body is reduced to a desirable and safe minimum.

This also explains why simple, easily digestible foods are important and why the foods that overburden the digestive organs must be eliminated.

## The Use of Oxygen

The oxygen used in the treatment of heart disease is a concentrated, irritating gas and not the same as the oxygen and nitrogen mixture we breathe. When used carelessly, it can cause harm. Nonetheless, when carefully employed in cases of heart failure it often provides dramatic relief. We have seen many cases where its cautious use overcame the decompensation in the heart, rid the body of excess fluids, and made the elimination of mercurial diuretics, even in advanced cases of heart disease, possible.

*Oxygen Therapy News,* September 20, 1950, referred to Dr. R. L. Levy who pointed out that with the use of oxygen, "pain is lessened or abolished, the heart rate falls, and respiration is slower and less labored. The patient is no longer restless. It is possible to curtail materially or stop entirely the use of opiates and sedatives."[2]

This is in line with our findings, and the fact that oxygen helps to limit or eliminate the use of the opiates and sedatives only adds value to it.

Our primary aim should be to maintain our health so as to avoid lapsing into a condition where this therapy becomes necessary, but when this point is reached the cautious use of oxygen can often save human life. Needless to say that its application must be carefully supervised by one who is thoroughly experienced in the handling of these cases.

The handling of a heart case is not a simple matter. Many problems may arise that may require the decision of one skilled in the handling of these emergency measures.

However, to ensure gratifying results, it is imperative that the doctor or practitioner in charge of the case possess a full grasp of hygienic principles and understands how to make the delicate adjustments necessary to help the patient recover.

[2] *Bulletin,* New York Academy of Medicine, June, 1950.

## 15

## PHYSICAL EXERCISE AND HEART DISEASE

Outdoor sports and physical exercises, when used in moderation, act as a valuable brake against the onset of heart disease. This is now being recognized by an ever greater number of authorities.

This does not mean that we can gorge ourselves on rich indigestible foods or that we can wear ourselves out in business or in social activities and hope that long walks or a Sunday spent on the greens will undo the harm. It merely means that the outdoor life and physical exercises, indulged in properly and used in conjunction with the other wholesome habits of living, will provide a well-rounded program of healthful living and serve as an added protection against the onset of these diseases.

Jean Mayer, Assistant Professor in the School of Public Health, Harvard University, in reporting on the physical fitness tests conducted by Dr. Hans Kraus and Mrs. Ruth Hirshland of the Institute of Physical Medicine, Bellevue Medical Center, pointed out that "several thousand American boys and girls attending public schools were compared to children of similar ages in Austria and Italy" and that the incidence of failure in muscular fitness among our youngsters was 78.3 per cent as against 8.5 per cent for the European children.

She stated further that "the mortality from the so-called degenerative diseases, particularly heart disease, is exceptionally high among Americans between the ages of thirty-five and fifty-five" and then mentioned that "accumulating evidence shows that lack of regular exercise is one of the factors involved."

We were glad to note that Jean Mayer mentioned that it was merely *one* of the factors, since it is important that none of the other factors that play a part should be overlooked or disregarded. She stated it very aptly when she said "that our motorized mechanized 'effort-saver' civilization is rapidly making us as soft as our processed foods, our foam rubber mattresses, and our balloon tires."[3]

Outdoor sports and physical exercises promote the intake of oxygen into the lungs, counteract stagnation, strengthen the abdominal muscles, and increase the blood supply to the heart, and in this way do much to strengthen the heart and blood vessels.

Dr. Ernest Simonson, Associate Professor of Physiological Hygiene at the University of Minnesota Medical School, asserted that exercise enables the heart and lungs to handle large volumes of oxygen without strain and protects the nervous system against fatigue.[4] Dr. Ernst Jokl, a leading European heart specialist, commented on the fact that many athletes are in peak form and able to participate in competitive activities "long past the years when they would have been too old to compete a few generations ago." He said that "one important explanation for this change is a life of healthful exercise."[5]

Dr. Julius Hofman, of Berlin and Bad Nauheim, when asked why the results obtained by exercise could not be obtained more simply and with equal certainty by drugs, said that while "drugs enable the heart to utilize more of its available strength" (in other words, act as stimulants), it is not known "whether by continued use they increase the sum total of the heart's strength.

"But baths and gymnastics we know, by the way they influence the heart, increase its strength."[6]

### Points to Remember

Here are a few points to be kept in mind in connection with physical exercise as it applies in heart diseases.

1. Never indulge in exercise indiscriminately. Make sure that you follow only those exercises which have been outlined for you to meet your particular needs.

2. A weak or debilitated person should exercise in a reclining position since this induces more complete relaxation and is least taxing to the heart.

3. Never exercise to the point of fatigue. Always stop

[3] *The New York Times Magazine,* November 6, 1954.
[4] *The New York Times,* April 17, 1954.
[5] *The New York Times,* March 20, 1953.
[6] Julius Hofman, *Remedial Gymnastics for Heart Affections.*

before you are tired. If tired, stop, take deep, slow breaths, and rest, before you continue your exercises.

4. Avoid competitive sports.

5. Whenever possible, perform your exercises on a hard surface or on the floor.

6. All exercises should be done slowly.

Here are a few of the simpler exercises that strengthen the heart and the circulation, and benefit the body as a whole.

## Deep Breathing Exercises

### Abdominal Breathing Exercises

1. Lie down on hard surface or floor. Inhale slowly and deeply, expanding the abdomen as you breathe in. Then exhale slowly and completely, drawing your abdomen in. Inhale and exhale through nose, with mouth closed. Relax and repeat.

2. Repeat the same exercise with each nostril separately.

### Chest Breathing Exercises

1. Take position as before. While inhaling through the nose, lift up your shoulders and collar bone, filling your chest with air, while the abdomen remains largely inactive.

2. Repeat the same exercise with each nostril separately.

A variation of these exercises is to lift and stretch your arms upward and above your head when inhaling and to lower the arms when exhaling.

A modification of this exercise is to keep both arms at the sides, then raise them slowly to a horizontal position when inhaling, and return them to the sides when exhaling.

## Leg Exercises

1. Assume reclining position and relax completely. Then, without bending the knees, raise both legs slowly as high as they will reach, then slowly lower them until they touch

the floor. Make sure to do this exercise slowly and in an even manner. Relax, and repeat.

2. Repeat the same exercise with each leg separately.

The following exercises are permissible when the patient's strength returns; but we repeat that all exercises should be done only under careful direction.

## Sitting-up Exercises

Continue in reclined position and relax. Keeping the knees and legs straight, fully touching the floor, sit up slowly, stretching the arms and hands in front in an effort to touch the legs with the hands. Then slowly return to reclined position.

## More Advanced Leg Exercises

1. Assume reclining position as in the simpler leg exercises, and relax. Then raise one leg slowly (knees straight), and when reaching the upright position, bend leg over first to the left side as far as it will reach; then to the right side as far as it will reach, then return to the center and lower leg to touch the floor again.

2. Repeat the same movements with the other leg.

3. Repeat the same movements with both legs together, turning both legs first to one side then to the other side, then bringing them back to the center and lowering them until they touch the floor.

Many other exercises can be added as the patient regains his strength, but they should be done only under careful supervision.

## Stretching Exercises

### Stretching Upward

Lie flat on the back and relax. Keep arms close to body. Then raise both arms slowly over the head and stretch—stretch—stretch. Return arms to side and repeat all over again.

### Stretching Sideways (Upper Part of Body)

Lie flat on the back and relax. Bend upper part of trunk slowly first to right side, then to left side. Return to position, rest, and repeat.

### Stretching Sideways (Lower Trunk)

Assume position as before. Bend lower part of trunk slowly first to right side then to left side. Return to straight position, rest, and repeat.

### Stretching Sideways (Whole Trunk)

Assume position as before. Keep arms close to body. Raise arms upward then bend body to left, then to right, and then return to normal position.

### The Cradle Exercise

Raise both legs upward. Then as the legs are lowered, raise upper part of body, rocking cradle fashion.

## 16

## A SAMPLE PROGRAM

The following is a program sent to a patient suffering from a chronic heart condition. While this program cannot be followed indiscriminately, since the measures employed in each case must be carefully evaluated, it nevertheless serves as an illustration of what must be the basic approach in such cases.

1. Eat sparingly. Small meals do not overtax the digestion and save the heart from overwork.
2. Eat simple meals. Avoid fancy desserts and sauces, all rich foods, and do not use too many dishes at any one meal.
   Omit completely all fat foods, all spices and condiments, all sweets, all white flour and white sugar products, coffee and tea. Eliminate fried foods and don't use chilled foods.
3. Do not take liquids or liquid foods with your meals.
4. Make sure to take a complete rest after each meal.
5. See that you get plenty of rest and sleep. A nap after the noon meal is of great help.
6. Relax completely. Avoid tension and emotional upsets.
7. Bowels must be kept functioning regularly. If necessary, small enemas should be used.
8. Warm baths before retiring induce relaxation and in most cases help bring on restful sleep. (Where for any reason the full bath cannot be used, the hot mustard foot bath, if permissible in the case, can be of great help.)
9. Do everything slowly and be of good cheer. Eat slowly, talk slowly, and do everything slowly. Never do anything to excess.
10. Always keep your feet warm and your head emotionally cool.

## A Seven-Day Menu

We have seen that the diet for the sufferer from heart and blood vessel diseases varies in accordance with the condition and the needs of the case. At times the diet has to be greatly restricted, while at other times a more liberal food intake is permissible. This is the reason we emphasize that the diet, as well as all other care, be subject to the supervision of the doctor who has an understanding of the patient's requirements and who is conversant with the latest nutritional concepts as well as the hygienic principles of healing.

In view of this, it should be apparent that the seven-day menu that we are presenting on these pages is not meant for those who require special care but is offered merely as an illustration to indicate what the diet should be where no special supervision is necessary.

### Sunday

BREAKFAST    Grated or shredded raw apple (slightly heated.)    Buckwheat groats.    Four to six ounces of raw skimmed milk.    Four or five medium-sized stewed prunes.

LUNCH    Waldorf salad of diced apple, pear, ripe pineapple, Pascal celery. Add a few natural raisins and strawberries in season. Served on lettuce leaves with three or four ounces of cottage cheese.    Stewed fresh peaches or soaked unsulphured dry peaches.

DINNER    Salad of grated carrots, chopped lettuce, grated or shredded cucumber, a sprig of watercress. Bowl of brown or converted rice with steamed pole beans or string beans.    Compote of fresh stewed fruits.

### Monday

BREAKFAST    Half grapefruit.    Heated apples and blueberries.    Baked banana.    Four to six ounces of skimmed milk, clabbered or soured milk or yoghurt (sipped slowly or eaten with a spoon).

LUNCH    Salad of letture, tomatoes, and shredded cucumber. Lentils steamed or baked with celery and carrots (with leak or onion for flavoring) and steamed string beans. Stewed fresh or soaked dry unsulphured apricots.

DINNER Salad of finely grated cabbage, grated beets, diced pascal celery with the addition of a few raisins. Vegetable stew of carrots, parsnips, squash, and string beans. Baked potato. Stewed pears.

## Tuesday

BREAKFAST Sliced peaches and blueberries, heated. Shredded wheat (eaten with stewed fruit). Four to six ounces of raw skimmed milk, clabbered or soured milk, or yoghurt.

LUNCH Salad of grated carrots, escarole, diced green pepper, grated parsnips, a sprig of watercress. Wild rice with sauce of stewed celery, green pepper, and onion, steamed green peas and carrots. Baked apple filled with raisins.

DINNER Salad of lettuce, grated beets, endive, sliced cucumber. Baked potato, steamed eggplant (with onion and celery for flavoring). Compote of fresh stewed fruits.

## Wednesday

BREAKFAST Raw apple and raspberries, heated. Brown or converted rice with diced apple and natural raisins. Four to six ounces of raw skimmed milk, clabbered or soured milk, or yoghurt.

LUNCH Fruit salad of diced honeydew, cantaloupe balls, diced ripe pineapple, balls of watermelon. Add a sprinkling of raisins. Served on a bed of lettuce leaves with three or four ounces of farmer cheese or ricotta cheese. Grated raw apple and raisins.

DINNER Salad of grated white turnips, grated half-cooked beets, grated raw carrots, served in balls on lettuce leaves. Baked yams, steamed okra (steamed with onion and tomato for flavoring), green peas and carrots. Baked pear.

## Thursday

BREAKFAST    Stewed blueberries and apple.    Baked banana.    Four to six ounces of raw skimmed milk, clabbered or soured milk, or yoghurt.

LUNCH    Lettuce, tomato, and chicory salad.    Steamed lentils (onions and celery for added flavor), steamed kale, baked butternut squash.    Stewed apricots or any other stewed fresh or soaked dry unsulphured fruit.

DINNER    Salad of lettuce, grated beets, escarole, strips of cucumber. Baked potato, steamed kale, steamed or baked pumpkin.    Any stewed fruit for dessert.

## Friday

BREAKFAST    Fruit salad of apples, bananas, pears, and blueberries.    Four to six ounces of raw skimmed milk or clabbered or soured milk, or yoghurt.

LUNCH    Spring salad of finely diced cucumbers, diced radishes (used sparingly, primarily to add color), diced green pepper, finely diced scallions, served on lettuce leaves with three or four ounces of farmer cheese or cottage cheese.    Steamed beets and steamed broccoli. Half grapefruit.

DINNER    Salad of finely grated cabbage, grated carrots, grated beets, strips of green pepper.    Young tender corn on cob, prepared as per instructions, steamed eggplant (steamed with celery and onion), steamed string beans. Baked apple.

## Saturday

BREAKFAST    Blueberries and sliced peaches, heated. Buckwheat groats.    Four to six ounces of raw skimmed milk.    Four or five medium sized prunes.

LUNCH    Tomatoes stuffed with cottage cheese, garnished with watercress and parsley, served on lettuce leaves, with strips of carrots and cucumber on the side.    Steamed beets, baked acorn squash.    Compote of fresh stewed fruits.

DINNER    Salad of grated raw cauliflower, finely diced green pepper, diced celery and apple.    Stew of white potato, yams, stewed prunes and raisins, steamed string beans.    Stewed pears.

As a rule, we prefer that no meat or fish be included in the diet. However, those who feel that they cannot do without these foods may use small portions of chicken, lamb chops, or lean fish, or any lean meat, in place of cheese or lentils. When meat or fish is included in the diet, it should be used at most three times a week.

Substitutions of vegetables or fruits in season for those not available or difficult to obtain will help vary the meals and make them more pleasurable.

The following steamed or baked vegetables may be substituted for one another: parsnips, carrots, beets, turnips, celery, leek, kale, okra, beet greens, zucchini, butternut squash, acorn squash, pumpkin, green peas, string beans, asparagus, artichokes, Swiss chard, broccoli.

No sugar should be added to the fruit. No salt or butter should be used. Steamed vegetables may be flavored by the addition of dill, tomato, onion, leek, garlic, celery, sage, anise, sweet basil, rosemary, caraway seeds. The use of these natural flavorings can be developed into an art. Use them sparingly, merely to enhance the natural flavors of the food, not to drown them out.

A dressing of lemon and honey may be added to the fruit and vegetable salads for flavoring purposes. A dressing of tomato juice, cottage cheese, lemon juice and honey, with or without the addition of garlic, will enhance the flavor of the raw vegetable salad. Sweet paprika may also be used for garnishing purposes on either raw or steamed vegetables.

If still hungry, one may take a yam or baked banana with the stewed fruit for dessert.

Milk, clabbered or soured, and yoghurt should be sipped slowly or taken with a spoon. Remove cream from clabbered milk. Acidophilus milk is an excellent milk food and could be used in place of the above. Use only raw skimmed milk whenever possible.

Remember that complete abstinence from food for a day or two or even a longer period often saves human life.

THE FOLLOWING RULES MUST BE CAREFULLY OBSERVED:

1. Eat slowly.
2. Eat only when hungry.
3. Do not overeat (small meals.)
4. Do not eat between meals.
5. Do not eat when disturbed or emotionally upset.

## Other Points of Importance

No smoking, no liquor, no carbonated drinks.

Small servings of apple juice, unsweetened grape juice, or any freshly squeezed unsweetened fruit juice may be taken between meals if desired and if conditions allow it.

A sound health-building program must be followed consistently if good results are to be attained. However, it is imperative that the program outlined in the individual case conform to the needs of the case. This is why we stress the need of careful supervision.

A menu presented in print, even if it is a good one, is but a poor substitute for a diet worked out to suit the temperament, the habits, and the needs of the individual paient. Guidance, furthermore, helps to do a more thorough job and removes some of the uncertainties as well as the difficulties that may present themselves to one who is not acquainted with this way of living.

However, those who are not in position to avail themselves of personal care will, provided they have no special problems requiring individual attention, benefit tremendously by changing from the conventional diet to the menu presented above.

It is evident that the meals outlined in the above menu are different from those served in the average home. Some may wonder how satisfying they are, as well as how difficult they are to prepare. In reply to this, we wish to point out that much less time is required for the preparation of these meals; while so far as taste is concerned, most persons find them extremely satisfying and pleasurable. Just give them a good try and see how enjoyable these meals can be; they will pay off immeasurably in improved health!

# 17

## A DECALOGUE OF HEALTH FOR
## THE HEART SUFFERER

By way of reminder, let us state that the body possesses vast recuperative powers which, if not abused, are of tremendous help even in the most difficult cases of heart disease. Here is a summary of the essentials that must be followed if we are to obtain maximum benefits in these cases:

1. Plenty of rest and sleep is imperative. In heart disease we are dealing with an overworked and badly injured heart, and its work must be reduced to a minimum if it is to become strengthened and rebuilt.

2. The food of the sufferer from heart disease must be carefully controlled. The meals should be composed of simple, natural foods, the live foods, the foods that contain all the protective elements, including vitamins, minerals, and enzymes, in addition to all other essential nourishing elements required by the body. All processed and preserved foods, rich, concentrated, fat foods, seasoned foods, as well as all foods of a stimulating or irritating nature must be strictly excluded.

Furthermore, the combinations must be the simplest possible, since a mixture of too many foods at any one meal interferes with digestion, overtaxes the digestive organs, and places an added burden on the heart.

3. The quantity of food must be limited in these cases since this lessens the work of the heart and gives the body a chance to control weight, a factor of great importance in these cases. We are in complete agreement with the French proverb quoted by Bogomoletz, that "to get fat is to get old."

4. Regular bowel functioning must be maintained. The many dietetic abuses extending over many years have made us a nation of constipated people. It is well to remember that the bowels act as an important organ of elimination, and when unable to function normally lead to the retention of waste products that produce putrefactive

poisons and cause the formation of gas. This leads to pressure against the diaphragm, which is directly underneath the heart, producing a strain on the heart as well as all other adjacent organs.

5. The use of drugs to induce sleep should be avoided since natural physiological methods can induce restful sleep without imparing our vital functions.

6. That a happy and cheerful disposition can do much to prolong life and keep us healthy is now well appreciated. Fear, insecurity, depression impair the functions of our body, create much unhappiness and increase the burden on the heart. Cheerfulness, contentment, and a peaceful outlook, on the other hand, promote good digestion and keep the body young and healthy.

7. Avoid all habits of a dissipating and health-destroying character. This includes the discontinuance of tobacco, liquor, an overindulgence in sweets, overeating, late hours, overstimulation, excitement of various kinds, and excesses of all types.

8. Choose a sensible and relaxing hobby. It contributes to a serene and contented outlook and promotes a well-balanced life.

9. Don't overlook the benefits of exercise. While total or complete rest may be necessary during the acute stage of the disease or when the heart is at a very low ebb, properly regulated exercises or activities adjusted to the needs and the ability of the patient can be of great help in strengthening and rebuilding the heart and circulation.

10. Finally, when in need of help, make sure that you avail yourself of the services of a doctor who is versed in the physiological approach and who possesses the knowledge, experience, and skill to help you through the difficult period successfully. In addition, he must also recognize the importance of teaching you to adhere to a sensible, well-balanced way of living, as protection against the possibility of a recurrence of the condition.

## 18

## PREVENTION POSSIBLE

If the problem of heart disease is really to be solved, all the factors entering the picture must receive serious attention.

The fact that nearly 50 per cent of our young men were found unfit for military service is history. *U.S. News & World Report*[1] reported that out of 3.6 million American men under twenty-six years of age examined for military service between July, 1950 and September, 1953, 1.7 million, or nearly half, were rejected as unfit.

Further investigation will disclose that 9.3 per cent of those rejected suffered from heart disease while another 5 per cent suffered from high blood pressure.

Furthermore, we have seen from the report of Major General Dan C. Ogle that an examination of our boys who were killed in the Korean War, average age twenty-two, disclosed that 77.3 per cent were suffering from diseased arteries.

It all adds up to one thing. With a poor beginning and a continuance of an unhealthful although rich standard of living, no better results can be expected. No wonder investigations revealed that we have the highest rate of heart disease of any nation in the world.

Blake Clark[2] in *Reader's Digest*, November 1955, pointed out that Dr. Ancel Keys, in a study of coronary heart disease in many parts of the world and its relation to the consumption of fat, found that the mortality in Italy "from degenerative heart disease in men is less than a third of ours," that in occupied Norway, where the fat supply was low as compared with unoccupied Sweden whose fat supply was near normal standards, "the coronary heart disease rate declined most," that the incidence of seriously diseased coronaries in Japan proved to be about

[1] *U.S. News & World Report,* October 4, 1955.
[2] "Is This The Number One Villain in Heart Disease?"

one tenth of that in the United States, and that checks in other countries proved that wherever the consumption of fat is high, a correspondingly high mortality from coronary heart disease exists, and that our mortality is highest because of the high consumption of fat in our diet.

While Dr. Keys's study stressed primarily the high level of fat consumption, we must not make the mistake of concentrating our attention on one factor only, disregarding all the other factors.

## Problem Not Insoluble

From all the facts disclosed in this encyclopedia, it should be clear that the problem is not insurmountable, but that only when all the deleterious influences are recognized and removed can it be brought under control.

We are happy to see Dr. Paul Dudley White, who is Dean of American heart specialists, point out that many of the factors "about which we can do something have received much too little study." He mentions "diet, tobacco, alcohol, exercise, stress and strain, and local customs" among them. These factors must receive attention not when we are already advanced in years and when the foundation for the disease has already been laid, although they will be of help even then, but must become an integral part of our existence throughout life.

We cannot do better than quote Dr. Alexis Carrel, who many years ago stated that "any true prolongation of life will require not only protection against disease but improvement of the quality of tissues and blood,"[3] and Dr. Edmund V. Cowdry of the Washington School of Medicine, who said that what we need is not only medical help for aging persons but also new measures which will help us prevent "a sizable number of ills and handicaps that otherwise will beset increasing millions of people."[4]

While we are interested in handling the diseases of the heart and blood vessels most efficiently, our major problem is to prevent their development and this can easily be

[3] "Carrel Urges Fund for Study of Aging," *The New York Times,* Demember 4, 1937.
[4] "Geriatrics Urged in Medical Schools," *The New York Times,* August 28, 1953.

done through a reorganization of our daily habits of living.

We can do no better at this point than quote Dr. Shirley W. Wynne, who, as early as 1930, stated: "The cause of arteriosclerosis is not at all clear. Some authorities claim that it results from the infectious diseases, especially syphilis. Others blame tobacco. Others put it down to a diet containing too much protein and salt. . . . As it is frequently associated with chronic diseases of the heart and the kidneys, the well-regulated life which tends to prevent these diseases may likewise prevent this ailment."[5]

## Conclusion: Fifty Years Ahead of Our Time

Dr. Irvine H. Page[6] warned against discouraging people by stressing too many "don'ts" such as do not smoke and do not drink, or eliminate this thing or that thing from the diet since "we don't want to make invalids, but to help these people to live lives that are longer and happier and more useful."

On the other hand, noted authorities everywhere are becoming ever more aware that nutrition, exercise, smoking, and alcohol play a part in the onset of these diseases and must be controlled if effective results are to be attained. White[7] reaffirmed this point when at a clinical meeting of the American Medical Association he declared that "diet and exercise might be important factors in the disease" and that tobacco, alcohol, and climate also play a part, although to a lesser degree.

Dr. Page would be right if the "don'ts" he mentioned were based on mere speculation, and not on scientific reasoning. It seems to us that the elimination of health-destroying habits and the substitution of a sensible way of living actually prevent people from becoming invalids and provide their only assurance they may have for long, happy, and useful lives.

There is no question that all healing professions will ultimately recognize the soundness of the physiological ap-

5 *New York World,* May 25, 1930.
6 *Time,* October 31, 1955.
7 *The New York Times,* December 3, 1955.

proach in the treatment of these diseases, and that all doctors will resort to the measures conforming to this approach. The statements of such a man as White show in which direction we are traveling. We are merely fifty years ahead of our time, and we wish to say, in all humility, that those who seek the most of health and the best of life are most certain to succeed by traveling our path.

We have traveled, then, the path of wisdom that has brought us to where we might see the causes and principles of correction of man's great afflictions: digestive disease, respiratory ailments, diabetes, arthritis, and now in this section, heart ailments. There remains but to spell out in detail the program of nutrition and plan for life that will permit good health to belong to you and your family.

## 19

# EATING FOR HEALTH

It has been suggested that a menu for one or two weeks would be a fitting ending to this encyclopedia. We are not sure that this is necessary, or even advisable. Eating habits vary, and what may appear as a full nourishing meal for one may be too much or too little for the other.

Some people may desire only a token breakfast, while others may not be satisfied with less than a heavy meal in the morning. Variations may be necessary for those who, because of ill health, follow special diets.

We shall, nevertheless, attempt to present a sample of what we consider to be a satisfactory menu for average circumstances:

BREAKFAST    If not hungry for breakfast, do not eat. Do not eat just for eating's sake. If a light breakfast will satisfy you, raw and stewed fruits are ideal. We favor the no-breakfast plan or, at most, a light breakfast, but no large breakfast except where one is hungry enough to require a large meal in the morning.

For those who feel the need for a large breakfast, we would recommend:

A fruit juice (either freshly squeezed or of the unsweetened variety, taken preferably ½ hour before rest of meal); a service of raw fruits (unsweetened); a cereal, eaten dry, with stewed fruits or berries (sweetened with honey, if desired); a cold cereal preferably, a cooked whole-grain cereal if one feels the need; a glass of milk or buttermilk or yoghurt or any of the hot herb or vegetable drinks listed in this volume.

LUNCH    A vegetable or fruit salad; cottage or pot or farmer cheese or young green soybeans or avocado or any easily digestible protein food; 1 or 2 steamed vegetables or vegetable soup; fruit or berries for dessert.

Or a vegetable salad; a few whole grain crackers or 1

or 2 slices whole wheat toast; 1 or 2 steamed vegetables or vegetable soup; fruit or berries for dessert.

If you have to pack a lunch for your man at work or for your school child follow the suggestions offered in the chapter on lunches.

In connection with lunch, it is well to bear in mind that when working, it is best to eat a light meal, and that the heavier meal should be eaten at night when you are able to rest after it.

In many European countries the custom is to take the main meal at midday, but then two hours are taken for the occasion and most people relax or take a nap after the meal.

DINNER    For a nice satisfying dinner, we recommend:

A large raw vegetable salad; baked white potatoes or sweet potatoes or corn on cob or any other starch food one day, to be alternated with cheese, soybeans, or any other protein food the next day; 1 or 2 steamed vegetables or occasionally a vegetable soup; fruit or berries or any of the desserts listed above.

Among the concentrated starch foods we list potatoes, yams, sweet corn, fresh lima beans, bananas, all grain foods.

The concentrated proteins include meat, fish, eggs, cheese, nuts, soybeans.

When cheese or other protein is taken with the lunch meal, it is advisable that a starch be taken at night.

## 20

## A FINAL SUMMARY:
## THE DO'S AND DON'T'S OF CORRECT EATING

A correct diet is particularly important for those with a health problem, especially for those who suffer from digestive disorders, diabetes, high blood pressure, heart disease, arthritis or other rheumatic diseases, anemia, nervous disorders, bronchial and asthmatic conditions.

However, prevention, which is the job of everyone, dictates that all, the sick and the healthy alike, follow these rules:

1. *We must never eat unless really hungry.* This rule is important. Our body is its own finest barometer as to when food or drink is needed. We rarely go wrong when we follow our natural instincts with regard to the taking of food or liquid.

This may exclude the taking of three regular meals a day. You may not be hungry when you get up in the morning. When this is the case, you may omit breakfast altogether.

Again, you may feel the need for a substantial breakfast, and may not be hungry for lunch. Do not force yourself to eat just because it is meal time. If you are not hungry at noon, skip your meal completely or take only a glass of juice or a piece of fruit.

The majority of people think that unless they eat three regular meals a day they are not well fed. In reality this is not the case. If you force yourself to eat when you are not hungry, you do yourself untold harm.

2. *Make it a practice to eat slowly, and chew your food thoroughly.* Many people gulp their food down and often do not even take time to sit down for their meals. What an abuse to the stomach and to the digestion! Food should be eaten slowly and chewed thoroughly to break it up into small particles and mix it with the saliva. This is the first step for good digestion. It lightens the work of the stomach and provides maximum nourishment.

3. *Never overeat.* We have pointed out that we should

eat or drink only when actually hungry or thirsty. In additon, we must also bear in mind that it is just as important to take only enough food or liquid to satisfy hunger or thirst. An excess of either food or drink overburdens the organs and is not conducive to good health.

4. *Do not eat when under emotional stress or when extremely fatigued.* When we are emotionally upset or when we are overtired, food cannot be properly digested. At such times, it is advisable that we first rest or relax before we take our meal.

5. *Always select simple dishes and make sure that your meals are prepared in as natural a way as possible.* Rich and complicated dishes overtax digestion, while refined and processed foods fail to provide adequate nourishment.

6. *The fewer the combinations at a meal the better.* A raw vegetable salad with either a baked potato, brown rice, buckwheat groats, one of the soft, mild cheeses, or any other easily digestible protein, and a steamed vegetable make a complete and highly satisfying meal, without overtaxing the digestion.

7. *Meals can be made appetizing and enjoyable even when you omit complicated or unwholesome dishes.* The flavor of our simple, wholesome dishes can be enhanced and made most inviting by the addition of a dash of lemon juice, lime juice, or tomato juice, or augmented by the skillful use of onion, garlic, leek, or scallions. The flavorful herbs such as dill, basil, sage, marjoram, caraway seeds, or chopped chives or parsley often do wonders even with the simplest dishes. Just use your imagination, and you will be proud of your accomplishments.

8. *Arrange vegetables attractively especially with regard to color and taste.* The many salad recipes in this volume offer a wealth of variety for zestful and inviting meals.

9. *It is a good policy not to take liquids with meals.* Liquids taken at mealtime often induce overeating. Food should be thoroughly chewed, not be washed down. When you take fruit juice, tomato juice, vegetable soup, or milk, take it as a food, not as a liquid. Take it with a spoon, or sip it slowly.

10. *Do not feel sorry for yourself when giving up foods not conducive to good health.* You are doing it for health's sake! Be proud that you have the good sense to do it. Be a leader, not a follower!

11. *Bear in mind the good that you derive from following a well-balanced diet.* Don't feel discouraged if, in a moment of weakness, you fall off the bandwagon. Old habits sometimes get the best of even the best of us. You simply have to try again. The encouragement and guidance of a good nutritionist or doctor who recognizes the importance of rational living principles, and who is conversant with your problem could be of considerable help to you at such times.

12. *When planning a diet for weight reduction, make sure that the food you eat does not merely take weight off, but also rebuilds and maintains good health.*

Just counting calories is not enough.

13. *Potatoes are a wonderful food and need not be shunned even by those who are trying to lose weight.* It is how much we eat that counts. Those who are calorie conscious will be interested to know that one medium-sized potato contains 100 calories. A raw vegetable salad, one medium-sized potato, and one steamed leafy vegetable make a perfect meal and do not add weight. Potatoes should be baked, boiled or steamed in the jacket. Salt should be omitted, for it increases the weight.

14. *Beginners may be helped by keeping a daily chart of the food they eat.* They can then compare their daily food intake and notice where they have slipped up.

15. *Make your dinner—any meal for that matter—an enjoyable occasion.* Be relaxed and enjoy every morsel of food you eat.

16. *Eat a raw vegetable salad at least once a day, and always eat the salad first.* Make it the most important course of the meal. It is filling and supplies the vitamins, minerals, and enzymes essential for good health. If you are unable to digest raw vegetables, consult a doctor who is conversant with your problem and has a thorough understanding of the subject of nutrition.

17. *This brings us to the question of health care.* When in need of such care, always choose a doctor who, in addition to his skill as a physician, is also versed in the subject of sound nutrition, so that he can guide you in the selection and preparation of the foods suitable in your case.

18. *An occasional fast day or a day on fruit juices or vegetable broth can do wonders for your health.* It gives your body a chance to catch up with its work and rests

your digestive organs. Take a glassful of orange juice, grapefruit juice or apple juice, or a cupful of vegetable broth every two hours or less often. It is well to make this a regular habit at least one day each week.

# INDEX OF NAMES AND TITLES

buse of Rest in Bed in Orthopedic Surgery," 238
cute Allergic Colitis Presenting the Clinical Picture of Acute Appendicitis," 89
gene Toxicity," 387
rens, Edward H., 365
en, Edgar V., 357
llergic Corditis," 427
nerican Association for the Advancement of Science, 383
nerican Cancer Society, 397
nerican Heart Association, 329
nerican Journal of Cardiology, 375
nerican Journal of Digestive Diseases, 140
nerican Journal of Orthodontics and Oral Surgery, 380
nerican Magazine, 387
nerican Medical Association, 330, 391, 410, 432, 465
nerican Medicine, 329
nerican Public Health Association, 131
nerican Society of Arteriosclerosis, 364
nderson, Dr., 427
re You Eating Your Way to Arteriosclerosis?", 364
rmstrong, Donald, 329, 407
rthritis and Allied Conditions, 310
rthritis—General Principles,

*Physical Medicine and Rehabilitation,* 254

"Backfire in the War Against Insects," 140
Banting, F. G., 195
Barnes, Mildred W., 104
Barr, David P., 431
Beck, Donald, 278
Beckman, Harry, 28
Beckman, Max, 405
Belding, L. J., 274
Belding, P. H., 274
*Berentning Til Indenrigsministeriet om Rationeringens Indvirkning Paa Sundhedstilstanden ved M. Hindhede,* 371
Berg, Ragnar, 271
Bernard M. Baruch Committee, 315
Best, C. H., 195
Bierers, B. W., 141
"Big Feeding Tests Give Disease Clue," 384
Bjerver, Kjell, 403
Blackfan, Dr., 261
Blond, Kasper, 101
Blumenthal, Herman T., 366
Boas, Ernest, 247, 310
Bogomoletz, A. A., 330, 374, 461
Bortz, Edward L., 330, 407
Boyd, William, 22, 65-66, 102, 105, 128, 159, 160, 193, 196, 207, 212, 347, 349, 352, 433
Brodie, Bernhard B., 138

*Bulletin, New York Academy of Medicine,* 449
Burchell, Howard B., 357
Byers, Sanford, 364

Cabot, Richard C., 83, 268, 309
Cameron, Charles, 399
*Cancer Therapy, A,* 101
Carrell, Alexis, 356, 464
"Case Against Poison Spray," 140
"Case Against Smoking," 397
*Century of Progress in Longevity, A,* 361
Chittenden, Dr., 370
Christone, Dr., 246
Clark, Blake, 463
Clendenning, Logan, 237
*Clinical Heart Disease,* 420, 429, 435
"Clinical Manifestations of Arterio-Sclerosis," 358
Cohen, Alfred E., 329
Collip, J. B., 195
Comroe, Bernard I., 248, 249, 251, 310
*Connecticut Wildlife Conservation Bulletin,* 142
"Contributions of the Pathologist to Present-Day Concepts of Gastric Ulcer," 67
Corcoran, Dr., 388
Corday, Eliot, 118
Cossar, Dr., 138
Cowdry, Edmund V., 464
Crampton, C. Ward, 447
Crawford, Charles W., 388
Cruickshank, Allen D., 141
Cutter, Irving S., 247, 386

*Daily Compass,* 364
*Daily Mirror,* 389
*Daily News,* 373, 395
"Dangers of Smoking," 396
Delaney, James J., 387, 390, 391

*Dental Cosmos,* 274
"Diabetic Neuropathy," 211
Dibble, Dr., 66
"Diet and Rest Help Sufferer from Rheumatoid Arthritis," 316
"Diet and Stress in Vascular Disease," 375
*Differential Diagnosis,* 310
"Digitoxin Intoxication," 42
Dresen, Karl Albert, 71
"Drug Fatalities," 433, 434
Dubos, Rene, 103-4, 157
Dublin, Louis I., 356, 405-6

"Effect of Heat Processed Foods and Metabolized Vitamin-D Milk on the Dento-Facial Structures of Experimental Animals," 38
Eisenhower, D. D., 98, 129, 358, 359
Emerson, Haven, 329
"Evaluation of Present-day Therapy in Rheumatoid Arthritis," 252
Evans, Howard, 390
Ewing, Dr., 66

Finland, Maxwell, 104
Flaxman, Dr., 433, 434
"Focal Infection in Relation to Rheumatic Diseases: A Critical Appraisal," 311
Foethout, W. D., 94
Food and Drug Administration, 137
Foster, James J., 113
Franklin, Benjamin, 385
Freeman, Smith, 278
French National Institute of Demographic Study, 404
Freyberg, Richard H., 254, 311
*Functional Pathology,* 402

Gailmor, William S., 363
Garrod, Dr., 260
George, John L., 141
Gersner, Franz, 144
Gerson, Max, 101
Ghormley, Ralph K., 238
Gofman, John W., 364, 398
Goldberg, Leonard, 403
Golding, J. R., 256
Goldman, Dr., 114
G. P., 378
Graham, Dr., 246, 315, 418
Green, Morris B., 405
Gregory, Dr., 427
Gumpert, Martin, 396

Hahnemann, Dr., 325
Hall, Dr., 427
Hammond, E. Cuyler, 397-98
Handbook of Digestive Diseases, 72
Harper's Magazine, 385, 406
Hart, F. D., 256
Hartung, Dr., 254
Hauser, Ernest O., 372-73
Hay, Dr., 315
"Hazards of Modern Diagnosis and Therapy," 431
"Health Department and the Food of the People," 389
Heart Disease, 246, 418, 420, 429
"Heart Disease Forty Years Ago and Now," 358
Heffernon, Elmer W., 71
Heiser, Victor G., 383, 427
Hindhede, Michael, 370, 371
Hirshland, Ruth, 450
Hofman, Julius, 451
Holiday, David, 324
Houssay, B. A., 194
Hueper, Wilhelm C., 364
Human Body, The, 237
"Human Poisoning by Chlordane," 391
Hutchinson, John J., 131

Hygeia, 355
Hypertension, A Manual for Patients with High Blood Pressure, 357

"Iatrogenic Jaundice," 103
Iglesias, Rigaberts, 144
Illson, Murray, 131
International League for the Control of Rheumatism, 314
"Intoxication Due to Chlordane," 390
"Is This the Number One Villain in Heart Disease?," 463
"It's No Fun to Be an Englishman," 372
Ivey, Dr., 114

Jackson, Dr., 261, 315
Jameson, Sir Wilson, 372
Jennings, Dr., 315
Johnson, Harry J., 395
Johnson, Lemmon, 397
Jokl, Ernst, 451
Jondorf, W. Robert, 138
Jones, Martha R., 274
Jones, Wilfred F., 104
Jordan, Sara M., 23, 64
Journal American Dental Association, 311
Journal of the American Medical Association, 67, 71, 89, 103, 105, 110, 114, 118, 119, 120, 124, 129, 138, 142, 211-12, 220, 238, 246, 255, 256, 257, 261, 278, 315, 358, 373, 375, 387, 389, 390, 392-93, 427, 429, 431, 434, 435
Journal of the American Veterinary Medical Association, 142
Journal of Studies on Alcohol, 403

Kaempffert, Waldemar D., 254-55, 364, 365
Kahn, Fritz, 224
Kanter, Dr., 72, 96
Kesich, Dr., 72, 96
Kaufman, Paul, 278
Kellogg, Harvey J., 315, 344, 447
Kempner, W., 376, 378
Kendall, Forest E., 364
Keys, Ancel, 359, 463-64
King, Charles Glenn, 383, 385
Kirkland, Henry, 359
Klein, Ernest, 435
Kling, Dr., 427
Knight, Granville, 144
Knudson, Donald L., 113
Kommerell, Dr., 119
Kountz, W. D., 363-64
Kratzer, Guy L., 71
Kraus, Hans, 450

Lancet, 397
Lapresa, Dr., 246
Larrick, George P., 27
Laseque, E. C., 417
Lautman, Maurice F., 374
Layman's Handbook of Medicine, A, 83, 268
Leary, Timothy, 363
Leavitt, Jacob M., 85, 127, 324, 383
Ledermann, Sully Charles Marcel, 404
Lee, Walter Estell, 316
Lehman, A. J., 390, 391
Lemmon, O. Bruce, 390
Lemon, Frank R., 374
Lensky, Paul, 390
Levenson, Sam, 409
Levin, Morton L., 395
Levine, Samuel, 420, 429, 435-36
Levy, Robert L., 329, 449
Lewis, Howard B., 373
Lichtwitz, Dr., 260, 402
Lieb, Clarence Williams, 398

Linsman, Joseph F., 118-19
Literary Digest, 274
"Lithium Poisoning from th Use of Salt Substitute," 38
Lowman, Dr., 254

MacCallum, W. G., 159, 266 402, 420
Macfadden, Dr., 315
Macleod, J. Wendel, 105
Maickel, Roger P., 138
Maisel, Albert G., 104
Man in Structure and Func tion, 224
Man the Unknown, 356
March, Dr., 432
Martin, W. Coda, 144
Marvel, Dr., 432
Master, Arthur M., 429, 430
Mayer, Jean, 450
McArthur, Charles E., 129-3(
McCann, Alfred W., Sr., 389
McCay, Clive, 370
McHardy, Gordon, 24-25, 13'
Meakins, Jonathan C., 329
"Medical Education Today," 315
Merkin, Leon, 431-32
Metropolitan Life Insuranc Company, 329
Miami Herald, 359
Middleton, William S., 256
Millhoun, William A., 71
Mirage of Health, 104, 157
Modell, Walter, 355
Moersch, F. P., 357
Moon, Henry D., 365
Moore, Normal L., 420, 421 427
Muir, Dr., 138
Mutual Life Insurance Com pany, 328

Naegels, Charles F., 403
Nation, The, 397
National Audubon Society 141, 142

National Heart Institute, 138

National Institute of Health, 406

"New Approach to the Rheumatic Fever Problem," 420

"New Drug Is Born, A," 256

New York Academy of Medicine, 396

*New York Globe,* 389

New York Heart Association, 329

*New York Herald Tribune,* 141, 274, 375, 395

*New York Medicine,* 252, 435

*New York Post,* 278

*New York State Journal of Medicine* 405, 420, 431

*New York Times, The,* 27, 105, 131, 139, 142, 143, 166, 195, 255, 274, 328, 329, 330, 356, 364, 366, 372, 384, 388, 394, 395, 403, 406, 419, 440, 451, 464, 465

*New York World,* 465

*New York World-Telegram,* 250, 396, 397

*New York World Telegram and The Sun,* 137

"Newer Concepts of the Causes and Treatment of Diabetes Mellitus," 194

"No Alcohol for Angina," 403

"Nutritional Contributions of Wheat," 373

"Obesity and Hypertension," 405

"Occurrence of Serious Bacterial Infections Since Introduction of Anti-Bacterial Agents," 105

Ochsner, Alton, 396

Ogle, Major General Dan C., 360

Ohringer, Leonard, 379

O'Neill, John J., 274

*Organic Gardening and Farming,* 140

*Orlando Sentinel,* 379

Osler, William, 103, 152, 167, 262, 312

*Out of My Life and Thought,* 323

"Overweight—America's No. 1 Health Problem," 405

*Oxygen Therapy News,* 449

Page, Irving H., 329, 357, 388, 465

Parker, Dr., 418

Pasteur, Louis, 103

*Pathology of Internal Diseases,* 22, 65, 102, 213, 347, 352

*Pathology for the Physician,* 66, 193, 197

Pearl, Raymond, 396

Pere, Dr., 432

"Peril on Your Food-Shelf," 387

Pierce, Commander Wilmot F., 390

"Possible Cancer Hazard Presented by Feeding Diethylstilbesterol in Cattle," 144

"Possible Risks in Anticoagulation Treatment of Cerebral Vascular Disease," 435

*Postgraduate Medicine,* 138

Pottenger, Francis M., 380-82, 384-85, 427

*Practice of Medicine,* 103

*Prevention,* 362

*Principles and Practice of Medicine,* 167

*Progressive Medicine,* 316

*Prolongation of Life, The,* 330, 374

Public Health Cancer Association, 394

*Quarterly Journal of Medicine,* 419

Radical Treatment of Hypertension and Arteriosclerotic Vascular Disease, Heart and Kidney Disease, 378
Rawls, William B., 252
Reader's Digest, 140, 463
Reference Handbook of the Medical Sciences, 402
Regan, Frederick D., 403
Remedial Gymnastics for Heart Afflictions, 451
Reston, James, 359
Rich, Dr., 427
Rihm, Alexander, Jr., 166
Riley, Robert, 389
Rinehart, James F., 365
Robbins, Stanley L., 66
Rodale, I. J., 362
Rorty, James, 385, 406
Rosen, Sidney W., 71
Rosenbloom, Samuel, 324
Roth, Grace, 395
Rudd, Dr., 254
Rusby, Henry H., 402
Russek, Henry I., 403
Russel, Dr., 432

Sackren, Harry, 324
Safer Smoking, 398
Saphir, Otto, 379
Saturday Evening Post, 138, 364, 372
Schaffner, Fenton, 102-3, 111
Schroeder, Henry A., 432
Schweitzer, Albert, 323
Sebrell, W. H., 406
Second Forty Years, The, 406
Selye, Hans, 352-54
Schaefer, Louis, 374
Sherman, H. C., 271, 370
Sherman, William B., 164, 177-78
Shullenberger, Dr., 432
Simonson, Ernest, 451
Sirovich, I., 389
Slocumb, C. H., 278
Smith, William E., 144

Society of Actuaries, 23, 13
Somogyi, Michael, 195
Spencer, Stephen M., 137, 36
"Spontaneous Disappearanc of Gallstones," 120
State Air Pollution Contro Board (New York), 166
Steinberg, V. L., 256
Steincrohn, Peter J., 401
Steiner, Alfred, 364
Stieglitz, Dr., 406
"Straight Facts About Hear Disease," 355
Stromont, Dr., 410
Sunday Compass, 330
Sunshine, Abraham, 375
"Surgery of the Extremities," 316

Taylor, Dr., 388
Textbook of Pathology, A 266, 402, 420
Textbook of Physiology, 94
"Thin Rats Bury the Fa Rats," 385, 406
Thomas, W. A., 375
"Thromboembolism Following Diureses," 432
Tildeu, Dr., 315
Time, 138, 329, 365, 465
Today's Health, 64, 104, 40.
Tomorrow, 396
Trall, Dr., 315
"Treatment of Arthritis," 22(
Treatment in General Practice, 29
Treatment of Patients Past Fifty, 310
Tuttle, W. W., 94

U. S. Dispensatory, 246, 248, 261-62, 419, 430
U. S. Food and Drug Administration, 387
U. S. News and World Report, 356, 360, 363, 391, 440, 463

"Untoward Effects of Treatment with Mercurial Diuretics," 431

Van Dellen, Theodore R., 316, 373, 394
Vaubel, Dr., 427
Vickers, C. L., 141

Walden, Richard, 374
Wallace, George, 141
Ward, Thomas G., 160
"Warning Flag for Wonder Drugs," 104
Wassersug, Joseph D., 357
Weinsier, Stanley C., 205, 324
Weinstein, Howard I., 137
Welsh, Henry, 137
Westergaard, Harold, 371-72

"What Air Force Is Doing to Ease Heart Attacks," 360
White, Paul Dudley, 246, 329-30, 358, 360, 420, 429, 430, 440, 464, 465
Wilbur, Ray Lyman, 315-6
Wiseman, Richard D., 278
Wolpers, Dr., 119
Wrights, Irving S., 395
Wynder, Ernest L., 375
Wynne, Shirley W., 465

*Yearbook of New York State Joint Legislative Committee on Problems of the Aging*, 477
"Young at Any Age," 447

Zohuam, Dr., 432

# INDEX OF SUBJECTS

acids
  amino, 31
  hydrochloric, 31, 53, 94, 392
ACTH, 254, 255, 256, 366
  and rheumatic fever, 419
additives and pollutants, chemical, 140-45, 387-93
  agene, 387
  Aldrin, 140
  aminotriazole, 143-44
  arsenic sprays, 389
  cranberries, unsafe, 143
  chlordane, 390-91
  danger to animals, 141-43
  D.D.T., 141, 390, 393
  Dieldrin, 140
  diethylstilbestrol, 144
  EDB, 142
  farming, organic, 392
  in food, 387-93
  Heptachlor, 141
  hydrochloride wash, to remove pesticides, 392-93
  lithium chloride, 388
  liver poisons, 140
  monochloro-benzene, 140
  paradichlorobenzene, 140
  polyoxyethylene monortearate, 388
  potassium bromate, 389
  stilbestrol, 390
  T.M.T.D., 142
adrenalin, and asthma, 177
Adventists, Seventh Day, diet of, 375
agar-agar in constipation, 80
agene, 387

alcohol
  and arthritis, 235
  and asthma, 177
  danger of, in angina, 403
  destroys thiamin reserve in liver, 403
  impairs driving ability, 403
  other dangers of, 403-4, 460, 462, 464
Aldrin, danger of, 140
allergy
  and catarrh, 186
  and hay fever, 186, 187
  and respiratory diseases, 185-89
  and rheumatic fever, 426-27
  and ulcerative colitis, 89-90
almond milk, 44, 186
aminopyrine, dangers of, 139
aminotriazole, and cranberries, 143
amyl nitrite, in angina, 433
amytal, in asthma, 178
Anacin, 102
anaphylaxis, 137-38
angina pectoris
  and alcohol, 403
  care of patient, 433-34
  coronary sclerosis, 346
  nitrites in, 433
  treatment for, 433-34
antacids, dangers of, 29
antibiotics
  and arthritis, 250
  in asthma, 178
  dangers from, 137-38
  destruction of favorable bacteria, 166

and digestion, 26, 28
harmful effects of, 26-27, 104
and new diseases, 174
and pneumonia, 165-66
anticholinergics, 25
apoplexy, 345
arsenic; 102
in insect sprays, 389
arsenicals, in gastrointestinal disorders, 25
arteries
    capillaries, 339
    cholesterol and hardening, 362-66
    hardening, 342-43
    hardening, in diabetes, 194
    hardening, in gout, 260
    hardening, and indigestion, 129
    hormone missing in hardening, 366-67
    and kidneys, in circulatory system, 340-41
    prevention of hardening, 359
    sequence of events in hardening, 362-67
    veins, 340
arteriosclerosis, 342-43
arthritis
    and alcohol, 235
    and aspirin, 245-46
    associated disorders, 226-27, 240
    atrophic or rheumatoid, 229
    carbohydrates and, 271-75
    case histories, 253, 257, 298-307
    change of climate and, 253
    changes in joints, 224-25
    chronic fatigue and, 240-41
    cinchophen and, 247
    cortisone and, 254-58
    development of, 226
    diet in, 235-36, 269-79, 285-88

drugs, effect of, 227, 245-53, 290
emotional factors, 236-37, 289
exercise and rest in, 237-38, 293
fats, 275-76
fever therapy, 265-67
food, abstinence from, 240-41, 292
fruits and vegetables, 276
general discussion, 222
gold therapy, 251-52
gout, 259-62
hypertrophic, 229
importance of clean body, 280-83
infection, theory of, 308-13
infectious, 229
injuries and, 233
Marie Struempel, 229, 304
menopause and, 232
a metabolic disease, 351
mineral baths and, 253
miracle drugs, 250-51
number afflicted, 222
nutrition and, 235-36, 269-79
and obesity, 406
and other rheumatic diseases, 217-319
overexposure and, 232-33
physiotherapy and, 238
poise, importance of, 243-44
principles relating to correction, 228
program of treatment, 284-95
proteins and, 269-71
readjustments required in recovery, 263-65, 284-95
reasons for persistence, 227-28
spiritual life and, 242-43
Still's disease, 229-30
symptoms, 223-24

vaccines and, 248-49
value of therapeutic fasting, 239-40, 292-93
Van Bechterow's disease, 229
vitamins and minerals, 276-79

ascorbic acid, stress and, 376
aspirin
dangers of, 138
in arthritis, 245-46
relation to gastroduodenal hemorrhage, 138
rheumatic fever, 418-19
asthma, bronchial, 176-84
atrophy of bronchial tubes, 176
care of patient, 181-82
case histories, 179-81, 183-84
in children, 183-84
diet in, 182
and gout, 260
medication, dangers of, 177-79
and penicillin, 178
scar tissue in, 176
atherosclerosis and carbohydrates, 130
Aureomycin and arthritis, 250
avitaminosis and health of nerves, 125

bacteria, intestinal, functions of, 34
Bahai, 243
baking of painful joint, in arthritis, 292
barbiturates
in arthritis, 227
in asthma, 177
dangers of, 138
baths; *see also* care of patient
hot, in arthritis, 281-82
hot, in heart disease, 448
bile, 32
bile duct

function of, 112
obstruction of, 113
biliousness, 107-8, 109-10
bird losses, from pesticides, 141-42
block, heart, 350
blood
amount, 334
clotting substances, 334
composition, 334
drugs that influence clotting, 434-36
pressure, high, and obesity, 405-6
pressure, low, 368
red and white cells, 333-34
body
importance of clean, 280-83
an interrelated organism, 367
powers of, 267-68
rehabilitation of, needed, 146-50
breathing, deep, exercises, 134
broth, vegetable, preparation, 38
bronchial asthma, *see* asthma
bronchitis, 172-75
diet for, 173
and influenza, 159-61
bronchopneumonia, and influenza, 159-60
bursitis, 230
butter, not to be added to vegetables, 40, 84, 100

cancer, 29, 65-66, 106
and smoking, 394-95
capillaries, 339
carbohydrates, *see also* diet; nutrition
in arthritis, 271-75
and atherosclerosis, 130
concentrated sugars, 271-72
grains, 273
in hardening of arteries, 365-66

metabolism, diabetes a disease of, 193
and tooth decay, 273-75
carcinogenic additives to food,
25-26
care of patient
arthritis, 280-97
asthma, 181-82
bronchitis, 172, 173
common cold, 158
constipation, 75
diabetes, 198-200, 209-11
gallbladder inflamation, 117
heart disease, 447-49
influenza, 160-61
nerves, weakened or de-
bilitated, 126-27
pneumonia, 167-69
rheumatic fever, 422
sinusitis, 171
ulcerative colitis, 86-88
case histories
arthritis, 253, 257-58, 298-
307
asthma, 179-81, 183-84
constipation, 75-77
diabetes, 197-98, 201-204,
204-206
gallbladder  inflamation,
120-21, 122-23
gastritis, 46-50
heart disease, 437-46
ileitis, 98-99
pneumonia, 169-70
rheumatic fever, 422-26
ulcer, 67
ulcerative colitis, 90-92, 92-
93, 96-97
cataracts
in diabetes, 194
and gout, 261
catarrh, 186
and arthritis, 226
gastric, 50-52
changes, in heart, 354
checkups, heart, value of, 129

cheese, *see also* diet; nutrition
arthritis and, 270
chemicals; *see also* additives
and pollutants
carcinogenic, 25-26
in food processing, toxicity
of, 25-26
children
asthma in 183-84
diabetes in, 207-208
chilling
and arthritis, 232-33
and common cold, 156
and  respiratory  diseases,
188
chloral hydrate, in asthma,
177
chlordane, 390, 391
chloroform, 102
Chloromycetin, and arthritis,
250
cholelithiasis, 114
cholesterol,
in artery, 343, 345
avoid, in ulcers, 59
food rich in, limit in heart
disease, 369, 379
in gallstones, 114
giant cell, 362-63
and hormones, 363-67
hormone missing that con-
trols, 362-67
hypercholesteremia, 130
chorea or St. Vitus dance,
417, 420
cinchophen, and arthritis, 247-
48
circulation; *see also* circulatory system
importance of, in arthritis,
282
and oxygen, 133-36
circulatory system, 333-41
arteries and veins, 338-41
blood, 333-34
diet in diseases of, 130-32
heart a pump, 334-38

kidneys, function in, 340-41
mortality rate higher among
doctors in diseases of,
129-30
cirrhosis, of liver, 106
clots, in arteries, 345, 346-48
codeine, in arthritis, 227, 248
coffee and respiratory diseases,
187-88
colchicum, dangers of, 261-62
cold, common, 155-58
cure for, 158
development of, 155-57
germs or viruses in, 157-58
colectomy, 96-97
colitis, ulcerative, 20, 82-99,
188
aftercare, 99
allergy in, 89-90
care of patient, 86-88
case histories, 90-92, 92-93,
95
diet, 83-86
diverticulitis, 95-96
drug-induced, 25
surgery in, 82-83, 88-89
symptoms, 82-83
colon, 34, 69-81, 82-99
spastic, 83, 95, 115
colostomy, 83
condiments,
and respiratory diseases,
constipation, 20, 69-81, 113,
461; *see also* care of patient
in arthritis, 226, 234, 280-
81
care of patient, 75
case history, 75-77
in diabetes, 211
diet, 72-75
types of, 70-71
with weakened or debili-
tated nerves, 126-27
cooking, effect of, on food,
382, 385

coronary or arteriosclerotic
heart disease, 346-48
coronary sclerosis, 346
coronary thrombosis, 346-
48
corticotropin, in asthma, 178
cortisone, 25, 366
asthma and, 177-79
dangers of, in arthritis, 254
related drugs, 254-58
reports on effects of, 255-58
rheumatic fever and, 419

D.B.I., 197, 204
D.D.T., dangers of, 140, 141,
390
degeneration, fatty, of liver,
106
Demerol, in asthma, 177
Denmark, health improve-
ment during World War
I, 370-72
diabetes, 193-213
arteries, hardening in, 194
care of patient, 198-200,
209-11
case histories, 197-98, 201-
204, 204-206
in children, 207-208
diet, 199, 203, 209-11
discussion, 193-95
gangrene and, 194
insulin, 195
a metabolic disease, 193,
194, 197, 211-12, 351
new remedies, 197
and obesity, 406
and pregnancy, 211
program for, 209-213
Diabinese, 197
Diamox and hepatic coma,
138
diastolic pressure, 343
dicoumarol, 434
Dieldrin, dangers of, 140, 141
diet
arthritis, 269-79, 285-88

asthma, 182
billiousness, 107-109
bronchitis, 173-74
catarrh, 186, 189
circulatory diseases, 129-30
common cold, 158, 189
constipation, 72
of Denmark, World War I, 370-72
diabetes, 199, 203, 210-11
faulty, and infectious disease, 311-12
gallbladder inflammation, 117
gastric catarrh, 50-51
gastritis, 38-39, 40
of Great Britain, World War II, 372
hay fever, 187
heart disease, 433-34, 436, 455-60
influenza, 160-61
nerves, weakened or debilitated, 126-27
pneumonia, 167-68
rheumatic fever and deficient, 421
rice, 376-78
sinusitis, 171
spastic constipation, 74
and stress, 375-76
ulcer, 54, 56-57, 58-59
ulcerative colitis, 83-86
underweight, 73-74
of U.S., World War II, 373-74
diethylstilbestrol, dangers of, 144
digestion
consequences of disorders, 28-30
development of disorders, 20-22
disagreements concerning improper, 15-18
disorders and arthritis, 226-33

a healthy, 15-152
impaired, and circulation, 130
improper, results of, 15-18
process of, 31-35
résumé and summary, 146-52
upset, mistaken for heart attack, 128-29
digitalis, in heart disease, 428-31
dinitrophenol, danger of, in reducing, 410
diseases, 239
affect normal range of metabolism, 314
brought on by faulty diet, 311-12
degenerative, shorten life, 331-32
developed by animals on imperfect diets, India, 383-85
paradox of, in World's richest and best-fed nation, 151-52
prevalence of, in cats fed cooked meat only, 380-82
resulting from constipation, 70-71
sound approach to, 139
diuretics, mercurial, in heart disease, 432-34
diverticulitis, 114
doctor, choice of right, 147-50
drinking and respiratory diseases, 187-88; see also alcohol
drip, postnasal, in sinusitis, 171
drugs; see also individual names of drugs
avoid, in heart disease, 462
that cause disorders, 24-25
digitalis, 428-31

disorders caused by, 24-25, 26-27
and health of nerves, 125
in heart disease, 428-36
as inducers of disease, 24-25
influencing blood clotting mechanism, 434-36
mercurial diuretics, 431-33
nitrites, 433-34
suppressive, in asthma and pneumonia, 164-65
symptom—relieving, and more disease, 137-39
symptom—suppressive, 174
widespread use of, 24-25
duodenum, 33

eating; *see also* diet; foods
faulty, and heart symptoms, 128-29
habits to observe, 288
eczema, and asthma, 183, 184
E.D.B., effect on eggs, 142
eggs, *see also* cholesterol
affected by fungicide-treated corn in diet of laying hens, 142
in arthritis, 270
in heart disease, 369
elimination and arthritis, 280
emotions, and health, 289
emphysema, bronchial, 176
empyema, 163
enema, 39, 42, 52, 58, 75, 80, 86-87, 117, 127, 158, 160-61, 168, 171, 182, 211, 281, 447
energy foods, *see also* carbohydrates
enzymes, 46, 59, 61, 436
amylopsin, 32
in greens, 161
lipase, 32
liver, storehouse for, 100-101
need for, 61

pepsin, 53
ptyalin, 31
rennin, 31
trypsin, 32
in uncooked foods, 379-80
Ephedrine in asthma, 177
epsom salt baths, in arthritis, 281-82
estrogens, natural, in foods, 144-45
exercise
abdominal muscles, 135
in arthritis, 237-38
deep breathing, 452
and heart disease, 450-54
knee-chinning, 135
leg, 134-35, 452-53
leg, advanced, 135, 453
and rest, 134-36
sitting-up, 135-453
stretching, 135-36, 453-54
value and kinds of, 133-36

facts worth knowing, résumé of, 146-50
farming, organic, 392-93
fasting, 386
arthritis, 241, 292
cold or catarrhal condition, 189
common cold, 158
constipation, 72-73
diabetes, 209
heart disease, 386, 436, 448
influenza, 160
pneumonia, 167
sinusitis, 171
ulcer, 56
ulcerative colitis, 83-84
fat; *see also* diet
and arthritis, 275-76
digestion of, 32-35
exclusion of, in heart and blood vessel diseases, 369, 463-64
increase of, in diet, 379

metabolism disturbed by smoking, 398
fatigue and arthritis, 240-41
fever
  increased metabolism, 266
  natural and induced, 266-67
  therapy, 266-67
fire ant control, 141, 142
fluids in constipation, 78-79
food; see also diet; nutrition
  absorption of, 31-35
  to be avoided, 46, 50, 58, 74, 107, 108, 109, 126, 130, 157, 173, 186, 187-88, 195, 209, 236, 271-76, 455, 461
  effect on blood pressure, 405-406
  natural, in convalescence, see care of patients; diet
  residue of, 34-35
  uncooked, superiority of, 379-83, 384-85
  wrong, effects of, 21-22
fruit juices, 37, 38, 73, 74, 85, 108, 110, 158, 160, 167, 182, 209
fruits, raw, see also diet
  and arthritis, 276
  and gastric catarrh, 51
  and constipation, 73, 74
  and gastritis, 44
  and ulcers, 56, 59-62
  and ulcerative colitis, 83-84, 88

gallbladder, 112-123
  attack mistaken for heart attack, 128
  bile duct, 112-13
  care of patient in acute attack, 117
  case histories, 120-21, 122
  diet, 117
  disease, 113-16
  disease of, and obesity, 406
  gallstones, 114-15

obesity and, 406
pain in gallbladder inflammation, 116
surgery for, 118, 120
composition of, 114, 118
dissolving of, 118-20
and gout, 260
passage of, through duct, 117
gangrene, in diabetes, 194
gastritis, 36-49, 113, 188
  care of patient, 38-40, 42, 45-46
  case history, 46-50
  diet, 38-39, 40, 44-45
  milk, 38, 43-44
  program for, 37-46
  raw fruits and raw vegetables, 44
gastroenteritis and colchicum, 261-62
glands, lymphatic
  detoxification by, 145
  in health, 225
  in respiratory diseases, 188-89
glaucoma and gout, 260-61
glycogen, role in diabetes, 193
gout, 259-62
  arteries, hardening and, 260
  colchicum, dangers of 261-62
  joints affected, 259-60
  and other diseases, 260-61
  poor man's, 261
  tophi, 260
  uric acid crystals, 259
gold
  complications, 252
  in treatment of arthritis, 221, 251-52
grains, responsibility for disease, 273-74
Great Britain, health improvement during World War II, 372

habits, injurious to health, 289
hardening of arteries, 342-43; *see* arteries
healing, power of, inherent, 139
health
  defined, 353-54
  must be maintained, 123
  within reach, 148-50
health and immunity to disease, stomach in, 102, 103
heart and heart disease, 20, 128-32, 323-466
  additives, chemical, in foods, 387-93
  arteries, hardening of, 129-30
  care of patient, 447-49, 461-66
  case histories, 437-46
  circulatory system, 333-41
  diseases associated with indigestion, 19-20
  drugs in, 428-36
  effects of alcohol, 402-404
  major types, 342-50
  mechanics of, 334-40
  metabolism a factor in disease, 351-68
  mortality from, 328-32
  nervous tension and, 413-16
  nutrition, role of, 369-86
  obesity, dangers of, 405-12
  oxygen in, 449
  physical exercise and, 450-54
  prevention of disease, 359-60
  program for, 455-60
  a pump, 334-38
  rheumatic fever and, 417-27
  smoking and, 394-401
  structure, 334-35
  surgery, 336
  surgery, unnecessary, in simulated abdominal conditions, 128-29
  work of, 334-38
hemorrhages
  in eyes, diabetes, 194
  of ulcers, 54-55
heparin, 434
hepatitis, 110
  and D.D.T., 140
  infectious, 106
Heptachlor, 141
herb flavorings, 45
herb teas, 37, 86
  in ulcer treatment, 56
  in ulcerative colitis, 86
hiatus hernia, 114
Hodgkin's disease, and D.D.T., 140
homeostasis, 354
hormone
  cortisone type, and ulcers, 138
  search for, involved in heart and blood vessel diseases, 362-64, 366-67
hydrochloric acid, 31, 53, 94, 392
  excessive in ulcer stomach, 65
  wash, to remove pesticides, 392-93
hydrocortisone, in asthma, 178
hypertensive heart disease, 342-45
  arteriosclerosis, 342-43
  blood pressure, 343-45
  clots, 345
  coronary thrombosis, 345, 346-48

ileitis, 98-99
ileostomy, 83
ileum, 33
India, diet experiments in, 383-85

indigestion, 19-30
  symptoms known as, 19-20
infection, theory of, 308-13
  care of local, 31-3
  faulty diet and infectious
    disease, 311-13
  germs, modification or
    change of, by environ-
    ment, 308-309
  Osler explanation, 312-13
  surgery, 310
  tonsils, 309-10
inflammation, beginning of
  stomach disease, 36
influenza, 159-61
  care of patient, 160-61
  diet, 160-61
  kinds of, 160
  rest in bed, 160
  vaccine, 160
  virus, 159-60
injuries, and arthritis, 233
insulin, 195-96, 202, 203, 204,
  206, 207, 208, 366
  shock 196-97
intestine
  large, 33-35
  small, 32-33
iritis and gout, 261
irritants of digestive system
  deep-tissue, 21
  superficial, 20-21
iproniazid, 25

jaundice, 25, 103, 106, 107,
  111, 250
  and pneumonia, 163
jejunum, 33
joints
  arthritis a disease of, 222-
    23, 226-27
  condition in health, 225
  gout and, 259-60
  kinds of, 224
  symptoms of arthritis in,
    223, 225
  in transitory period, 263-64

Karrell diet, 386, 436
kidneys
  and circulation, 340-41
  detoxification by, 145
  as filtering system, 351-53
knee-chin exercise, 135

Langerhans, islands of, 193,
  212
laxatives
  in constipation, 76
  dangers of, 77, 79
  foods, 79
leg, exercises for
  advanced, 135
  beginning, 134-35
leukemia, and D.D.T., 140
life
  length of, 354-55
  saving of, adult, 362
  saving of, children, 360-61
  span, longer, 331
lithium chloride, in food, 388
liver, 20, 25, 32, 35
  and cinchophen damage,
    247-48
  damage, in gold therapy,
    251-52
  detoxification by, 138, 145
  diet, 108-110
  difficulty of determining
    damage, 110-111
  and digestion, 100-111
  functions of, 100-101
  how damaged, 101-107
  importance of, 100-101
  poisons, insecticides, 140
  recovery and degree of
    damage, 107
  and toxins, 352-53
lumbago, 230
luminal, in asthma, 178
lymphatics, 32, 33

malabsorption syndrome, 124
malnutrition

contributory to rheumatic fever, 420-21
and health of nerves, 124-25

meals, small, importance of, 385

meat
and arthritis, 287-88
and metabolism, 287

medicines, do not cure, 323-24

medication, to be discarded by arthritic, 290

menopause, associated with arthritis, 232

Mercuhydrin, 431

mercupurin, 431

mercurial diuretics, in heart disease, 431-33

mercury, 102

metabolism; *see also* metabolism in heart disease
cholesterol, excess, disturbs, 275-76
diseases of kidney and liver, 351-52
disordered, of cholesterol, 364-66
disturbed, and disorders of heart and circulatory system, 130
faulty, cause of gallbladder inflammation, 113, 120
heart and blood vessel disease, outgrowth of disordered, 351-66
increased, indicated by fever, 266
meat and, 287
normal, 283
normal range of change in, 314
rheumatic diseases, outgrowth of disordered, 318
of sugars and fats, in diabetes, 194-95

metabolism in heart disease, 351-68
cholesterol, 362-66
entire organism involved, 367
hardening of arteries, prevention, 357-60
heart adaptations, 354
a hormone missing, 366-67
kidney system of filters, 351-53
length of life, 354-57
low blood pressure, 368
saving of life, 360-62
stress, theory of, 353-54

milk, 26-27, 38-39, 43-44, 56, 57, 62, 88, 115
in arthritis, 270
in gastritis, 38-39, 43-44
infants with catarrhal tendency, 186
in ulcer treatment, 56-57, 62
in ulcerative colitis, 88

metacorton, 257

methods
of healing, natural, increasing, 314-16
natural, in treatment of arthritis, 265

migraine and gout, 260

mineral oil in constipation, 77

minerals, 46, 58, 61-62, 240, 436
and arthritis, 276-77
concentrated, 277
in grains, 273-74
in greens, 210
liver a storehouse for, 101
need for, 61
in uncooked foods, 379

morphine, in asthma, 177

mortality
heart disease, 328-32
high, in pneumonia, 166, 167, 168

rapid increase in heart disease, 328

mothers, expectant, and newborn infants, drugs dangerous for, 139

muscles, abdominal, exercises for, 135

myalgia (myositis), 230

Natural Health, discussion of, *preface*

nature, only cure, 296-97

needs, spiritual, of man, 242-43

nephritis, glomerular, blood pressure, and heart disease, 352-53

nerves
and digestion, 124-27
health of, and avitaminosis, 124
health of, destroyed by faulty diet, 125
rehabilitation of unhealthy, 125-27

neuritis (neuralgia), 230

nicotine, action on blood vessels, 395

nitrites, in heart disease, 433-34

nitroglycerin, in angina, 433

*no nocere*, 137, 139

nutrients in well-balanced diet, 269

nutrition; *see also* diet; nutrition in treatment of arthritis; nutrition in treatment of heart and blood vessel diseases
faulty, and diseases of stomach, 21-22

nutrition in treatment of arthritis, 269-79
carbohydrates, 271-75
fats, 275-76
fruits and vegetables, 276

minerals and vitamins, 276-77
proteins, 269-71
Vitamin D and, 278-79

nutrition in treatment of heart and blood vessel diseases, 369-86
complete program essential, 379-80
diet and stress, 375-76
effects of wartime diet, 370-75
fasting, value of, 386
fat foods, exclusion of, 370
meals, small, importance of, 385
Pottenger experiments, 380-83
protein, 370-75
rice diet, 377-78
Rockefeller Foundation experiments, 288-85
table salt, exclusion of, 370
uncooked foods, superiority of, 379-82, 384
vegetarianism, 375

obesity, 405-412
and arthritis, diabetes, gallbladder disease, 406
case histories, 407-408
damage to cardiovascular system, 405-406
high blood pressure and, 405-406
how to overcome, 411-412
pregnancy and, 409-412

oil, mineral, objections to, 77-78

opiates, 25

organs, digestive, 31-35

Orinase, 197, 198

osmosis, 339

otitis media, 163

overeating, 50; *see also* obesity

and common cold, 157
and respiratory disease, 187
overexposure, and arthritis, 233
overfatigue
and catarrhal disorders, 187
and common cold, 156
contributory to rheumatic fever, 421
overweight; *see also* obesity
and arthritis, 235, 293-95
plus high blood pressure, in heart and blood vessel disease, 131
oxygen, 133-36
in heart disease, 449

pain
in angina, 346, 347
in arthritis, 230
in transition from arthritis, 265
in coronary thrombosis, 347
in gallbladder inflammation, 116
of ulcers, 54, 63, 64, 65
pancreas, 32, 193, 212
Paracelsus, and gold therapy, 251
penicillin
and arthritis, 250
and asthma, 178
fatalities from, 137
pericarditis, 163
peristalsis, 35
phenacetin, 102
dangers of, 139
phenolphthalein, dangers of, 139
phospholipids, level relative to cholesterol, 364
phosphorus, 102
physiotherapy, 315
physiotherapy, in arthritis, 238
pleurisy, 163

pneumonia, 162-171
antibiotics and, 165-66
care of patient, 167-69
case history, 169-70
complications, 163
jaundice and, 163
mortality, 164, 165, 167
progress of, 162-63
treatments, 163-64
types, two major, 163
pollutants and additives, chemical, 140-145; *see also* additives and pollutants
polycythemia and gout, 260
polyoxyethylene monostearate, bread softener, 388
polyps, in sinusitis, 171
prednisolene, 254
in asthma, 178
prednisone, 254
prevention of heart disease, 359-360
protein
and arthritis, 269-71
complete, 271
cheese and milk, 270
danger of excessive amount, 370-75, 379, 465
digestion of, 31-35
eggs, 270
in heart and blood vessel disease, 370-75
misconceptions concerning, 41
sources of, 374-75
sources other than meat, 41
and starches in same food, 32
vegetable, 210
wartime diets, 371-74
psoriasis, and arthritis, 303
psyllium seeds, in constipation, 80
ptyalin, 31
pylorospasm, 62-63

pyloric stenosis, 62-63
Pyramidon, 102

radiation, dangers of, 105
Rauwolfia compounds, 25
reactions in transition from arthritic condition, 263-64
residues
  food, 33-35
  insecticides and penicillin, hazards of, 26-27
resistance, lowered
  and common cold, 156-58
  and influenza, 159-60
  and rheumatic fever, 420-21
respiratory system, diseases of, 155-89
  and allergies, 185-89
  bronchial asthma, 176-84
  bronchitis, 172-75
  common cold, 155-58
  influenza, 159-61
  lymphatic glands in, 188-89
  pneumonia, 162-71
  sinusitis, 170-71
rest
  in arthritis, 237-38, 293
  in heart disease, 461
  in bed, in influenza, 160
rheumatic fever, 417-27
  allergy in, 426-27
  aspirin, cortisone, and A.C.T.H., 418-19
  best treatment for, 422
  case histories, 422-26
  chorea or St. Vitus dance, 417
  development of, 419-21
  parts of body affected, 417
Rockefeller Foundation experiments in diet, India, 383-85
rice
  diet, 376-78

saccum, 34
saliva, in digestion, 31
salt, table
  excluded in heart and blood vessel diseases, 370, 379
  not to be added to vegetables, 84
salyrgan, 431
sand fly control and aquatic damage, 141
sciatica, 230
sclerosis, coronary, and angina, 346
serum therapy, in pneumonia, 165-66
sinusitis, acute and chronic, 170-71
  occurrence of, 171
  polyps, 171
  postnasal drip, 171
Sister Kenny treatment, 315
sitting-up, exercises for, 135
smoking, 460, 462, 465
  and arthritis, 235
  cancer-producing factor in tobacco, 394-95
  economic aspects of, 397
  effects of, 396-98
  effects of stopping, 397
  fat metabolism disturbed by, 398
  heart disease death from, 398
  how to stop, 398-401
  nicotine, action of, 395
  and respiratory diseases, 187-88
soda, bicarbonate of, 28, 29, 227
sodium-potassium balance and mercurials, 432
soups
  in diet, 374
soybean
  milk, 43, 186
spinach, protein in, 271
starch, digestion of, 31, 32

starvation and health of nerves, 124

starvation, oxygen, results of, 133

steaming of painful joint, in arthritis, 292

stilbestrol, 390
as cancer hazard, 144, 390

stomach
bacteria destroyed in, 94
deformed ulcers of, 55
in digestion, 31
disorders of, 19-30
hourglass ulcers of, 55
inflammation of, 36-52
obstructions, 62-64
ulcers of, 53-68

stool, characteristics of, 35

streptomycin, and arthritis, 250

stress
and ascorbic acid, 376
theory of, 353-54

stretching, exercises for, 135-36

stroke, 345

sugars, concentrated, in arthritis, 271-72

sulfas, 102
in arthritis, 250
in pneumonia, 165-66

sunbaths, for arthritis, 289

surgery, 63, 309, 310
in colitis, 82-83, 88-89
in constipation, 71-72
in diabetes, 202
gallbladder, 118, 120
gallbladder in mistake for ulcers, 115-16
harmful effects of, 310
in heart attacks, 128
heart, 336
in spastic colitis, 115-16
tonsils and adenoids, 188
in ulcerative colitis, 82-83, 88-89

ulcers, 55

systolic pressure, 344

tea and respiratory diseases, 187-88

tensions
emotional problems, 415-16
how to readjust, 416
nervous and emotional, 21, 64
way of life can be altered, 413

Theosophy, 243

Thorazine and liver damage, 138

thrombosis, coronary, 345, 346-48

time, importance of, in arthritis treatment, 290-92

T.M.T.D., effect on eggs, 142

tonsils, 309-10

toxins
in arthritis, 263
circulating, 27-28
elimination of, 309
and liver, 102, 138, 144-45, 355

tranquilizers, in asthma, 177

treatment of pneumonia, 165

types of heart disease, 342-50
coronary or arteriosclerotic, 346-48
hypertensive, 342-45
valvular on rheumatic, 348-350

ulcers, 37, 42, 44, 53-68, 115, 138
and cancer, 65-66
care of patient, 58
case history, 67
diet, 54, 56-57, 58-62
drug-induced, 25
hemorrhages, 54-55
kind and size, 53-54
milk and, 56-57, 62
pain of, 54, 63, 64, 65

peptic, and drugs, 138
  stomach wall, deformity, 55
Unity groups, 243
uric acid crystals, 259-62
urticaria and gout, 260

vaccine
  for arthritis, 248-49
  for influenza, 160
valvular or rheumatic heart
    disease, 348-50
  heart block in, 350
vegetables,
  raw, in arthritis, 276
  raw, in constipation, 74, 77
  raw, in gastric catarrh, 50-
    51
  raw, in gastritis, 44
  raw, in ulcers, 56, 59-62, 86
  raw, in ulcerative colitis, 86,
    88
veins, 340; see arteries
villi, 33
virus
  and common cold, 157-58
  and influenza, 159-60
Vis medicatrix naturae, 139

vitamin D and calcification,
    278-79
vitamins, 46, 59, 61-62, 240,
    435
  and arthritis, 277-79
  body need for, 61
  concentrated, 277
  in grains, 273
  in greens, 210
  liver a storehouse for, 101
  in uncooked foods, 379-80

waste products, accumulation
    of toxic, cause of colds,
    155
water, drinking of, 78-79
weakness, in arthritis, 293
weight
  and health, 23-24
  ideal, 131

X-ray, gastrointestinal tract,
    patients with malnutri-
    tion, avitaminosis, starva-
    tion, 124

yoghurt, 73, 456, 457, 458,
    467